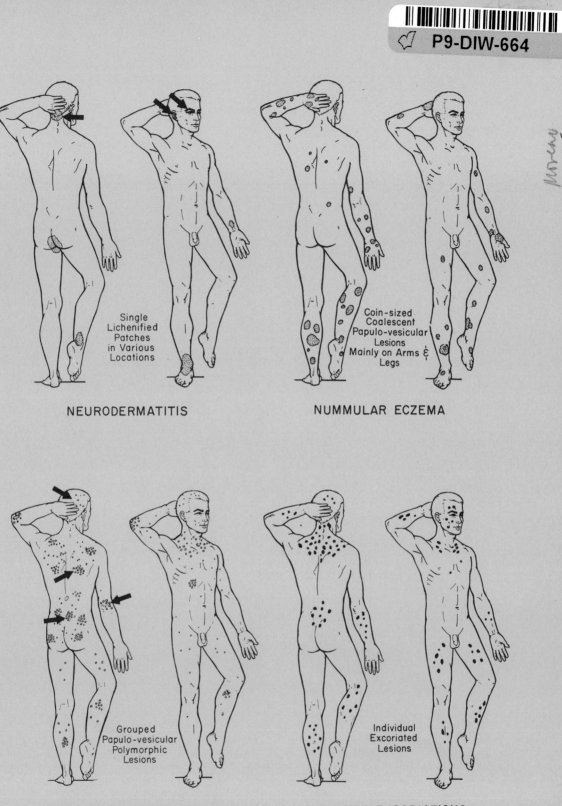

NEURODERMATITIS

Single
Lichenified
Patches
in Various
Locations

NUMMULAR ECZEMA

Coin-sized
Coalescent
Papulo-vesicular
Lesions
Mainly on Arms &
Legs

DERMATITIS HERPETIFORMIS

Grouped
Papulo-vesicular
Polymorphic
Lesions

NEUROTIC EXCORIATIONS

Individual
Excoriated
Lesions

Manual of
SKIN DISEASES

Manual of
SKIN DISEASES

Gordon C. Sauer, M.D.

Clinical Professor of Medicine (Dermatology)
University of Kansas School of Medicine; Attend-
ing Physician, Kansas City General Hospital and
Medical Center, Kansas City, Missouri.

THIRD EDITION

150 Figures and 60 Color Plates

J. B. Lippincott Company
Philadelphia • Toronto

Library of Congress Cataloging in Publication Data

Sauer, Gordon C
    Manual of skin diseases.

    Includes bibliographies.
    1. Skin—Diseases. I Title [DNLM: 1. Skin diseases. WR 140 S255m 1973]
    RL71.S2 1973   616.5   73-2568
        ISBN 0-397-52061-1

Dedicated to
My Wife
Mary Louise

Preface to the Third Edition

It is gratifying that my "Skin Manual" continues to serve the medical students and physicians for whom it is intended. Many have told me that they consult it frequently for diagnostic clues or therapeutic suggestions.

To further enhance the diagnostic value, this third edition contains 15 additional color plates and distinct chapters on pediatric and geriatric skin problems. The many therapeutic suggestions have been up-dated and continue to be listed 1-2-3.

To reflect recent changes in medical emphasis, new chapters have been added to cover more extensively the sunlight effect on the skin and hereditary skin diseases.

Moreover, the type was completely reset to accommodate the numerous further changes, additions and deletions that were made throughout the entire book.

The Dictionary Index section continues to expand to satisfy the needs for a comprehensive dictionary-type coverage of all the field of dermatology.

GORDON C. SAUER, M.D.

Preface to the First Edition

The motivation for this book was a question asked of me by a senior medical student: "Where can I find a good 50-page book on dermatology?" This book is written as an answer to those students and practitioners who have asked that same general question. This book is not 50 pages long, but it is one of the shortest and most concise books published on diseases of the skin.

Approximately 15 per cent of all patients who walk into the general practitioner's office do so for care of some skin disease or skin lesion. It may be for such a simple treatment as the removal of a wart, for the treatment of athlete's foot or for something as complicated as severe cystic acne. There have been so many recent advances in the various fields of medicine that the medical school instructor can expect his students to learn and retain only a small percentage of the material that is taught them. I believe that the courses in all phases of medicine, and particularly the courses of the various specialties, should be made as simple, basic and concise as possible. If the student retains only a small percentage of what is presented to him, he will be able to handle an amazing number of his walk-in patients. I am presenting in this book only the material that medical students and general practitioners must know for the diagnosis and the treatment of patients with the common skin diseases. In condensing the material many generalities are stated, and the reader must remember that there are exceptions to every rule. The inclusion of these exceptions would defeat the intended purpose of this book. More complicated diagnostic procedures or treatments for interesting or problem cases are merely frosting on the cake. This information can be obtained by the interested student from any of several more comprehensive dermatologic texts.

This book consists of two distinct but complementary parts.

The first part contains the chapters devoted to the diagnosis and the management of the important common skin diseases. The chapter on a dermatologic formulary has been especially marked for easy reference. In discussing the common skin diseases, a short introductory sentence is followed by a listing of the salient points of each disease in outline form. All diseases of the skin have primary lesions, secondary lesions, a rather specific distribution, a general course which includes the prognosis and the recurrence rate of the disease, varying subjective complaints and a known or unknown cause. Where indicated, a statement follows concerning seasonal incidence, age groups affected, family and sex incidence, contagiousness or infectiousness, relationship to employment and laboratory findings. The discussion ends with a paragraph on differential diagnosis and treatment. Treatment, to be effective, has to be thought of as a chain of events. The therapy outlined on the first visit is usually different from that given on subsequent visits or for cases that are very severe. The treatment is discussed with these variations in mind. The first part of the book concludes with a chapter on basic equipment necessary for managing dermatologic patients.

The second part consists of a very complete dictionary-index to the entire field of dermatology, defining the majority of rare diseases and the unusual dermatologic terms. The inclusion of this dictionary-index has a twofold purpose. First, it enables me to present a concise first section on *common* skin diseases unencumbered by the inclusion of the rare diseases. Second, the dictionary-index provides a rather complete coverage of all of dermatology for the more interested student. In reality, two books are contained in one.

Dermatologic nomenclature has always been a bugaboo for the new student. I heartily agree with many dermatologists that we should simplify the terminology, and that has been attempted in this text. Some of the changes are mine, but many have been suggested by others. However, after a diligent effort to simplify the names of skin diseases, one is left with the appalling fact that some of the complicated terms defy change. One of the main reasons for this is that all of our field, the skin, is visible to the naked eye. As a result, any minor alteration from normal has been scrutinized by countless physicians through the years and given countless names. The liver or heart counterpart of folliculitis ulerythematosa reticulata (ulerythema acneiforme, atrophoderma reticulatum symmetricum faciei, atrophodermie vermiculée) is yet to be discovered.

What I am presenting in this book is not specialty dermatology but general practice dermatology. Some of my medical educator friends say that only internal medicine, pediatrics and obstetrics should be taught to medical students. They state that the specialized fields of medicine should be taught only at the internship, residency or postgraduate level. That idea misses the very important fact that cases from all of the so-called specialty fields wander in to the general practitioner's office. The general practitioner must have some *basic* knowledge of the varied aspects of all of medicine so that he can properly take care of his general everyday practice. This basic knowledge must be taught in the undergraduate years. The purpose of this book is to complement such teaching.

GORDON C. SAUER, M.D.

Acknowledgments

For the most realistic presentation of skin diseases, color photography is essential. However, the cost of color reproduction is so great that it is almost impossible to enjoy the advantages of color plates and still keep the price of the book within the range where it will have the broadest appeal. This problem has been solved for the three editions of this book through the generosity of several pharmaceutical companies which contributed the cost of the color plates credited to them.

For this third edition the following drug companies contributed money for additional new color plates:

Burroughs Wellcome & Co., Inc. (2 plates)
Derm-Arts Laboratories
Dermik Laboratories, Inc. (in part)
Duke Laboratories, Inc.
G. S. Herbert Laboratories
Johnson & Johnson
Owen Laboratories, Inc. (in part)
Schering Corporation
Syntex Laboratories, Inc.
Texas Pharmacal Co.
Westwood Pharmaceuticals (2 plates)

While the majority of photographs are from my own private collection, I gratefully acknowledge assistance from the several photographers at the University of Kansas School of Medicine under the direction of Burton Johnson and from Roger Odneil, photographer at the Kansas City General Hospital. The line drawings were done by Jo Ann Clifford. The physician or institution that furnished illustration material is acknowledged under the respective picture with appreciation.

Dr. James Kalivas, head of the section of dermatology at the University of Kansas, gave considerable advice on revision of the chapter on Structure of the Skin and wrote the chapter on Photosensitivity Dermatoses.

Mrs. Ruby Steele and Mrs. Natalie Graves typed and retyped the many drafts that were necessary to complete this edition, and I am grateful.

In the first and second editions further acknowledgments were made, but it would be redundant to repeat them here. Finally a great deal of credit again goes to the medical department of J. B. Lippincott Co. and especially Mr. J. Stuart Freeman, Jr. The book and I profited by our association with them.

Contents

List of Color Plates

Manual of
SKIN DISEASES

1

Structure of the Skin

The skin is the largest organ of the human body. It is composed of tissue that grows, differentiates and renews itself constantly. Since the skin is a barrier between the internal organs and the external environment, it is uniquely subjected to noxious external agents and is also a sensitive reflection of internal disease. An understanding of the cause and the effect of this complex interplay in the skin begins with a thorough understanding of the basic structure of this organ.

LAYERS OF THE SKIN

The skin is divided into 3 rather distinct layers. From inside out they are the subcutaneous tissue, the dermis and the epidermis (Fig. 1-1).

Subcutaneous Tissue. This layer serves as a receptacle for the formation and the storage of fat, is a locus of highly dynamic lipid metabolism, and supports the blood vessels and the nerves that pass from the tissues beneath to the dermis above. The deeper hair follicles and the sweat glands originate in this layer.

Dermis (Corium). This layer is made up of connective tissue, cellular elements and ground substance. It has a rich blood and nerve supply. The sebaceous glands and the shorter hair follicles originate in the dermis. The corium can anatomically be divided into papillary (upper) and reticular (lower) layers.

The *connective tissue* consists of collagen fibers, elastic fibers and reticular fibers. All of these, but most importantly the collagen fibers, contribute to the support and the elasticity of the skin.

The collagenous fibers are made up of eosinophilic acellular proteins responsible for nearly a fourth of man's over-all protein mass. Under the electron microscope the fibers are seen to be composed of thin nonbranching fibrils held together by a cementing ground substance. These fibrils are composed of covalently cross-linked and overlapping units called *tropocollagen* molecules. When tannic acid or the salts of heavy metals, such as dichromates, are combined with collagen, the result is leather.

Elastic fibers are thinner than most collagen fibers and are entwined among them. They are composed of the protein elastin. Elastic fibers do not readily take up acid or basic stains such as hematoxylin and eosin (H & E) but can be stained with Verhoeff's stain.

Reticular fibers are thought to be immature collagen fibers, since their physical and chemical properties are similar. They can be stained with silver (Foot's stain). Reticulum fibers are sparse in normal skin but are abundant in certain pathologic conditions of the skin such as the *granulomas* of tuberculosis, syphilis and sarcoidosis, and in the *mesodermal tumors* such as histiocytomas, sarcomas and lymphomas.

The *cellular elements* of the dermis consist of 3 groups of mesodermal cells, a reticulohistiocytic group, a myeloid group and a lymphoid group. Under pathologic conditions, the potentiality of these cells can change.

The reticulohistiocytic group consists of fibroblasts, histiocytes and mast cells. Immature cells of the reticulohistiocytic group are known as reticulum cells.

Fibroblasts form collagen fibers and may be the progenitor of all other connective tissue cells.

Histiocytes normally are present in small numbers around blood vessels but in pathologic conditions can migrate in

1

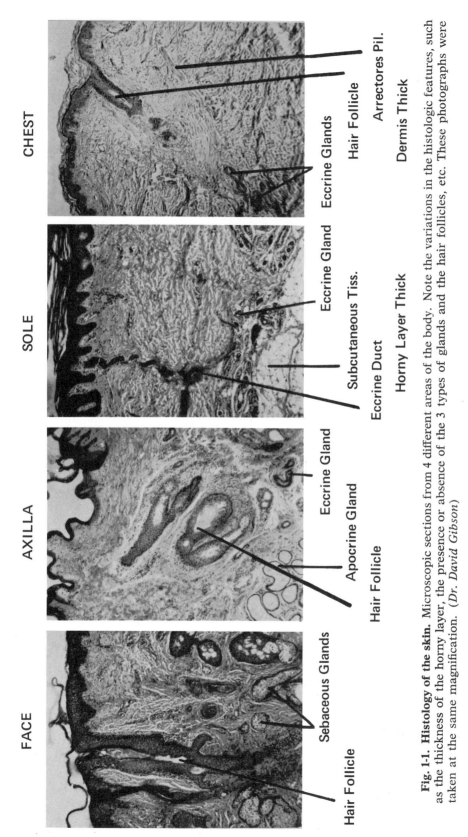

Fig. 1-1. Histology of the skin. Microscopic sections from 4 different areas of the body. Note the variations in the histologic features, such as the thickness of the horny layer, the presence or absence of the 3 types of glands and the hair follicles, etc. These photographs were taken at the same magnification. *(Dr. David Gibson)*

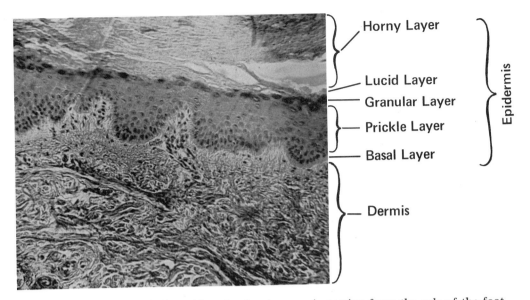

Horny Layer

Lucid Layer

Granular Layer

Prickle Layer

Basal Layer

Epidermis

Dermis

Fig. 1-2. Histology of the epidermis. A microscopic section from the sole of the foot. (*Dr. David Gibson*)

the dermis as *tissue monocytes.* They can also form abundant reticulum fibers. When they phagocytize bacteria and particulate matter, they are known as *macrophages.* Histiocytes, under special pathologic conditions, can also change into epithelioid cells which in turn can develop into so-called giant cells.

Mast cells are also histiocytic cells. Mast cells have intracytoplasmic basophilic metachromatic granules containing heparin and histamine. The normal skin contains relatively few mast cells, but their number is increased in many different skin conditions, particularly the itching dermatoses such as *atopic eczema, contact dermatitis* and *lichen planus.* In *urticaria pigmentosa* the mast cells occur in tumorlike masses.

Plasma cells, rarely seen in normal skin sections, occur in small numbers in most chronic inflammatory diseases of the skin and in larger numbers in granulomas. The origin of plasma cells is unknown, but they are thought to arise from reticulum cells.

In the myeloid group of cells, the polymorphonuclear leukocyte and the eosinophilic leukocyte occur quite commonly with various dermatoses, especially those with an allergic etiology.

In the lymphoid group, the lymphocyte is commonly found in inflammatory lesions of the skin. The myeloid and the lymphoid groups of cells are also found in their specific neoplasms of the skin.

The *ground substance* of the dermis is a gel-like, amorphous matrix not easily seen histologically, but it is of tremendous physiologic importance, since it contains proteins, mucopolysaccharides, soluble collagens, enzymes, immune bodies, metabolites and many other substances.

Epidermis. This is the most superficial of the 3 layers of the skin and averages in thickness about the width of the mark of a sharp pencil or less than 1 mm. There are 2 distinct types of cells in the epidermis, the keratin-forming cells and the melanin-forming cells. These latter cells synthesize melanin, the principal pigment of the epidermis. The keratin-forming cells are found in the basal layer and give rise to all the other cells of the stratified epidermis.

The epidermis is divided into 5 layers from within outward (Fig. 1-2).

1. Basal layer ⎫
2. Prickle layer ⎬ Living epidermis
3. Granular layer ⎪
4. Lucid layer ⎭
5. Horny layer—Dead end-product

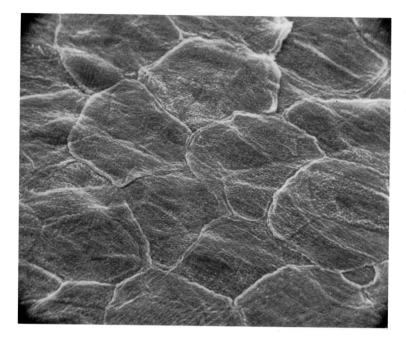

Fig. 1-3. Underside of top layer of epidermal horny layer cells on Scotch tape stripping seen with Cambridge Mark II Stereoscan at 1000 ×. (*Drs. J. Arnold, W. Barnes and G. Sauer*)

The *basal layer* of cells lies next to the corium and contains both the keratin-forming and the melanin-forming cells. The keratin-forming cells can be thought of as stem cells which are capable of progressive differentiation into the cell forms higher up in the epidermis. It normally requires 3 or 4 weeks for the epidermis to replicate itself by the process of division and differentiation. This cell turnover is greatly accelerated in such diseases as *psoriasis* and *ichthyosiform erythroderma.*

The melanin-forming cells, or melanocytes, are sandwiched between the more numerous keratin-forming basal cells. These melanocytes are *dopa positive* because they stain darkly following contact with a solution of levorotatory, 3,4-dihydroxyphenylalanine, or *dopa.* This laboratory reaction closely simulates physiologic melanin formation in which the amino acid tyrosine is oxidized by the enzyme tyrosinase to form dopa. Dopa is then further changed through a series of complex metabolic processes to melanin.

Melanin pigmentation of the skin, whether increased or decreased, is influenced by many local and systemic factors (see p. 198). The melanocyte-stimulating hormone from the pituitary is the most potent melanizing agent.

The *prickle layer,* or stratum malpighii, is made up of several layers of epidermal cells, chiefly of polyhedral shape. This layer gets its name from the existence of a network of cytoplasmic threads called prickles, or intercellular bridges, that extend between the cells. These prickles are most readily visible in this layer but, to a lesser extent, are present between all the cells of the epidermis.

The third layer is the *granular layer.* Here the cells are flatter and contain protein granules, called keratohyaline granules.

The *lucid layer* is next and appears as a translucent line of flat cells. This layer of the skin is present only on the palms and the soles. The granular and the lucid layers make up the transitional layer of the epidermis and act as a barrier to the inward transfer of noxious substances and outward loss of water.

The outermost layer of the epidermis is the *horny layer.* It is made up of stratified layers of dead keratinized cells that are constantly shedding (Fig. 1-3). The chemical protein in these cells—keratin—is capable of absorbing vast amounts of water. This is readily seen during bathing when the skin of the palms and the soles becomes white and swollen.

The normal oral mucous membrane does not have any granular layer or horny layer.

VASCULAR SUPPLY

A continuous arteriovenous meshwork perforates the subcutaneous tissues and extends into the dermis. Blood vessels of varying sizes are present in all levels and all planes of the skin tissue and appendages. In fact, the vascularization is so intensive that it has been postulated that its main function is to regulate heat and blood pressure of the body, with the nutrition of the skin as a secondary function.

A special vascular body, the glomus, deserves mention. The glomus body is most commonly seen on the tips of the fingers and the toes and under the nails. Each one of these organs contains a vessel segment which has been called the Sucquet-Hoyer canal. This canal represents a short-circuit device that connects an arteriole with a venule directly without intervening capillaries. The result is a marked increase in the blood flow through the skin. When this body grows abnormally, the result is a very painful red *glomus tumor*, commonly occurring underneath a nail, that has to be removed by surgical means.

NERVE SUPPLY

The nerve supply of the skin consists of sensory nerves and motor nerves.

Sensory Nerves. The sensory nerves mediate the sensations of touch, temperature or pain. The millions of terminal, apparently nonspecific, free nerve endings have more to do with the specificity of skin sensation than the better-known highly specialized nerve endings, such as the Vater-Pacinian and the Wagner-Meissner tactile corpuscles.

Itching is certainly the most important presenting symptom of an unhappy patient. It may be defined simply as the desire to scratch. Itching apparently is a mild painful sensation that differs from pain in having a lower frequency of impulse stimuli. The release of proteinases (as follows itch powder application) may be responsible for the itch sensation. The pruritus may be of a pricking type or of a burning type and can vary greatly from one individual to another. Sulzberger called those abnormally sensitive individuals "itchish," analogous to the "ticklish" person. Itching can occur without any clinical signs of skin disease, or from circulating allergens or from local superficial contactants.

Motor Nerves. The involuntary sympathetic motor nerves control the sweat glands, the arterioles and the smooth muscles of the skin. Adrenergic fibers carry impulses to the arrectores pilorum muscles which produce goose flesh when they are stimulated. This is due to traction of the muscle on the hair follicles to which it is attached.

APPENDAGES

The appendages of the skin include both the cornified appendages (hairs and nails) and the glandular appendages.

Hairs are derived from the hair follicles of the epidermis. Since no new hair follicles are formed after birth, the different types of body hairs are manifestations of the effect of location and of external and internal stimuli. Hormones are the most important internal stimuli influencing the various types of hair growth. This growth is cyclic, with a growing (anagen) phase and a resting (telogen) phase. The average period of scalp hair growth ranges from 2 to 6 years. However, systemic stresses such as childbirth, may cause hairs to enter a resting stage prematurely. This *postpartum effect* is noticed most commonly in the scalp when these resting hairs are depilated during combing or washing; and the thought of approaching baldness causes sudden alarm on the part of the woman.

TYPES. The adult has two main types of hairs: the vellus hairs (lanugo hairs of the fetus) and the terminal hairs. The vellus hairs ("peach fuzz") are the fine, short hairs of the body, whereas the terminal hairs are coarse, thick and pigmented. The latter hairs are developed most extensively on the scalp, the brows and the extremities.

HAIR FOLLICLES. The hair follicle may be thought of as an invagination of the epidermis with its different layers of cells. These cells make up the matrix of the hair follicle and produce the keratin of the mature hair. The protein-synthesizing capacity of this tissue is enormous when one considers that at the rate of scalp hair growth of 0.35 mm. per day, over 100 linear feet of scalp hair is produced daily. The density of hairs in the scalp varies from 175 to 300 hairs per square centimeter.

FACTS ABOUT HAIR AND ITS GROWTH. Certain facts should be stated concerning hair and its growth. (1) Shaving of excess hair on the extremities does not promote more rapid growth of coarse hair. The shaved stubs appear more coarse but, if allowed to grow normally, they would appear no different than before shaving. (2) The value of intermittent massage to stimulate scalp hair growth has not been proved. (3) Hair cannot turn gray overnight. The melanin pigmentation, which is distributed throughout the length of the nonvital hair shaft, takes weeks to be shed through the slow process of hair growth. (4) The common male type of baldness cannot safely be influenced by local and systemic measures, including hormones. Heredity is the greatest factor predisposing to baldness, and an excess of male hormone may contribute to hair loss in these people. Male castrates do not become bald.

Nails. The second cornified appendage, the nail, consists of a nail plate and the tissue that surrounds it. This plate lies in a nail groove which, similar to the hair follicle, is an invagination of the epidermis. Unlike hair growth, which is periodic, nail growth is continuous. Nail growth is about one third the rate of hair growth, or about 0.1 mm. per day. It takes approximately 3 months to restore a removed fingernail and about 3 times that long for the regrowth of a new toenail. Nail growth can be inhibited during serious illnesses or in old age, increased through nail-biting or occupational stress, and altered because of hand dermatitis or systemic disease.

Topical treatment of nail disturbances is very unsatisfactory due to the inaccessibility of the growth-producing areas.

Glandular Appendages. TYPES. The glandular appendages of the skin are divided into 2 types: the sebaceous glands and the sweat glands (Fig. 1-4). The sebaceous glands form their secretion through disintegration of the whole glandular cell, whereas the sweat glands eliminate only a portion of the cell in the formation of secretion.

The *sebaceous glands* are present everywhere on the skin except the palms and the soles. The secretion from these glands is evacuated through the sebaceous duct to a follicle that may or may not contain a hair. This secretion is not under any neurologic control but is a continuous outflowing of the material of cell breakdown. These glands produce sebum, which covers the skin with a thin lipoidal film that is mildly bacteriostatic and fungistatic and retards water evaporation. The scalp and the face may contain as many as 1,000 sebaceous glands per square centimeter. The activity of the gland increases markedly at the age of puberty and, in certain individuals, becomes plugged with sebum, debris and bacteria to form the *blackheads* and the *pimples* of acne.

The *sweat glands* are found everywhere in the human skin. They appear in greatest abundance on the palms and the soles and in the axillae. There are two main types of these glands. The eccrine or small sweat glands open directly onto the skin surface; the apocrine or large sweat glands, like the sebaceous gland, usually open into a hair follicle.

The *apocrine sweat glands* are found chiefly in the axillae and the genital region and do not develop until the time of puberty. These glands in man have very little importance except for the production of odor (the infamous "B.O."). Any emotional stresses which cause adrenergic sympathetic discharge produce apocrine sweating. This sweat is sterile when excreted but undergoes decomposition when contaminated by bacteria from the skin surface, resulting in a strong and characteristic odor. The purpose of the many

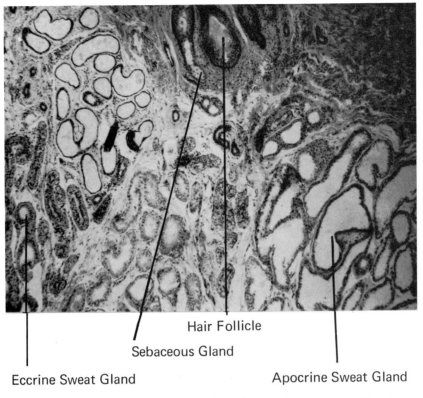

Hair Follicle

Sebaceous Gland

Eccrine Sweat Gland   Apocrine Sweat Gland

Fig. 1-4. Histology of the glands of the skin. A microscopic section from the axilla. (*Dr. David Gibson*)

cosmetic underarm preparations is to remove these bacteria or block the gland excretion. The main disease of the apocrine glands is *hidradenitis suppurativa.* This uncommon, chronic infection of these glands is caused by blockage of the duct which usually occurs in patients with the *acne-seborrhea complex.*

The *eccrine sweat glands* and the cutaneous blood vessels are key factors in the maintenance of stable internal body temperatures despite marked environmental temperature changes. The eccrine glands flood the skin surface with water for cooling, and the blood vessels dilate or constrict to dissipate or to conserve body heat. The eccrine sweat glands are distributed everywhere on the skin surface, with the greatest concentration on the palms, the soles and the forehead. The prime stimulus for these small sweat glands is heat. Their activity is under the control of the nervous system, usually through the hypothalamic thermostat. Both adrenergic and cholinergic fibers innervate the glands. Blockage of the sweat ducts results in the disease entity known as *prickly heat* (*miliaria*). When the sweat glands are congenitally absent, as in *anhidrotic ectodermal dysplasia,* a life-threatening hyperpyrexia may develop.

BIBLIOGRAPHY

Lever, W. F.: Histopathology of the Skin, ed. 3. Philadelphia, J. B. Lippincott, 1967. Consult pages 7 through 56 for the histopathologic aspect of this introductory material.

Montagna, W.: The Structure and Function of Skin, ed. 2. New York, Academic Press, 1962. A reading of this book will dispel any innuendos concerning lack of basic research in dermatology.

2

Laboratory Procedures and Tests

In addition to the usual laboratory procedures used in the workup of medical patients, certain special tests are of importance in the field of dermatology. These include *skin tests, fungus examinations, biopsies,* and *cytodiagnosis.*

SKIN TESTS

There are 3 types of skin tests:
1. Intracutaneous
2. Scratch
3. Patch

The *intracutaneous tests* and the *scratch tests* can have two types of reactions: an immediate wheal reaction and a delayed reaction. The immediate wheal reaction develops to a maximum in 5 to 20 minutes. This type of reaction is elicited in testing for the cause of urticaria, atopic dermatitis and inhalant allergies. This immediate wheal reaction test is seldom used for determining the etiology of skin diseases.

The delayed reaction to intracutaneous skin testing is exemplified best by the tuberculin skin test. Tuberculin is available in two forms: Old Tuberculin Koch (OTK) or Purified Protein Derivative (PPD). Using OTK, the procedure is to start with 0.1 ml. of the 1:10,000 dilution (0.01 mg.) injected intracutaneously. This test is read in 48 hours and is positive if the redness at the site of the injection is 5 mm. greater than that at the control test site. If negative, the test can be repeated using a 1:1,000 dilution (0.1 mg.).

The PPD test is performed by using tablets that come in two strengths and injecting a solution of either one intracutaneously. If there is no reaction following the PPD No. 1 test, then the second strength may be employed.

The Tuberculin Tine Test (Rosenthal) is a simple and rapid procedure utilizing OTK. Four prongs or tines covered with OTK are pressed into the skin. If, at the end of 48 or 72 hours, there is over 2 mm. of induration at the site of any prong insertion, the test is positive.

Other intracutaneous skin tests with delayed reactions include the Ducrey vaccine test (Lederle) for the diagnosis of chancroid; the trichophytin test, which if positive shows an allergy to fungi of that type; and the Lygranum (Squibb) or Frei antigen (Lederle) skin tests which are used in the diagnosis of lymphogranuloma venereum.

Patch tests are used rather commonly in dermatology and offer a simple and accurate method of determining whether a patient is allergic to any of the testing agents (Figs. 2-1 and 2-2). There are two different reactions to this type of test: a primary irritant reaction and an allergic reaction. The primary irritant reaction occurs in the majority of the population when they are exposed to agents that have skin-destroying properties. Examples of these agents include soaps, cleaning fluids, bleaches, "corn" removers and counter-irritants. The allergic reaction indicates that the patient is more sensitive than normal to the agent being tested. It also shows that the patient has had a previous exposure to that agent.

The technic of the patch test is rather simple. For example, consider that a patient comes in with a dermatitis on the top of his feet, and shoe leather or some chemical used in the manufacture of the leather is suspected as causing the reaction. The procedure for a patch test is to cut out a ½-inch-square piece of the material from the inside of the shoe, moisten

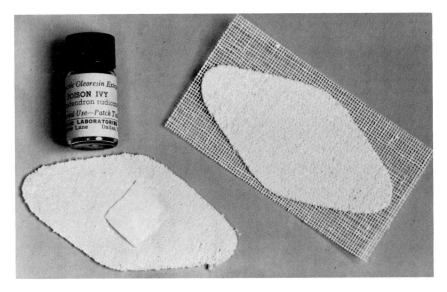

Fig. 2-1. Patch test material. Diagnostic oleoresin extract of poison ivy (Graham) and Elastopatch (Duke). The Elastopatch is ready for application to the skin in the lower left-hand of the figure. The extract is placed on the square piece of sheeting. (*K.U.M.C.*)

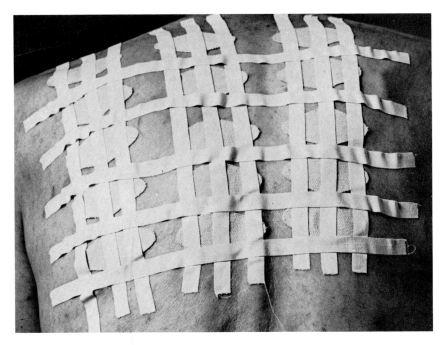

Fig. 2-2. A series of patch tests on the back of a patient to establish the cause of chronic contact dermatitis in a farmer. (*K.U.M.C.*)

the material with distilled water, place it on the skin surface, and cover with an adhesive band or some patch-test dressing. The patch test is left on for 48 hours to 72 hours. When the test is removed the patient is considered to have a positive patch test if there is any redness or vesiculation under the site of the testing agent.

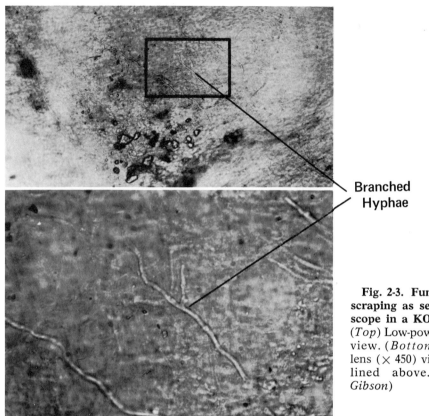

Branched
Hyphae

Fig. 2-3. Fungi from a skin scraping as seen with microscope in a KOH preparation. (*Top*) Low-power lens (× 100) view. (*Bottom*) High-power lens (× 450) view of area outlined above. (*Dr. David Gibson*)

The patch test can be used to make or confirm a diagnosis of poison ivy dermatitis, ragweed dermatitis, or contact dermatitis due to medications, cosmetics or industrial chemicals. Sulzberger and Baer[1] and Adams[2] have compiled a list of chemicals, concentrations and vehicles to be used for eliciting the allergic type of patch test reaction. However, most tests can be performed very simply, as in the case of the shoe-leather dermatitis. One precaution is that the test must not be allowed to become wet in the 48-to-72-hour period.

A method of testing for allergy when food is suspected is to use the Rowe elim-ination diet.[3] The procedure is to limit the diet to the following basic foods which are known to be hypo-allergenic: lamb, lemon, grapefruit, pears, lettuce, spinach, carrots, sweet potato, tapioca, rice and rice bread, cane sugar, maple syrup, sesame oil, gelatin and salt. The patient is to remain on this basic diet for 5 to 7 days. At the end of that time one new food can be added every 2 days. The following foods may be added early: beef, white potatoes, green beans, milk along with butter and American cheese, and white bread with puffed wheat. If there is a flare-up of the dermatitis, which should occur within 2 to 8 hours after ingestion of an offending food, the new food should be discontinued for the present. More new foods are added until the normal diet, minus the allergenic foods, is regained.

[1] Sulzberger, M. B., and Baer, R. L.: Office Immunology, pp. 312-330. Chicago, Year Book Publishers, 1947. Baer, R. L.: and Witten, V. H.: Year Book of Dermatology and Syphilology, 1957-1958 Series, pp. 29-45. Chicago, Year Book Publishers, 1958.

[2] Adams, R. M.: Occupational Contact Dermatitis, pp. 219-236. Philadelphia, J. B. Lippincott, 1969.

[3] Sulzberger, M. B., and Baer, R. L.: Office Immunology, p. 63. Chicago, Year Book Publishers, 1947.

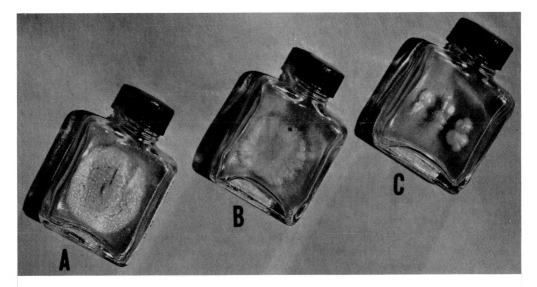

Fig. 2-4. Fungus cultures. Cultures grown on disposable bottles of Sabouraud's media (Mycosel, Derm Medical). The three fungi are (A) *Trichophyton mentagrophytes*, (B) *Microsporum canis*, (C) *Candida albicans*. (*K.U.M.C.*)

FUNGUS EXAMINATIONS

Fungus examinations are a simple office laboratory procedure. They are accomplished by (1) scraping the diseased skin and examining the material directly under the microscope, (2) culturing the material and (3) examining the grown culture under the microscope. The skin scrapings are obtained by abrading a scaly diseased area with a knife blade, depositing the material on a slide, covering this residue with a 20 per cent aqueous potassium hydroxide solution and a cover slip. A diagnostically helpful pale violet stain can be imparted to the fungi if the 20 per cent aqueous potassium hydroxide solution is mixed with an equal amount of Parker Super Quink, Permanent Black Ink. The preparation on the slide can be heated, or allowed to stand for 15 to 60 minutes, to allow the keratin particles to dissolve and reveal the fungi more clearly. The slide is then mounted on a microscope stage and examined for fungus elements with the low-power and the high-power lenses (Fig. 2-3).

For a culture preparation, a part of the material from the scraping can be implanted in a test tube containing Sabou-raud's media.* In 1 to 2 weeks a whitish or variously colored growth will be noted (Fig. 2-4). The species of fungus can be determined grossly by the color and the characteristics of the growth in the culture tube, and microscopically by study of a small amount of the culture material that has been removed, mixed with a solution of Lacto Phenol Cotton Blue and placed on a microscope slide. Most species of fungi have a characteristic microscopic appearance.

BIOPSIES

The biopsy of a questionable skin lesion and microscopic examination of the biopsy section is another important laboratory procedure. The histopathology of many skin conditions is quite diagnostic, particularly when the biopsy specimen is

---

* Tubes with this media can be obtained from most hospitals or from Derm Medical Co., P. O. Box 78595, W. Adams Station, Los Angeles, California, or Jim Pipkin, Dermatologic Supplies, 108 Tendicks, San Antonio, Texas, or Case Laboratories, 1407 N. Dayton, Chicago, Illinois 60622, or Fungus Diagnostic Services, 9 Watchung Ave., Plainfield, New Jersey. For cultures that will usually be contaminant-free, order the special Sabouraud's media that contains cyclohexamide and chloramphenicol, known as Myocosel Agar.

studied by a pathologist who has some knowledge of dermatologic lesions.

The instruments and the materials needed to perform a skin biopsy are listed on page 336 and are shown in Figure 32-1.

There are 3 principal technics for performing skin biopsies, namely, by *surgical excision with suturing*, by *punch* and by *scissors*. The decision in favor of one method depends on such factors as the site of the biopsy, the cosmetic result desired, the type of tissue to be removed, for instance flat or elevated, and last, simplicity.

The technic of performing *surgical excision biopsies with suturing* of the skin is well known. In general, this type of biopsy is performed when a good cosmetic result is desired and when the entire lesion is to be removed. The disadvantage is that this procedure is the most time-consuming of the 3 technics.

Punch biopsies can be done rather rapidly with or without suturing of the wound. A special punch-biopsy instrument of appropriate size is needed. A local anesthetic is usually injected at the site. The operator rotates the instrument until it penetrates to the desired depth, then the circle of tissue is excised. Bleeding can be stopped with pressure or the use of 1 or 2 sutures. An elliptical wound instead of a circular wound can be produced by stretching the skin perpendicular to the desired suture line before the punch is rotated. The resultant scar following suturing is neater.

The third way to remove skin tissue for a biopsy specimen is to excise the piece with sharp-pointed *scissors* (*scissors biopsy*) and stop the bleeding with light electrosurgery. This latter procedure is useful for certain types of elevated lesions and in areas where the cosmetic result is not too important. The greatest advantage of this procedure is the speed at which it can be done, and the simplicity.

The biopsy specimen must be placed in appropriate fixative solution, usually 10 per cent formalin. If the specimen is long and tends to curl, it can be stretched out on a piece of paper. Then paper and tissue can be dropped in the fixative solution.

The stain most routinely used is hematoxylin and eosin. With this stain the nuclei stain blue, and collagen, muscles and nerves stain red. A table of special stains can be found in Lever's book listed at the end of this chapter.

CYTODIAGNOSIS

The cervical *pap smear* is the commonest form of cytodiagnosis. In dermatology, cytodiagnosis is useful in bullous diseases (pemphigus), vesicular virus eruptions (herpes), and basal-cell epitheliomata. The technique and choice of lesions is important. A concise review of this subject is presented in Rook, Wilkinson and Ebling's book, p. 32.

In addition to the above 4 special skin procedures (skin testing, fungus examination, biopsies, and cytodiagnosis), there are certain tests for specific skin conditions that will be discussed in connection with the respective diseases.

BIBLIOGRAPHY

SKIN TESTS

See Sulzberger and Baer, and Adams references on p. 10.

FUNGUS EXAMINATIONS

Wilson, J. W., and Plunkett, O. A.: The Fungus Diseases of Man. Berkeley, University of California Press, 1965.

BIOPSIES

Baer, R. L., and Kopf, A. W.: Dermatologic office surgery, Year Book of Dermatology 1963-64. Chicago, Year Book, 1964. A comprehensive article covering patient selection asepsis, wound infection, surgical instruments, local anaesthesia, scalpel surgery and "wrinkle lines," emergencies during office surgery and emergency supplies.

Epstein, E.: Skin Surgery, ed. 3. Springfield, Charles C Thomas, 1970.

Lever, W. F.: Histopathology of the Skin, ed. 4, pp. 1-2 and 41-45. Philadelphia, J. B. Lippincott, 1967.

CYTODIAGNOSIS

Rook, A., Wilkinson, D. S., and Ebling, F. J. G.: Textbook of Dermatology. Vol. 2, p. 32. Philadelphia, F. A. Davis, 1968.

3

Dermatologic Diagnosis

To aid in determining the diagnosis of a presenting skin problem, this chapter will be concerned with discussions of primary and secondary lesions; also, diagnosis by location. It will contain lists of seasonal skin diseases, military dermatoses and dermatoses of Negroes.

PRIMARY AND SECONDARY LESIONS

No two skin diseases look alike, but most of them have some characteristic *primary* lesions and it is very important to examine the patient closely to find them. Commonly, however, the primary lesions have been obliterated by the *secondary* lesions of overtreatment, excessive scratching, or infection. Even in these cases it is usually possible by careful examination to find ·some primary lesions at the edge of the eruption or on other less irritated areas of the body. (Plates 1-3.)

A complete examination of the entire body is a necessity when confronted with a diffuse skin eruption or an unusual localized eruption.

PRIMARY LESIONS

A description of the basic primary lesions follows:

Macules are up to 1 cm. in size, circumscribed, flat, discolorations of the skin. Examples: freckles, flat nevi.

Patches are larger than 1 cm., circumscribed, flat, discolorations of the skin. Examples: vitiligo, senile freckles, measles rash.

Papules are up to 1 cm. in size, circumscribed, elevated, superficial, solid lesions. Examples: elevated nevi, warts, lichen planus.

A *wheal* is a type of papule that is edematous and transitory. Examples: hives, insect bites.

Plaques are larger than 1 cm., circumscribed, elevated, superficial, solid lesions. Examples: mycosis fungoides, localized neurodermatitis.

Nodules range to 1 cm. in size and are solid lesions with depth; they may be above, level with, or beneath the skin surface. Examples: nodular secondary or tertiary syphilis, epitheliomas, xanthomas.

Tumors are larger than 1 cm. solid lesions with depth; they may be above, level with, or beneath the skin surface. Examples: tumor stage of mycosis fungoides, larger epitheliomas.

Vesicles range to 1 cm. in size and are circumscribed elevations of the skin containing serous fluid. Examples: early chickenpox, zoster, contact dermatitis.

Bullae are larger than 1 cm., circumscribed elevations containing serous fluid. Examples: pemphigus, second-degree burns.

Pustules vary in size and are circumscribed elevations of the skin containing purulent fluid. Examples: acne, impetigo.

Petechiae are up to 1 cm. in size and are circumscribed deposits of blood or blood pigments. Examples: certain insect bites and drug eruptions.

Purpura is a larger than 1 cm. circumscribed deposit of blood or blood pigment in the skin.

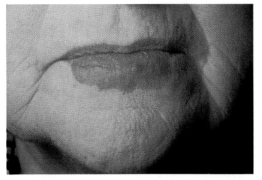

(A) Macule, on lip (port-wine hemangioma)

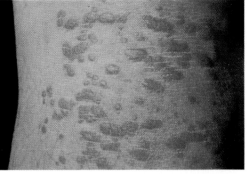

(B) Papules, on knee (lichen planus)

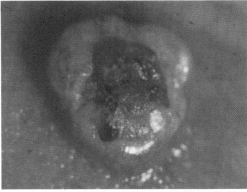

(C) Nodule, on lower eyelid
(basal cell epithelioma)

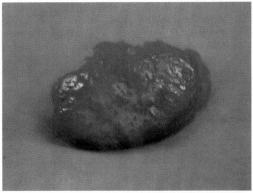

(D) Tumor, of abdomen (mixed hemangioma)

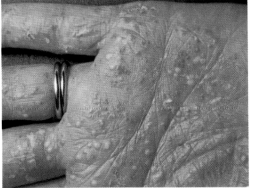

(E) Pustules, on palm (pustular psoriasis)

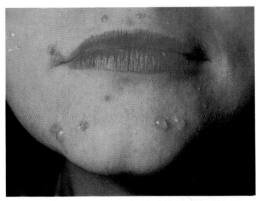

(F) Vesicles, on chin (pemphigus)

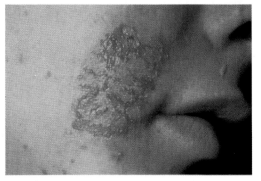

(G) Crust, on cheek (impetigo)

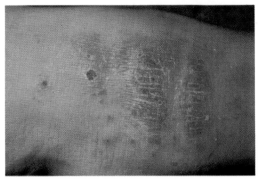

(H) Lichenification, on dorsum of ankle
(neurodermatitis)

Plate 1. Primary and secondary lesions. (*Geigy Pharmaceuticals*)

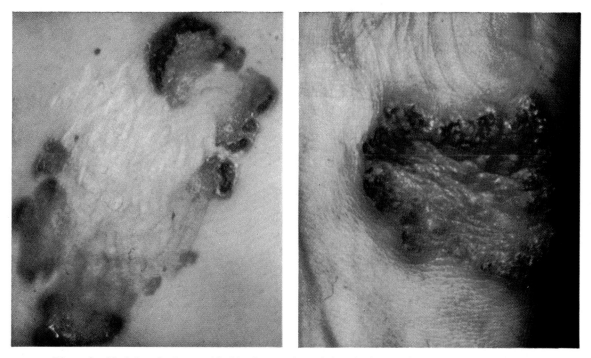

Plate 2. Nodular lesions. (*Left*) Grouped nodular lesions with central scarring (tertiary syphiloderm). (*Right*) Grouped warty, nodular lesions with central scarring (tuberculosis verrucosa cutis). (*Marion B. Sulzberger: Folia Dermatologica, No. 1, Geigy Pharmaceuticals*)

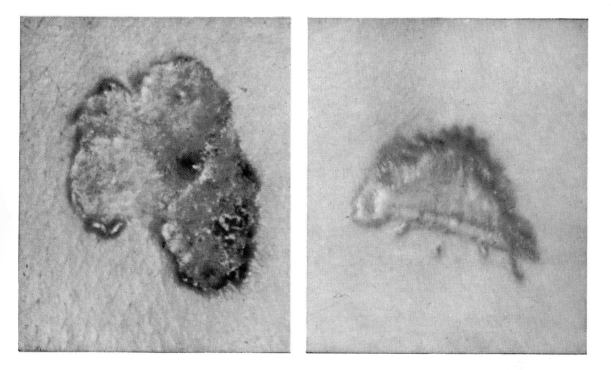

Plate 3. Nodular lesions. (*Left*) Polycyclic nodular lesion (superficial basal epithelioma). (*Right*) Keloid. (*Marion B. Sulzberger: Folia Dermatologica, No. 1, Geigy Pharmaceuticals*)

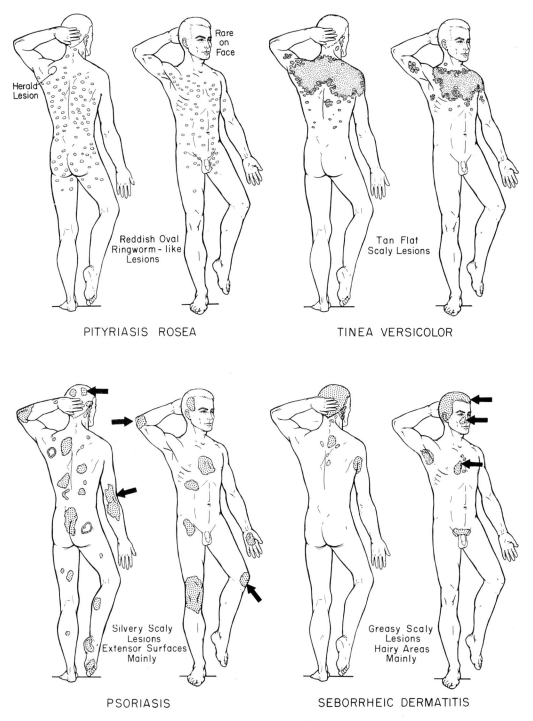

Fig. 3-1. Dermatologic silhouettes.

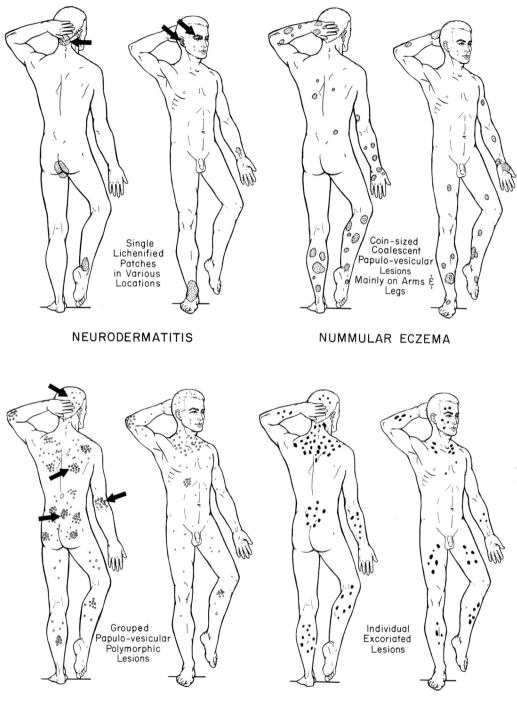

NEURODERMATITIS

Single Lichenified Patches in Various Locations

NUMMULAR ECZEMA

Coin-sized Coalescent Papulo-vesicular Lesions Mainly on Arms & Legs

DERMATITIS HERPETIFORMIS

Grouped Papulo-vesicular Polymorphic Lesions

NEUROTIC EXCORIATIONS

Individual Excoriated Lesions

Fig. 3-2. Dermatologic silhouettes.

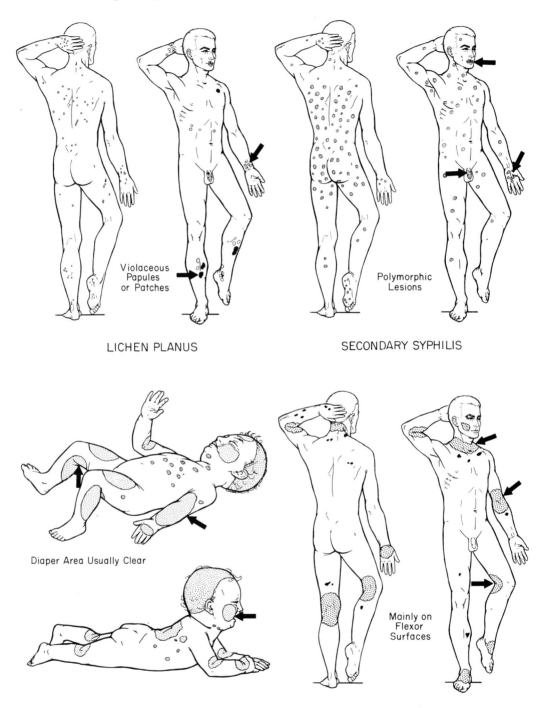

LICHEN PLANUS

Violaceous
Papules
or Patches

SECONDARY SYPHILIS

Polymorphic
Lesions

Diaper Area Usually Clear

Mainly on
Flexor
Surfaces

INFANTILE FORM of ATOPIC ECZEMA   ADULT FORM of ATOPIC ECZEMA

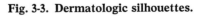

Fig. 3-3. Dermatologic silhouettes.

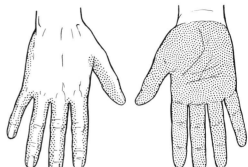

CONTACT DERMATITIS (Housewife)   DYSHIDROSIS or ID (Due to Tinea of Feet)

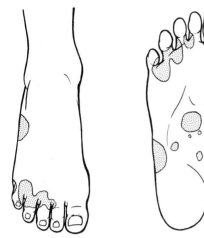
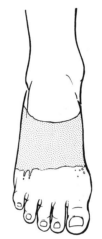
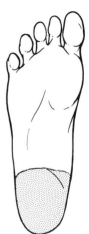

FUNGUS INFECTION   CONTACT DERMATITIS (Shoes)

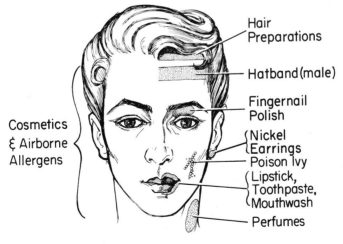

Hair Preparations

Hatband (male)

Fingernail Polish

Nickel Earrings
Poison Ivy

Lipstick, Toothpaste, Mouthwash

Perfumes

Cosmetics & Airborne Allergens

CONTACT DERMATITIS

Fig. 3-4. Dermatologic silhouettes.

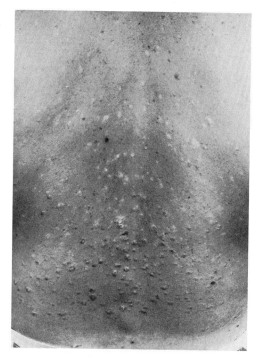

Psoriasis

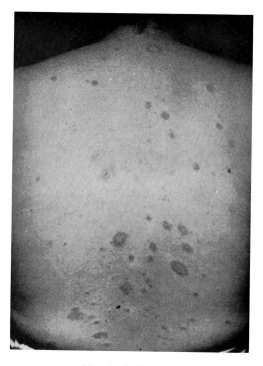

Pityriasis Rosea

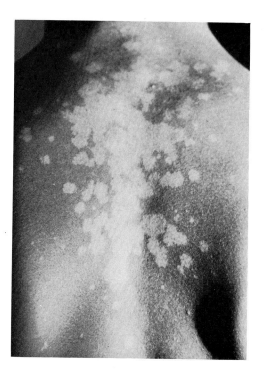

Tinea Versicolor (Negro)

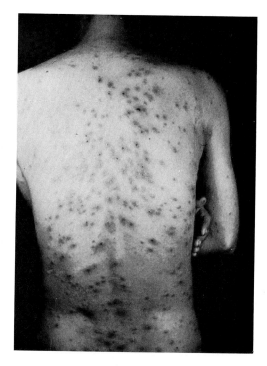

Secondary Syphilis

Fig. 3-5. Papulosquamous diseases on the back.

SECONDARY LESIONS

Scales (squamae) are shedding, dead epidermal cells which may be dry or greasy. Examples: dandruff, psoriasis.

Crusts are variously colored masses of skin exudates. Examples: impetigo, infected dermatitis.

Excoriations are abrasions of the skin, usually superficial and traumatic. Examples: scratched insect bites, scabies.

Fissures are linear breaks in the skin, sharply defined with abrupt walls. Examples: congenital syphilis, athlete's foot.

Ulcers are irregularly sized and shaped excavations in the skin extending into the corium. Examples: stasis ulcers of legs, tertiary syphilis.

Scars are formations of connective tissue replacing tissue lost through injury or disease.

Keloids are hypertrophic scars.

Lichenification is a diffuse area of thickening and scaling with resultant increase in the skin lines and markings.

Several combinations of primary and secondary lesions commonly exist on the same patient. Examples: papulosquamous lesions of psoriasis, vesiculopustular lesions in contact dermatitis, and crusted excoriations in scabies.

SPECIAL LESIONS

There are also some primary lesions, limited to a few skin diseases, that can be called specialized lesions.

Comedones or blackheads are plugs of whitish or blackish sebaceous and keratinous material lodged in the pilosebaceous follicle usually seen on the face, the chest or the back, rarely on the upper part of the arms. Example: acne.

Milia or whiteheads are whitish nodules, 1 to 2 mm. in diameter, that have no visible opening onto the skin surface. Examples: in healed burn or superficial traumatic sites, healed bullous disease sites, or newborn babies.

Telangiectasias are dilated superficial blood vessels. Examples: spider hemangiomas, chronic radiodermatitis.

Burrows are very small and short (in scabies) or tortuous and long (in creeping eruption) tunnels in the epidermis.

In addition, there are distinct and often diagnostic changes in the nail plates and the hairs that are discussed in the chapters relating to these appendages.

DIAGNOSIS BY LOCATION

A physician is often confronted by a patient with skin trouble localized to one part of the body (Figs. 3-1 to 3-4). The following list of diseases with special localizations is meant to aid in the diagnosis of such conditions, but this list must not be considered as being all-inclusive. Generalizations are the rule, and many of the rare diseases are omitted. For further information concerning the particular diseases consult the Dictionary-Index.

Scalp: Seborrheic dermatitis, contact dermatitis, psoriasis, folliculitis, pediculosis and hair loss due to the following: male or female pattern, alopecia areata, tinea, chronic discoid lupus erythematosus, postpregnancy or trichotillomania.

Ears: Seborrheic dermatitis, psoriasis, infectious eczematoid dermatitis, senile keratoses and, very rarely, fungal infection.

Face: Acne, rosacea, impetigo, contact dermatitis, seborrheic dermatitis, folliculitis, herpes simplex and, less commonly, lupus erythematosus and actinic dermatitis.

In diagnosing a rather generalized skin eruption, the following 3 mimicking conditions must be considered first and ruled in or out by appropriate history or examination:
(1) Drug eruption   (2) Contact dermatitis   (3) Secondary syphilis

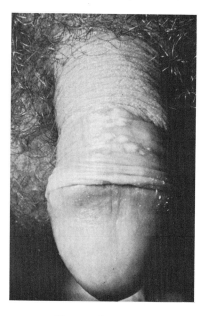

Herpes Simplex

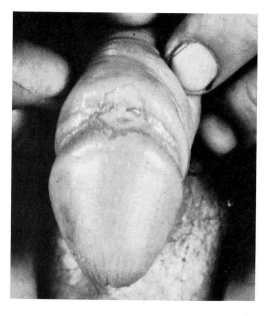

Primary Syphilis

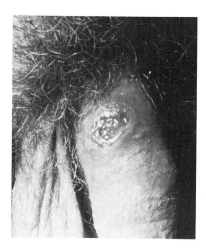

Furuncle

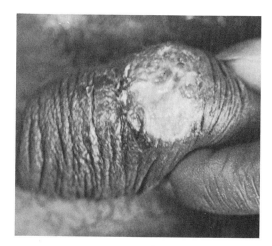

Chancroid

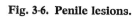

Fig. 3-6. Penile lesions.

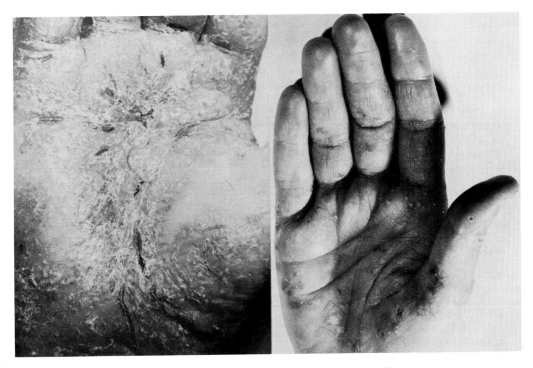

Contact Dermatitis   Tinea

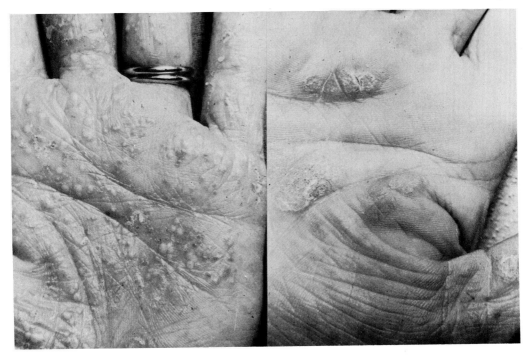

Pustular Psoriasis   Psoriasis

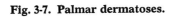

Fig. 3-7. Palmar dermatoses.

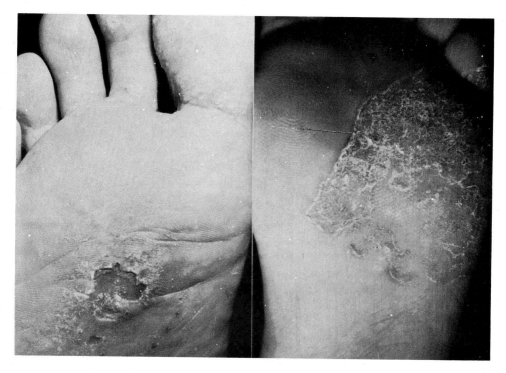

Acute Tinea   Chronic Tinea

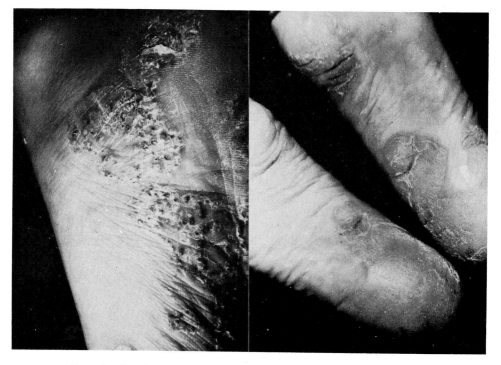

Pustular Psoriasis   Psoriasis

Fig. 3-8. Plantar dermatoses.

Eyelids: Contact dermatitis due to fingernail polish or hair sprays, seborrheic dermatitis or atopic eczema.

Posterior Neck: Neurodermatitis, seborrheic dermatitis, psoriasis or contact dermatitis.

Mouth: Aphthae, herpes simplex, geographic tongue, contact dermatitis and, less frequently, syphilis, lichen planus and pemphigus.

Axillae: Contact dermatitis, seborrheic dermatitis, hidradenitis suppurativa and, less commonly, erythrasma, acanthosis nigricans and Fox-Fordyce disease.

Chest and Back (Fig. 3-5): Tinea versicolor, pityriasis rosea, acne, seborrheic dermatitis, psoriasis and secondary syphilis.

Groin and Crural Areas: Tinea infection, monilial infection, bacterial intertrigo, scabies, pediculosis and granuloma inguinale.

Penis (Fig. 3-6): Contact dermatitis, fusospirochetal balanitis, chancroid, herpes simplex, primary and secondary syphilis and, less frequently, scabies and balanitis xerotica obliterans.

Hands (Fig. 3-7): Contact dermatitis, dyshidrosis, id reaction to fungal infection of the feet, atopic eczema and, less commonly, pustular psoriasis, nummular eczema, erythema multiforme, secondary syphilis and fungal infection.

Cubital Fossae and Popliteal Fossae: Atopic eczema, contact dermatitis and prickly heat.

Elbows and Knees: Psoriasis, xanthomas and, occasionally, atopic eczema.

Feet (Fig. 3-8): Fungal infection, primary or secondary bacterial infection, contact dermatitis from footwear or footcare and, less frequently, psoriasis, atopic eczema, erythema multiforme and secondary syphilis.

SEASONAL SKIN DISEASES

Certain dermatoses have an increased incidence in various seasons of the year. In a busy dermatologist's office one sees literal "epidemics" of atopic eczema, pityriasis rosea, psoriasis and winter itch, to mention only a few. Knowledge of this seasonal incidence is helpful from a diagnostic standpoint. It will be sufficient simply to list these seasonal diseases, since more specific information concerning them can be found elsewhere in the book. Remember that there are exceptions to every rule.

Winter

Atopic eczema
Contact dermatitis of hands
Psoriasis
Seborrheic dermatitis
Nummular eczema
Winter itch and dry skin (xerosis)
Ichthyosis (rare)

Spring

Pityriasis rosea
Dyshidrosis
Erythema multiforme (Hebra)
Acne (flares)

Summer

Contact dermatitis due to poison ivy
Tinea of the feet and the groin
Monilial intertrigo
Miliaria or prickly heat
Impetigo and other pyodermas
Actinic dermatitis
Insect bites
Tinea versicolor (noticed after suntan)
Darier's disease (uncommon)
Epidermolysis bullosa (uncommon)

Fall

Winter itch
Senile pruritus
Atopic eczema
Pityriasis rosea
Contact dermatitis due to ragweed
Tinea of the scalp (school children)
Acne (flares)

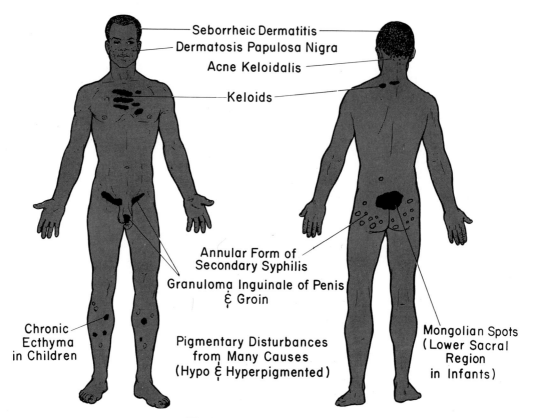

Fig. 3-9. Negro Dermogram.

MILITARY DERMATOSES

While the major part of the world is now at nominal peace, under the ravages of previous wars lack of good personal hygiene, lack of adequate food, presence of overcrowding, injuries and pestilence, resulted in the aggravation of any existing skin disease and an increased incidence of the following skin diseases:

Scabies
Pediculosis
Syphilis and other venereal diseases
Bacterial dermatoses
Jungle rot in tropical climates:
  Tinea of the feet and the groin
  Pyoderma
  Dyshidroses
  Miliaria

DERMATOSES OF NEGROES

The following skin diseases are seen with greater frequency in the black race as compared with the white race (Fig. 3-9 and 3-10):

Keloids
Dermatosis papulosa nigra
Pyodermas of legs in children
Pigmentary disturbances from many causes, both hypopigmented and hyperpigmented
Traumatic marginal alopecia (from braids, and heated irons used in hair straightening)
Seborrheic dermatitis of scalp aggravated by grease on hair
Ingrown hairs of beard
Acne keloidalis
Annular form of secondary syphilis
Granuloma inguinale
Mongolian spots
On the other hand, certain skin conditions are rarely seen in the Negro:
  Prickle cell or basal cell epitheliomas
  Senile keratoses
  Psoriasis

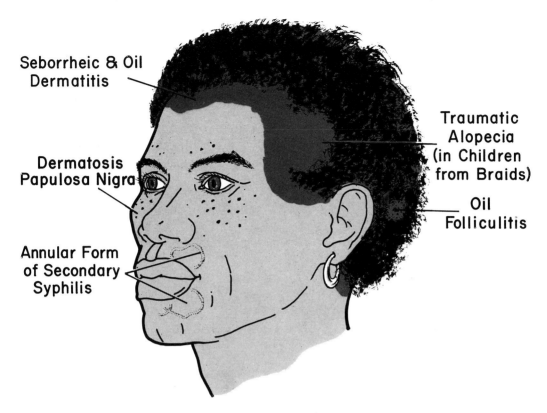

Seborrheic & Oil
Dermatitis

Traumatic
Alopecia
(in Children
from Braids)

Dermatosis
Papulosa Nigra

Oil
Folliculitis

Annular Form
of Secondary
Syphilis

Fig. 3-10. Negro Dermogram, head of woman.

BIBLIOGRAPHY

Fitzpatrick, T. B., and Walker, S. A.: Dermatologic Differential Diagnosis. Chicago, Year Book Publishers, 1962.

Kenney, J. A.: Management of Dermatoses Peculiar to Negroes. Arch. Derm., *91*:126, 1965.

——: Dermatoses Seen in American Negroes. Internat. J. Derm., *9*:110, 1970.

4

Your Introduction to the Patient

After the usual conversation of introducing yourself to the new patient, the following might transpire.

DOCTOR: "What can I do for you, Mrs. Jones?"

MRS. JONES: "I have a bad breaking out on my hands."

DOCTOR (Writes on his chart under present complaint "hand dermatitis"): "How long have you had this breaking out?"

MRS. JONES: "Well, I've had this before, but what I have now has been here for only 3 weeks."

DOCTOR (Writes "duration, 3 weeks."): "When did you have this before, Mrs. Jones?"

MRS. JONES: "Let me see. I believe I had this twice before. The first time I had this breaking out was shortly after our wedding and I thought that it had to do with the fact that I had my hands in soap and water more than before. It took about a month to heal up. l treated it with salves that I had at home. It certainly wasn't bad then. The next time I broke out it was a little bit worse. This was after my first child was born. Johnnie is 3 years old now. I suppose I should have expected my hands to break out again now because I just had my second baby 3 months ago."

DOCTOR (Has just finished writing down the following, "The patient states that she has had this eruption on two previous occasions. Home treatment only. Both eruptions lasted approximately 1 month. Present eruption attributed to care of baby born 3 months ago."): "Mrs. Jones, what have you been putting on your hands for this breaking out?"

MRS. JONES: "Let me take off my bandages and I'll show you how my hands look."

DOCTOR: "Let me help you with those bandages. However, I want to ask you a few more questions before I look at your hands."

MRS. JONES: "Well, first I used a salve that I got over at the corner drugstore that said on the label it was good for athlete's foot. One of my neighbors told me that she used it for her hand trouble, and it had cured her hands. I don't think that her hands looked like mine though and I sort of feel that the salve made my hands worse. Then I decided I would burn out the infection, so I soaked my hands in some bleaching solution. This helped some with the itching, but it made the skin too dry. Then I remembered that you had given me some salve for Johnnie's 'infantigo,' so I put some of that on. That softened up my hands but didn't seem to help with the itching. So here I am, Doctor."

DOCTOR (Writing, "Treated with athlete's foot R, bleach soaks, Johnnie's impetigo R."): "How much itching are you having?"

MRS. JONES: "Well, my hands sting and burn when I get any soap and water on them, but I can sleep without them bothering me."

DOCTOR (Notes "mild itching."): "Are you taking any medicine by mouth now for anything? I even want to know about laxatives, vitamins, or aspirin. Have you had any shots recently?"

MRS. JONES: "No, I'm not taking any medicine."

DOCTOR: "Now, are you sure?"

MRS. JONES: "Well, I do take sleeping medicine at night occasionally, and, oh yes, I'm taking some reducing pills that Dr. Smith gave me about 2 months ago."

DOCTOR (Writes, "Drugs—takes sleeping medicine h.s. and reducing pills."): "Mrs. Jones, does anyone in your family have any allergies? Does anyone have any asthma, hayfever, or eczema? Your parents, brothers, sisters, children, etc.?"

MRS. JONES: "No, not that I can recall, Doctor."

DOCTOR: "Have you ever had any of those conditions? Any asthma, hayfever, or eczema?"

MRS. JONES: "No, I haven't had any of those. Sometimes I have a little sinus trouble though."

DOCTOR (Writes, "No atopy in patient or family."): "Now, let me have a good look at those hands. I also want you to remove your shoes and hose so that I can get a good look at your feet." (The doctor then examines the patient's hands and feet very carefully.) "Now are you sure that you don't have this anywhere else, Mrs. Jones?"

MRS. JONES: "No, I am positive I don't because I looked all over my skin this morning when I took a bath. However, I do have a mole on my back that I want you to look at, Doctor."

DOCTOR: "Has it been bothering you recently?"

MRS. JONES: "Well, no, but my bra strap rubs it occasionally."

DOCTOR (Examines the mole on Mrs. Jones's back.): "That certainly is a small mole, Mrs. Jones. It doesn't have any unusual color, and I see no reason for having it removed. It could be removed if you wish, but I don't think it is necessary."

MRS. JONES: "Well, I don't want it removed if you don't think it is necessary. Now, what do you think about my hands?"

DOCTOR: "Let me make a few notes about what I saw and then I'll tell you about your hands and the treatment."

The doctor writes, "Physical exam.: (1) A crusting, vesicular dermatitis is seen mainly in the webs of the fingers of both hands, worse on the right hand. There is no sharp border to the eruption. The nail of the right ring finger has several transverse furrows. The feet are clear. (2) In the mid-line of the upper back is a 3 x 3 mm. flat, faintly brownish lesion. Diagnosis: (1) Contact dermatitis, prob-ably due to excess soap and water. (2) Pigmented compound nevus."

DOCTOR: "Mrs Jones, you have a very common skin condition, commonly called housewives' eczema or housewives' dermatitis. I feel sure that it is aggravated by having your hands in soap and water so many times a day. Most housewives don't even have enough time to dry their hands carefully every time they are wet. Some people seem to be more sensitive to soaps than others. It isn't a real allergy but just a sensitivity due to the fact that the soap and the water have a tendency to remove the normal skin protective oils and fats. Some of those blisters are infected, and we will have to take care of that infection along with the other irritation. Here is what we will do to treat your hands." (The doctor then gives very careful instructions to Mrs. Jones, particularly with regard to the hand soaks, the way the salve is to be applied, advice concerning avoidance of excess soap and water, the use of rubber and cotton gloves, etc.)

In the above play-by-play description, which is repeated many times a month in any busy practitioner's office, I have attempted to show some of the basic points in history-taking. The following factors should be stressed again:

1. *Local Treatment History.* Find out how much treatment and what kind of treatment has been given by the patient or by doctors.

2. *Drug History.* It is important to know if the patient is taking any medicine for any other disease for two reasons. First, you learn something about your patient from the drugs taken. For example, it is certainly important to know if a person is taking insulin for diabetes or digitalis for heart disease. This information can well influence your treatment of the patient. Secondly, drugs can cause many skin eruptions, and your index of suspicion of a drug eruption will be higher if you consistently request that information.

3. *Allergy History.* A family or a patient history of allergies can aid you in making a diagnosis of atopic dermatitis. Also if there is a positive allergy history,

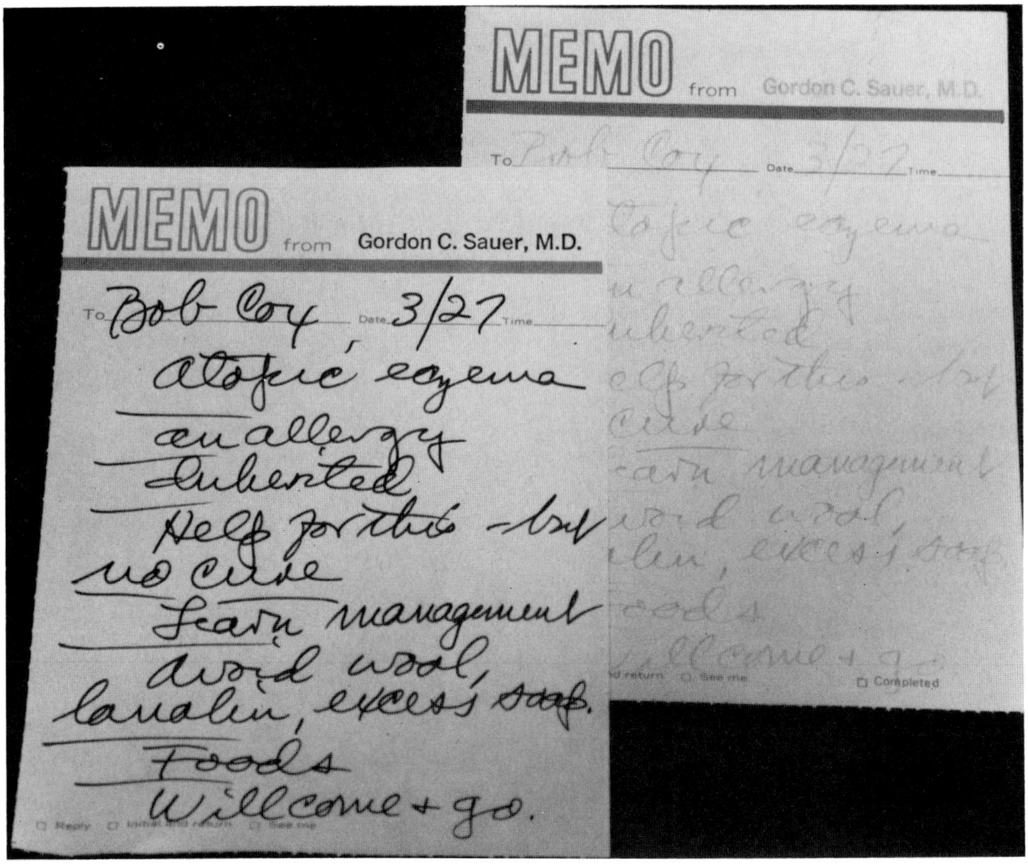

Fig. 4-1. Non-carbon form useful for both patient and physician to provide record of information and instructions given in office.

usually you can predict to the patient that her skin trouble will be slower in responding to treatment than a similar dermatitis in a nonallergenic patient. Atopic patients are more "itchish."

A careful history is followed by a complete examination of the skin problem, and this in turn is followed by therapy, or what I prefer to call management. For good management of the patient, I have found it helpful to write out the diagnosis, other information and instructions on non-carbon-paper forms. (The Drawing Board, Dallas, Texas 75221 calls them Mem-O-Grams, Fig. 4-1). Advantages to the patient and doctor are multiple. The patient has an individualized short note about the diagnosis, cause if known, what you as a physician can or cannot do (if there is "no cure" as for atopic eczema or psoriasis, say so), and instructions as to diet, bathing, therapy, etc.

For the doctor, the advantage is that you have a copy to keep in your chart that could be used later to help you refresh your patient's mind on instructions, or it could even be used advantageously in a medicolegal problem regarding information given.

5

Dermatologic Therapy

Many hundreds of medications are available for use in treating skin diseases. However, most doctors have only a few favorite prescriptions that are prescribed day in and day out. These few prescriptions may then be altered slightly to suit an individual patient or disease.

The treatment of the majority of the common skin conditions can be made simpler if the doctor is aware of three basic principles.

1. The *type of skin lesion*, more than the cause, influences the kind of local medication used. The old adage, "If it's wet, use a wet dressing, and if it's dry use a salve," is true for a majority of cases. For example, to treat a patient with an acute oozing, crusting dermatitis of the dorsum of the hand, whether due to poison ivy or soap, the doctor should prescribe wet soaks and a lotion. For a chronic-looking, dry, scaly patch of psoriasis on the elbow an ointment is indicated, since a lotion or a wet dressing would only be more drying. Bear in mind, however, that *the type of skin lesion can change rapidly under treatment*. The patient must be followed closely at the beginning of therapy. An acute oozing dermatitis treated with a lotion can change in 2 to 3 days to a dry scaly lesion that requires a paste or an ointment. Conversely, a chronic dry patch may become irritated with too strong therapy and begin to ooze.

2. The second basic principle in treatment is *never do any harm* and never overtreat. It is important for the physi-

---

THERAPY PEARLS

1. The type of skin lesion (oozing, infected, or dry), more than the cause, should decide the local medication that is prescribed.

2. Do no harm. Begin local therapy of a particular case with mild drugs. The concentration of ingredients can be increased as the acuteness subsides.

3. Carefully instruct the patient or the nurse regarding the local application of salves, lotions, wet dressings and baths.

4. Prescribe the correct amount of medication for the area and the dermatosis to be treated. This knowledge comes with experience.

5. Change the therapy as the response indicates. If a new prescription is indicated and the patient has some of the first ℞ left, use this up by instructing the patient to alternate using the old with the new prescription.

6. If a prescription is going to be relatively expensive, explain this fact to the patient.

7. Instruct the patient to telephone you if there are any questions, or if the medicine seems to irritate the dermatosis.

For New or Favorite Prescriptions of Your Own

cian to know which of the chemicals prescribed for local use on the skin are the greatest irritants and sensitizers. It is no exaggeration to say that the most commonly seen dermatitis is the overtreatment contact dermatitis. The overtreatment is often at the hands of the patient who has gone to his neighborhood drugstore or friend and used any and many of the medications available for the treatment of skin diseases. It is certainly not unusual to hear the patient tell of using a strong athlete's foot salve for the treatment of the lesions of pityriasis rosea.

3. The third principle is to *instruct the patient adequately regarding the application* of the medicine prescribed. The patient does not have to be told how to swallow a pill but does have to be told how to put on a wet dressing. Most skin patients are ambulatory, so there is no nurse to help them. They are their own nurse. The success or the failure of skin therapy rests upon adequate instruction of the patient or person responsible for the care. Even in hospitals, particularly when wet dressings or lotions are prescribed, it is wise for the doctor to instruct the nurse regarding the procedure.

With these principles of management in mind let us now turn to the medicine used. It is important to stress that I am endeavoring to present here only the most basic material necessary to treat the majority of skin diseases. For instance, there are many solutions for wet dressings, but boric acid solution is my preference. Other physicians have preferences different from the drugs listed, and their choices are respected; but to list all of them will not serve the purpose of this book. Two factors have guided me in the selection of medications presented in this formulary. First, the medication must be readily available in most drugstores; secondly, it must be a very effective medication for one or several skin conditions. The medications listed in this formulary will also be listed in a complete way in the treatment section concerning the particular disease. However, instructions for the use of the medications will be more nearly complete in this formulary.

One side of each page in this section has been left blank so that you can insert new or favorite prescriptions of your own.

FORMULARY

A certain topical medication is prescribed to produce a specific beneficial effect.

EFFECTS OF LOCALLY APPLIED DRUGS

1. **Antipruritic agents** relieve itching in various ways. Commonly used chemicals and strengths include menthol (0.25%), phenol (0.5%), camphor (2%) and coal tar solution (2 to 10)%. These chemicals are added to various bases for the desired effect. Numerous safe and unsafe proprietary preparations for relief of itching are also available. The unsafe preparations are those that contain antihistamines, benzocaine and related "caine" derivatives.

2. **Keratoplastic agents** tend to increase the thickness of the horny layer. Salicylic acid (1 to 2%) is an example of a keratoplastic agent, whereas stronger strengths of salicylic acid are keratolytic.

3. **Keratolytics** remove or soften the horny layer. Commonly used agents of this type include salicylic acid (4 to 10%), resorcinol (2 to 4%), and sulfur (4 to 10%). A *strong* destructive agent is trichloracetic acid, full strength.

4. **Antieczematous agents** remove oozing and vesicular excretions by various actions. The common antieczematous agents include 2 percent boric acid solution packs or soaks, coal tar solution (2 to 5%), and hydrocortisone (0.5 to 2%) and derivatives incorporated in lotions or salves.

5. **Antiparasitics** destroy or inhibit living infestations. Examples include Eurax lotion and cream for scabies, and Kwell cream and lotion for scabies and pediculosis.

6. **Antiseptics** destroy or inhibit bacteria and fungi. Commonly used examples include Vioform (3%), Sterosan (3%), ammoniated mercury (3 to 10%), and antibiotics such as Neomycin (0.5%), Aureomycin (3%) and Terramycin (3%). Antifungal agents include Whitfield's oint-

For New or Favorite Prescriptions of Your Own

ment, Desenex preparations, Tinactin preparations, Halotex preparations, and sulfur and ammoniated mercury in various bases.

7. **Emollients** soften the skin surface. Nivea oil, mineral oil and white petrolatum are good examples.

TYPES OF TOPICAL DERMATOLOGIC MEDICATIONS

1. **Baths:**

A. Tar Bath
   Coal tar solution, U.S.P. (liquor carbonis detergens)   120.0
   Sig: 2 tablespoons to the tub of lukewarm water 6 to 8 inches deep
   Actions: Antipruritic, antieczematous

B. Starch Bath
   Linit or Argo Starch, small box
   Sig: ½ box of starch to the tub of cool water 6 to 8 inches deep
   Actions: Soothing, antipruritic
   Indications: Generalized itching and dryness of skin, winter itch, urticaria

C. Aveeno Colloidal Oatmeal Box (Cooper)
   Sig: 1 cup to the tub of water.
   Actions: Soothing and cleansing
   Indications: Generalized itching and dryness of skin, and winter and senile itch.

D. Oil Baths (See Oils and Emulsions, p. 37)

2. **Soaps and shampoos:**

A. Oilatum Soap Unscented (Stiefel)
   Actions: Mild cleansing agent that leaves an oily film on the skin
   Indications: Dry skin, winter itch

B. Dial Soap (Armour)
   Actions: Cleansing, antibacterial
   Indications: Acne, pyodermas

C. Selsun Suspension Shampoo (Abbott)   120.0
   Sig: Shampoo hair with 3 separate applications and rinses. Can leave the last application on the scalp for 5 minutes before rins-

ing off. Do not use another shampoo as a final cleanser.
   Actions: Cleansing, antiseborrheic
   Indications: Dandruff, or itching scalp. Not toxic if used as directed.

D. Tar Shampoos: X Seb T (Cummins), Sebutone (Westwood), Ionil-T (Owen), Vanseb-T (Herbert) etc.
   Sig: Shampoo as necessary, even daily
   Actions: Cleansing and antiseborrheic
   Indications: Dandruff, psoriasis, or atopic eczema of scalp

3. **Wet dressings or soaks:**

A. Boric Acid Solution, 2%
   Sig: 1 level tablespoon of boric acid crystals to 1 quart of tap water. Cover affected area with sheeting wet with solution and tie on with gauze bandage or string. Do not allow any wet dressing to dry out. Can also be used as a solution for soaks.
   Actions: Acidifying, antieczematous, antiseptic
   Indications: Oozing or vesicular skin conditions. Do not use over a large area of the body and do not use on children.

B. Burow's Solution, 1:20
   Sig: 1 Domeboro tablet (Dome) or 1 Blueboro Packet (Derm-Arts) to 1 pint of tap water.
   For wet dressing or soaks as above.

C. Vinegar Solution
   Sig: ½ cup of white vinegar to 1 quart of water.
   For wet dressings or soaks as above.

4. **Powders:**

A. Purified Talc (U.S.P.)   60.0
   Sig: Dust on locally b.i.d. (Supply in a powder can)
   Actions: Absorbent, protective, cooling
   Indications: Intertrigo, diaper dermatitis

For New or Favorite Prescriptions of Your Own

B. Tinactin Powder (Schering)
or Desenex Powder (Pharma-craft)
Sig: Dust on feet in A.M.
Actions: Absorbent, antifungal
Indications: Prevention or treatment of tinea pedis, tinea cruris

C. Mycostatin Powder (Squibb) 15.0
Sig: Dust on locally b.i.d.
Actions: Antimonilial
Indications: Monilial intertrigo

5. **Shake lotions:**

A. Calamine Lotion (U.S.P.) 120.0
Sig: Apply locally to affected area t.i.d. with fingers or brush.
Actions: Antipruritic, antieczematous
Indications: Widespread, mildly oozing inflamed dermatoses

B. Nonalcoholic White Shake Lotion
Zinc oxide 24.0
Talc 24.0
Glycerin 12.0
Distilled water q.s.ad. 120.0

C. Alcoholic White Shake Lotion
Zinc oxide 24.0
Talc 24.0
Glycerin 12.0
Distilled water
95% alcohol āā q.s.ad. 120.0

D. Colored Alcoholic Shake Lotion
To 5C above add: Almay Neutra-color (brunette shade) 2.4

E. Aveeno Lotion (Cooper) 120.0

F. Acticort 100 Lotion (Cummins) 120.0
To the above lotions you can add sulfur, resorcinol, menthol, phenol, etc., as indicated.

6. **Oils and emulsions:**

A. Zinc Oil
Zinc oxide 40%
Olive oil q.s. 120.0
Sig: Apply locally to affected area by hand or brush t.i.d.
Actions: Soothing, antipruritic and astringent
Indications: Acute and subacute eczematous eruptions

B. Bath Oils
Nivea Skin Oil (Duke) or
Lubath (Texas) or
Alpha-Keri (Westwood) or
Domol (Dome) or
Geri Bath (Dermik)
Sig: 1 to 2 tablespoonfuls to the tub of water. Be careful to prevent slipping in tub.
Actions: Emollient, lubricating
Indications: Winter itch, dry skin, atopic eczema

C. Hand and Body Emulsions
Allercreme Special Formula Skin Lotion (Texas) (without lanolin)
Nivea Creme (Duke)
Keri Lotion (Westwood)
Nutraderm (Owen) (without lanolin)
Ultra-Derm Moisturizer (Cummins)
Sig: (No prescription required) Apply locally as necessary.
Actions: Emollient, lubricating
Indications: Dry skin, winter itch, atopic eczema

7. **Tinctures and aqueous solutions:**

A. Gentian Violet Solution
Gentian Violet 1%
Distilled Water q.s. 30.0
Sig: Apply with swab b.i.d.
Actions: Antifungal, antibacterial
Indications: Moniliasis, leg ulcers

B. Sodium Thiosulfate Solution
Sodium Thiosulfate 20%
Distilled Water q.s. 180.0
Sig: Apply nightly after bath
Actions: Mildly antifungal
Indications: Tinea versicolor

8. **Pastes:**

Zinc Oxide Paste (U.S.P.)
Sig: Apply locally b.i.d.
Actions: Protective, absorbent, astringent
Indications: Localized crusted or scaly dermatoses

9. **Creams and ointments:**

A physician can write prescriptions for creams and ointments in 2 ways. He can (1) formulate his own pre-

For New or Favorite Prescriptions of Your Own

scriptions by adding medications to certain bases as especially indicated for the particular patient being treated, or (2) he can prescribe proprietary creams and ointments already compounded by pharmaceutical companies.

For the physician who uses the first method, there are 2 different types of bases used.

A. Water-washable cream bases. These bases are pleasant for the patient to use, are nongreasy, and are usually always indicated when treating intertriginous and hairy areas. Their disadvantage is that they can be too drying. A multitude of medications, as specifically indicated, can be added to these bases—e.g., menthol, sulfur, tars, hydrocortisone, antibiotics, etc.
 a. Unibase (Parke-Davis)
 b. Neobase (Burroughs Wellcome)
 c. Acid Mantle Cream (Dome)
 d. Unscented cold cream (not water-washable)

B. Ointment bases. These "Vaseline" type bases are, and should be, the most useful in dermatology. While not as pleasant for the patient to use as the cream bases, their greasy quality alleviates dryness, removes scales and enables the medicaments to penetrate the skin lesions. Any local medicine can be incorporated in these bases.
 a. White Petrolatum (U.S.P.)
 b. Zinc Oxide Ointment (U.S.P.)

For the physician who wishes to prescribe ready-made proprietary preparations, these are listed in groups.

C. Antifungal Ointments and Creams
 a. Enzactin Cream (Ayerst)
 b. Desenex Ointment (Pharmacraft)
 c. Tinactin Cream (Schering)
 d. Halotex cream (Mead Johnson)
 e. Verdefam Cream (Texas)
    Actions: Antifungal, keratolytic

f. Benzoic and Salicylic Acid Ointment, U.S.P. (Whitfield's Ointment)

 Actions: Antifungal, keratolytic. Use full or double strength. Be sure to specify "U.S.P." or you may get the older and stronger 12% Benzoic and 6% Salicylic Acid Ointment.

D. Antibiotic Ointments
 a. Neosporin Ointment (Burroughs Wellcome)
 b. Neo-Polycin Ointment (Dow)
 c. Mycitracin Ointment (Upjohn)
    The following do not contain neomycin, so can be used in neomycin-sensitive patients.
 d. Polysporin Ointment (Burroughs Wellcome)
 e. Chloromycetin Ointment (Parke-Davis)
 f. Garamycin Cream (Schering)

E. Corticosteroid Ointments and Creams

 Hydrocortisone Preparations
 a. Cortef Acetate Ointment (½%, 1% & 2% strengths) (Upjohn)
 b. Cort-Dome Cream (½% & 1% strengths) (Dome)
 c. Texacort Cream (½% & 1% strengths) (Texas)

 Triamcinolone Preparations
 a. Kenalog Ointment and Cream (Squibb)
 b. Aristocort Ointment and Cream (Lederle)

 Fluorinated Corticosteroid Preparations
 a. Synalar Cream (0.01% and 0.025%) (Syntex)
 b. Cordran Cream (0.025% and 0.05%) (Lilly)
 c. Florinef Ointment (0.1% and 0.2%) (Squibb)
 d. Valisone Cream and Ointment (Schering)
 e. Fluonid Cream (0.025% and 0.01%) and Ointment (Dermarts)

For New or Favorite Prescriptions of Your Own

f. Lidex Cream and Ointment (Syntex)
and others

F. Corticosteroid-Antibiotic Ointments and Creams
   a. Neo-Cortef Ointment (Upjohn)
   b. Neo-Cort-Dome Cream (Dome)
   c. Cortisporin Ointment (Burroughs Wellcome)
   d. Humacort Ointment (Parke-Davis)
   e. Kenalog-S Ointment and Cream (Squibb)
   f. Cordran-N Cream (Lilly)
   g. Neo-Hydeltrasol Ointment (Merck Sharp & Dohme)
   h. Terra-Cortril Ointment (Pfizer)
   and many others.

G. Antipruritic Ointments
   a. Quotane Ointment (Smith Kline & French)
   b. Perazil Cream (Burroughs Wellcome)
   c. Eurax Cream (Geigy)
   d. Lida-Mantle Creme (Dome)

H. Miscellaneous Creams and Ointments
   a. Vioform Ointment or Cream, 3% (Ciba) or Sterosan Ointment or Cream, 3% (Geigy)
      Actions: Antiseptic, antiseborrheic
   b. Pragmatar (Smith Kline & French) contains 3% sulfur, 3% salicylic acid and a tar, 4%
      Actions: Antifungal, keratolytic, antipruritic

I. Scabicidal and Pediculocidal
   a. Eurax Cream and Lotion (Geigy)
      Actions: Scabicidal
   b. Benzyl Benzoate Emulsion, U.S.P.
      Benzyl Benzoate Emulsion (Burroughs Wellcome)
   c. Kwell Lotion & Cream (Reed & Carnrick)
      Actions of b and c: Scabicidal and pediculocidal

J. Sun Screen Creams
   a. Skole (Williams)
   b. A-fil (Texas)
   c. R.V.P. Ointment (Elder)
   d. Uval (Dome)
      Sig: Apply to exposed areas before going outside.
      Actions: Screen out ultraviolet rays.
      Indications: Actinic dermatitis, acute and chronic lupus erythematosus, possible prevention of skin cancers in light complexioned individuals. (These agents prevent skin tanning.)

10. **Aerosols and foams**

Various local medications have been incorporated in aerosol and foam-producing containers. These include corticosteroids, antibiotics, antifungal agents, antipruritic medicines, etc.

Kenalog spray (150 Gm. can) (Squibb) and Valisone Aerosol (85 Gm. can) (Schering) are effective corticosteroid preparations for scalp psoriasis and seborrhea.

11. **Medicated tape**
    A. Cordran Tape (Lilly)
       Indications: for small areas of psoriasis, neurodermatitis or lichen planus

12. **Fluorouracil preparations**

See section on actinic keratosis therapy, p. 265.

13. **Local agents for office use**
    A. Podophyllum in alcohol
       Podophyllum Resin
       (U.S.P.)   25%
       Alcohol q.s.ad.   30.0
       Indications: For removal of venereal warts
       Directions: Apply small amount to warts with cotton-tipped applicator every 4 to 5 days until warts are gone. Excess amount may be washed off in 6 hours after application to prevent irritation.

B. Chrysarobin Tincture

Chrysarobin	3%
Chloroform q.s.	30.0

Indications: Tinea of nails, tinea cruris.

Directions: Apply in office with cotton-tipped applicator every 5 to 7 days. It stings on crural area. Caution patient not to touch eyelids with treated fingers.

C. Trichloracetic Acid Solution (Saturated)

Indications: For removal by chemical cautery of warts on children, seborrheic keratoses and xanthelasma (with caution)

Directions: Apply with caution with cotton-tipped applicator. (Have water handy to neutralize.)

D. Modified Unna's Boot
  a. Dome Paste Bandage (Dome)
  b. Gelocast (Duke)

Indications: For stasis ulcers, localized neurodermatitis

E. Ace Bandage, 3 inches in width (Becton, Dickinson)

Indications: For stasis dermatitis and leg edema

LOCAL THERAPY RULES OF THUMB

Students and general practitioners state that they are especially confused by the dermatologists' reasons for using one chemical for one skin lesion and not another, or one chemical for unrelated skin diseases. The answer to this dilemma is not easily given. More often than not the major reason for our preference is that experience has taught us, and those before us, that the particular drug works. Some drugs do have definite chemical actions, such as antipruritic, antifungal or peeling actions, and these have been listed on page 33. But there is no definite scientific explanation for the beneficial effect of some of the other drugs, such as tar or sulfur on cases of psoriasis, etc.

In an attempt to solve this apparent confusion, here are some generalizations summarizing my experience.

NOTE: When prescribing one of these chemicals, always begin with the lower percentage of the drug and increase the percentage only when a stronger action is desired.

Tars

Coal Tar Solution (L.C.D.)	3-10%
Crude Coal Tar	1-5%
Oil of Cade	1-5%

Consider for use in cases of:
  Atopic eczema
  Psoriasis
  Seborrheic dermatitis
  Neurodermatitis, localized
Avoid in intertriginous areas (can cause a folliculitis)

Sulfur (Sulfur, precipitated, 3-10%)

Consider for use in cases of:
  Tinea of any area of body
  Acne vulgaris and rosacea
  Seborrheic dermatitis
  Pyodermas (combine with antibiotic salves)
  Psoriasis
Avoid: Do not mix with mercury (causes black mercuric sulfide deposit on skin)

Mercury (Ammoniated Mercury, 1-10%)

Consider for use in cases of:
  Psoriasis
  Pyodermas
  Seborrheic dermatitis
Avoid: Do not mix with sulfur (see above)

Resorcinol (Resorcinol monoacetate, 1-5%)

Consider for use in cases of:
  Acne vulgaris and rosacea (usually with sulfur)
  Seborrheic dermatitis
  Psoriasis

Salicylic Acid (1-5%, higher with caution)

Consider for use in cases of:
  Psoriasis
  Neurodermatitis, localized thick form
  Tinea of feet or palms (when peeling is desired)
  Seborrheic dermatitis
Avoid in intertriginous areas

Menthol (¼%); Phenol (½-2%); Camphor (1-2%)

Consider for use in any pruritic dermatoses

Avoid use over large areas of body

Hydrocortisone and Related Corticosteroids (Hydrocortisone powder, ¼-2%)

Consider for use in cases of:

Contact dermatitis of any area

Seborrheic dermatitis

Intertrigo of axilla, crural or inframammary regions

Atopic eczema

Neurodermatitis

Avoid use over large areas of body because of expense, and possible, but unlikely, internal absorption.

Fluorinated Corticosteroids Locally (Synalar preparations, Cordran preparations, Fluonid preparations, Locorten preparations, Lidex preparations)

These chemicals are not available as powders for personal compounding.

Consider for use with or without occlusive dressings in cases of:

Psoriasis, localized to small area (see p. 97)

Neurodermatitis, localized (see p. 72)

Lichen planus, especially hypertrophic type

Also anywhere that hydrocortisone is indicated

SPECIFIC INTERNAL DRUGS FOR SPECIFIC DISEASES

As in all fields of medicine, there are certain diseases that can be treated best by certain specific systemic drugs. These drugs may not be curative, but they should be considered when you begin to outline a course of management for a particular patient. Many factors will influence your decision to use or not use such a specific drug. Here follows a list of skin diseases and some systemic medicines considered specific (or as specific as specific can be) for the disease. For proper dosage and contraindications, check the appropriate sections in this book or in current books on therapy.

Acne vulgaris or rosacea in the scarring stage: antibiotics, sulfas and female hormones

Alopecia areata: occasionally corticosteroids in any of 3 forms—oral, parenteral and intralesional

Blastomycosis: Amphotericin B, administered in hospital

Creeping eruption: thiabendazole

Darier's disease: vitamin A, for controlled periods of time

Dermatitis herpetiformis: Diasone and sulfapyridine

Granuloma annulare: intralesional corticosteroids

Granuloma inguinale: streptomycin

Inflammation of the skin from many causes: antibiotics are indicated in some cases when local therapy is inadequate for control. Oral corticosteroids also indicated for mild cases of inflammation.

Keloids: intralesional corticosteroids

Lichen planus: bismuth (but not in children)

Lupus erythematosus (especially chronic discoid type): antimalarials for controlled periods of time. For systemic lupus erythematosus, use corticosteriods, and, in some mild cases, antimalarials.

Mycosis fungoides: corticosteroids, and nitrogen mustard and related drugs

Necrobiosis lipoidica diabeticorum: intralesional corticosteroids

Neurodermatitis, localized: intralesional corticosteriods

Pemphigus: corticosteroids

Pruritus from many causes: antihistamines and tranquilizerlike drugs. Selected cases can be treated with oral corticosteroids.

Psoriasis, localized: intralesional corticosteroids

Pyodermas of skin: systemic antibiotics are valuable when indicated

Sarcoidosis: possibly corticosteroids

Sporotrichosis: saturated aqueous solution of potassium iodide

Syphilis: penicillin or other antibiotics

Tinea of scalp, body, crural area, fingernails (not feet or toenails): griseofulvin

Tuberculosis of the skin: dihydrostreptomycin, isoniazid and para-aminosalicylic acid

Urticaria: antihistamines and corticosteroids

BIBLIOGRAPHY

Conn, H. F.: Current Therapy. Philadelphia, W. B. Saunders, published yearly.

Lerner, M. R., and Lerner, A. B.: Dermatologic Medications. Chicago, Year Book Publishers, 1960.

Pascher, F.: Dermatologic Formulary. New York, Hoeber, 1953.

Physician's Desk Reference (PDR). Oradell, Medical Economics, published yearly.

Sternberg, T. H., Newcomer, V. D., Calnan, C. D., Rostenberg, A., Jr., and Rothman, S.: The Evaluation of Therapeutic Agents and Cosmetics. New York, McGraw-Hill, 1964.

6

Physical Dermatologic Therapy

The field of physical medicine embraces therapy with a variety of agents which include massage, therapeutic exercise, water, air, radiations (which include heat, light, ultraviolet, x-rays and radium), vibrations, refrigeration, and electricity of various forms. Many of these agents are used in the treatment of skin diseases.

HYDROTHERAPY

The physical agent most commonly used for dermatoses is hydrotherapy in the form of medicated or nonmedicated wet compresses and baths. Distilled water or tap water are the vehicles and may contain any of the following chemicals in varying strengths: sodium chloride, boric acid, aluminum acetate (Burow's solution), potassium permanganate, silver nitrate, tar, starch, oatmeal (Aveeno) and colloid (Soyaloid). The instructions and the dilutions for boric acid compresses, starch baths and tar baths are listed in the Formulary.

WET DRESSINGS

Wet dressings can be applied as open or closed dressings. The *open* compresses are used most frequently, since excessive maceration of tissue occurs when the dressings are "closed" with wax paper or rubber sheeting. The compresses can be *hot, cold* or at *room* temperature. Instructions to the patient or the nurse concerning correct application of the compresses should be explicit and detailed. For most conditions the area to be treated should be wrapped with 2 or 3 layers of clean sheeting or muslin. Then gauze 3 inches wide should be wrapped around the sheeting to hold it firmly in place. After that the dressing can be moistened with the solution by pouring it on or by squirting it on with a bulb syringe. In most instances the dressing is wet with the solution before it is wrapped on the affected area. The compresses should never be allowed to dry out and should be left on only for the time specified by the doctor. The solution used should be made fresh every day. For treating the face, the hands and the genitalia, special masks, gloves and slings can be improvised. The indications for wet compresses are any oozing, crusting, or pruritic dermatoses regardless of etiology.

MEDICATED BATHS

Medicated baths should last from 15 to 30 minutes. Cool baths tend to lessen pruritus and are prescribed most frequently. Baths can be used for a multitude of skin diseases except those conditions where excessive dryness is to be avoided, such as for patients with atopic eczema, senile or winter pruritus and ichthyosis.

ELECTROSURGERY

Electrosurgery is employed very commonly in treating or removing a multitude of skin lesions. One of several different types of available current or instrument is employed to achieve a desired result. Five forms of electrosurgery are available.

ELECTRODESICCATION OR FULGURATION

Electrodesiccation or fulguration is produced by an Oudin current of high voltage and low amperage, using a single or monoterminal electrode. The high frequency current wave is damped. Such a current is produced by the Hyfrecator and by the larger Bovie or Wappler units, using the spark-gap part of the machine. The effect on the skin is a charring of the tissues.

45

ELECTROCOAGULATION

Electrocoagulation is produced by a d'Arsonval current of relatively low voltage and high amperage, using biterminal electrodes. This current also is damped and can be obtained from the Bovie and the Wappler combination units, using the spark-gap part of the machine. Electrocoagulation is more destructive than electrodesiccation, due to the intense heat.

ELECTROSECTION

Electrosection or cutting is produced by a current which is undamped when delivered by a vacuum tube apparatus and moderately damped from a spark-gap apparatus. Biterminal electrodes are used. The large Bovie and Wappler combination units produce a moderately damped current from the spark-gap part of the machine and an undamped current from the vacuum tube part. When the vacuum tube cutting current is used the cut is clean with practically no coagulation, whereas the current from a spark-gap machine produces some coagulation of the cut skin edge. Any coagulation can be minimized by making a rapid stroke. Tissue skillfully removed in this manner can be studied histologically if necessary.

ELECTROCAUTERY

Electrocautery is simply produced by applying heat to the skin. This can be supplied by many instruments, one of which is the Post Electric Cautery (Andover, N. J.). Many operators prefer this form of electrosurgery to electrodesiccation or electrocoagulation.

ELECTROLYSIS

Electrolysis utilizes a direct galvanic current to produce chemical cauterization of tissue due to the formation of sodium hydroxide in the tissues with liberation of free hydrogen at the negative electrode. Battery machines or rectified direct current instruments accomplish this. Electrolysis is used mainly to remove superfluous hair. A faster and less painful technic of hair epilation is to use the high frequency current set at a very low intensity where it will deliver a small electrodesiccation spark.

The dermatoses most commonly treated by electrosurgery are warts of all kinds, senile and seborrheic keratoses, leukoplakia, pigmented nevi, spider hemangiomas, hypertrichosis, and basal cell and prickle cell epitheliomas. The skill and the experience of the therapist will be the factor determining the scope of his use of the surgical diathermy machine.

CRYOSURGERY

Therapeutic refrigeration for the skin can be accomplished by the use of solid carbon dioxide, liquid nitrogen, or Freon 114.

Solid carbon dioxide is used most commonly because it is readily available from a tank of carbon dioxide, or as blocks from ice cream manufacturers, or from the Kiddie Dry Ice Apparatus (see p. 337). The temperature of solid carbon dioxide is $-78.5°$ C. The solid carbon dioxide is shaped into an appropriately sized "pencil" for treatment of superficial skin growths, warts or seborrheic keratoses.

Liquid nitrogen, which provides freezing at $-195.8°$ C., has recently become more readily available for office use. Many dermatologists now have a 25 liter refillable container in their office. This amount will last for three to four weeks with normal usage. A loosely wound large cotton applicator stick is used to hold the smoking liquid (Fig. 6-1). The applicator is applied to the skin for only a few seconds to freeze warts, seborrheic keratoses, actinic keratoses and other superficial skin growths. The pain varies from moderate to quite marked. A blister forms within 24 hours after the application and, hopefully, the growth comes off entirely when the dead skin peels away in ten to fourteen days. Additional liquid nitrogen applications may be indicated.

Freon 114 is used mainly to freeze and immobilize the skin for the dermabrasion removal of acne scars, tattoos, or senile keratotic skin.

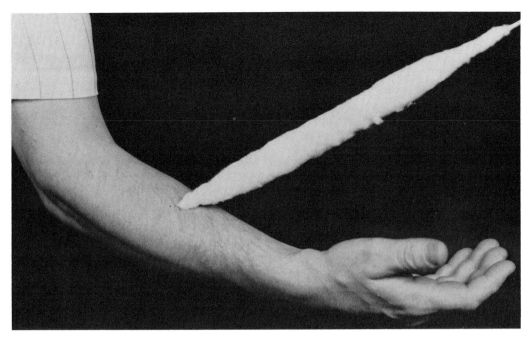

Fig. 6-1. Technique of applying liquid nitrogen to skin lesion with large cotton applicator.

RADIATION

Radiation agents are important in the field of skin diseases.

ULTRAVIOLET THERAPY

Ultraviolet therapy is most commonly utilized and available. The two sources of artificial ultraviolet radiation are the hot quartz mercury arc lamp, which operates at a high vapor pressure and relatively high temperature, and the cold quartz lamp which operates at a low vapor pressure and low temperature.

The *hot quartz lamp* is used mainly for the effect from its radiations at 2,900 to 3,200 Ångström units. These rays cause erythema and tanning of the skin. Modifications of these lamps are sold as sun lamps for use in the home. The dermatoses most commonly treated with the hot quartz lamp are psoriasis, acne, pityriasis rosea and seborrheic dermatitis, particularly when the last is of the generalized type on the body.

The *cold quartz lamp* has mainly disinfecting and desquamating effects on the skin, due to the predominance of rays at 2,537 Ångström units. Its use in dermatology and in general is limited.

X-RAY THERAPY

Another of the physical therapeutic agents commonly used for skin diseases is x-ray therapy. A detailed discussion of x-ray therapy is not within the scope of this book, since it is a specialized subject of considerable magnitude. Radiation therapy should be administered only by an adequately trained dermatologist or radiologist. If correct shielding and dosage are observed, x-ray therapy is quite safe, as has been proved by many well-controlled studies.

X-ray or radium therapy finds its greatest use in the treatment of skin cancers, acne, various pruritic dermatoses, and cutaneous lymphoblastomas (particularly mycosis fungoides). X-ray therapy is contraindicated in the management of light-sensitive eruptions (acute or chronic lupus erythematosus, actinic dermatitis), radiodermatitis, hypertrichosis and localized excessive perspiration.

For the majority of dermatoses, excluding malignancies, the physical factors of superficial x-ray therapy are 70 to 100 kilovolt-peak, 2 to 5 milliamperes, 20 to 30 cm. focal skin distance and no filter. The half-value layer with these factors varies with the machine from 0.6 to 1.0 mm. of aluminum. The average superficial x-ray therapy dose for dermatoses is 75 r per week. This weekly dose can be given up to a maximum total of 600 to 1,200 r if absolutely indicated. The top maximum dose depends on many factors, such as seriousness of the lesion being treated, response of the dermatosis to therapy, complexion of the individual, and age of the individual. *Under no circumstances should such a maximum course of x-ray therapy ever be repeated.* Grenz ray therapy is an even more superficial form of radiation therapy and therefore it is potentially less harmful.

BIBLIOGRAPHY

Cipollaro, A. C., and Crossland, P. M.: X-rays and Radium in the Treatment of Diseases of the Skin, ed. 5. Philadelphia, Lea & Febiger, 1967.

Epstein, E.: Skin Surgery, ed. 3. Springfield, Ill., Charles C Thomas, 1970.

Wansker, B. A.: X-ray and Radium in Dermatology. Springfield, Ill., Charles C Thomas, 1959.

7

Dermatologic Allergy

Contact dermatitis, industrial dermatoses, atopic eczema and drug eruptions are included in this chapter because of their obvious allergenic factors. Nummular eczema is also included because it resembles some forms of atopic eczema and may even be a variant of atopic eczema.

CONTACT DERMATITIS
(Plates 4 to 7)

Contact dermatitis, or dermatitis venenata, is a very common inflammation of the skin caused by the exposure of the skin either to primary irritant substances, such as soaps, or to allergenic substances, such as poison ivy resin. Industrial dermatoses will be considered at the end of this section.

Primary Lesions. See any of the stages from mild redness, edema or vesicles to large bullae with a marked amount of oozing.

Secondary Lesions. Crusting from secondary bacterial infection, excoriations and lichenification.

Distribution and Etiology. Any agent can affect any area of the body. However, certain agents commonly affect certain skin areas.

FACE AND NECK (Fig. 7-1): Cosmetics, soaps, insect sprays, ragweed, perfumes or hair sprays (sides of neck), fingernail polish (eyelids), hatband (forehead), mouthwashes, tooth paste or lipstick (perioral), nickel metal (earlobes), industrial oil (facial chloracne)

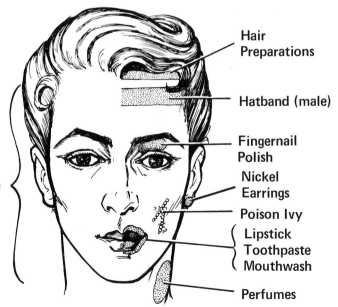

Fig. 7-1. Contact dermatitis of the face.

49

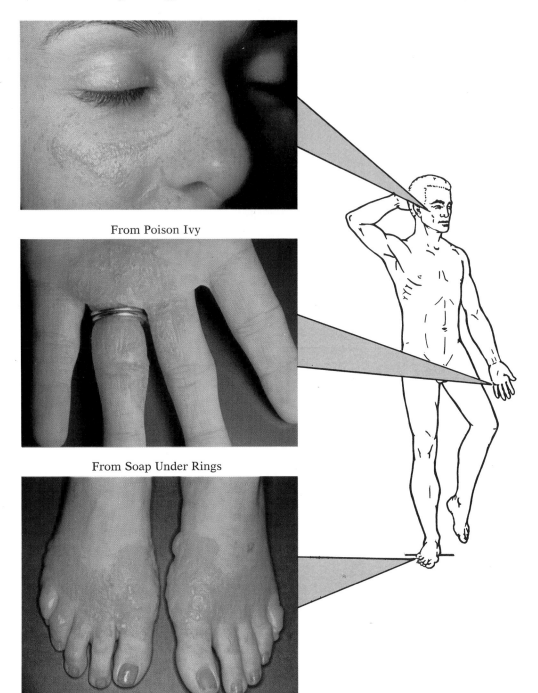

From Poison Ivy

From Soap Under Rings

From Shoe Material

Plate 4. Contact dermatitis. (*Burroughs Wellcome & Company, Inc.*)

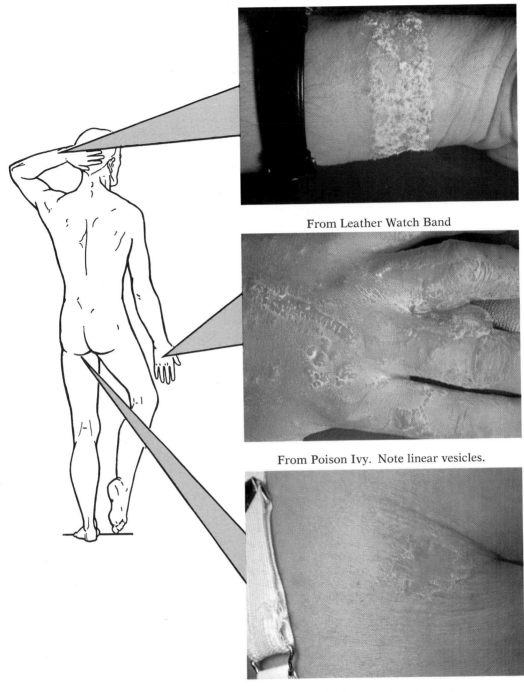

From Leather Watch Band

From Poison Ivy. Note linear vesicles.

From Nickel Metal in Garter Strap

Plate 5. Contact dermatitis. (*Burroughs Wellcome & Company, Inc.*)

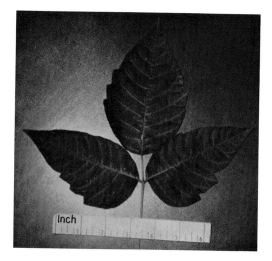

Fig. 7-2. Large leaves of the poison ivy plant.

HANDS AND FOREARMS: Soaps, hand lotions, wrist bands, industrial chemicals, poison ivy and a multitude of other agents. Irritation from soap often begins under rings.

AXILLAE: Deodorants, dress shields, or dry cleaning solutions

TRUNK: Clothing (new, not previously cleaned), rubber or metal attached to or in clothing

ANOGENITAL REGION: Douches, dusting powder, contraceptives, colored toilet paper, poison ivy, or too strong salves for treatment of pruritus ani and fungal infections

FEET: Shoes, foot powders, too strong salves for "athlete's feet" infection

GENERALIZED ERUPTION: Volatile airborne chemicals (paint spray, ragweed), medicaments locally applied to large areas, both powder, or clothing

Determine the site of the INITIAL eruption and think of the agents that touch that area.

Course. Duration very short to very chronic. As a general rule, successive recurrences become more chronic (i.e., seasonal ragweed dermatitis can become a year-round dermatitis). An established hypersensitivity reaction is never lost. Also, certain individuals have greater susceptibility for allergic and irritant contact dermatitis.

Season. A very careful seasonal history of the onset in chronic cases may lead to discovery of an unsuspected causative agent, such as ragweed.

Family Incidence. Not evident.

Contagiousness. The eczematous reaction, for instance the blister fluid of poison ivy, contains no allergen that can cause the dermatitis in another individual. However, if the poison ivy oil or other allergen remains on the skin of the affected person, contact of the allergen with a susceptible individual could cause a dermatitis.

Laboratory Findings. Patch tests (p. 9) are of value in eliciting the cause in a problem case. Careful interpretation is a necessity.

Differential Diagnosis. A contactant reaction must be thought of and ruled in or out in any case of eczematous dermatitis on any body area.

Treatment. Two of the commonest contact dermatoses seen in the doctor's office are *poison ivy dermatitis* and *hand dermatitis*. The treatment of these two conditions will be discussed.

TREATMENT OF CONTACT DERMATITIS
DUE TO POISON IVY

A patient comes into your office with a linear, vesicular dermatitis of the feet, the hands and the face. He states that he spent the weekend fishing and that the rash broke out the next day. The itching is rather severe but not enough to keep him awake at night. He had "poison ivy" 5 years ago (Fig. 7-2).

Treatment on First Visit

1. Assure the patient that he cannot give the dermatitis to his family or spread it on himself from the blister fluid.

2. Suggest that the clothes worn while fishing be washed or cleaned to remove the allergenic resin.

3. Débridement. The blisters should be opened with manicure scissors and not by sticking with a needle. Cutting the top open with the scissors will prevent that blister from re-forming.

4. Boric acid solution (2%) wet packs

Sig: 1 tablespoon of boric acid crystals to 1 quart of cool water. Apply sheeting or toweling, wet with the solution, to the blistered areas for 20 minutes twice a day. The wet packs need not be removed during the 20-minute period.

(For a more widespread case of poison ivy dermatitis, cool starch baths, ½ box of soluble starch to the tub, give considerable relief from the itching.)

5. Nonalcoholic white shake lotion q.s.   120.0

(See Formulary section, p. 37, for complete formula.)

Sig: Apply 3 times a day to the affected areas.

(The patient probably has been to the corner drugstore and obtained calamine lotion, so the nonalcoholic white shake lotion has the added value of being of a different color.)

6. Pyribenzamine tablets, 50 mg., or Temaril, 2.5 mg.   #30

Sig: 1 tablet t.i.d. a.c. (For relief of itching.)

Subsequent Visits

1. Continue the wet packs only as long as there are blisters and oozing. Extended use is too drying for the skin.

2. After 3 to 4 days of use the lotion may be too drying. Substitute:

Hydrocortisone   0.5%
Menthol   0.25%
Water-washable cream q.s.   30.0

Sig: Apply small amount locally t.i.d., or more often if itching is present.

Severe Cases of Poison Ivy Dermatitis

1. Triamcinolone (Kenacort or Aristocort), 4 mg.   #26

Sig: 1 tablet q.i.d. for 3 days then 1 tablet b.i.d for 7 days.

2. Hospitalization of a severe case might be indicated for more intensive wet packs, ACTH injections, etc.

The use of poison ivy vaccine orally or intramuscularly is contraindicated during an acute episode. Desensitization may occur following a long course of oral ingestion of graduated doses of the allergen. Desensitization does not occur following a short course of intramuscular injections of the vaccine.

TREATMENT OF CONTACT DERMATITIS OF THE HAND DUE TO SOAP

A young housewife states that she has had a breaking-out on her hands for 5 weeks. The dermatitis developed about 4 weeks after the birth of her last baby. She states that she had a similar eruption after her previous two pregnancies. She has used a lot of local medication of her own, and the rash is growing worse instead of better. The patient and her immediate family never have had any asthma, hay fever or eczema.

Examination of her hands reveals small vesicles on the sides of all of her fingers with a 5-cm.-sized area of oozing and crusting around her left ring finger.

Treatment on the First Visit

1. General instructions must always be given to these patients.

A. Assure the patient that the hand eczema is not contagious to her family.

B. Inform the patient that soap irritates the dermatitis and that it must be avoided as much as possible. A housewife will find this avoidance very difficult. One of the best remedies is to wear protective gloves when extended soap-and-water contact is unavoidable. Rubber gloves alone produce a considerable amount of irritating perspiration, but this is absorbed when thin white cotton gloves are worn under the rubber gloves. Lined rubber gloves are not as satisfactory, because the lining eventually becomes dirty and soggy and cannot be cleaned easily.

C. For body cleanliness any mild soap can be used, or the following:

Oilatum Soap (Stiefel)
Basis Soap (Duke)

D. Tell the patient that the above prophylactic measures will have to be adhered to for several weeks after the eruption has apparently cleared or there will be a recurrence. Injured skin is sensitive and needs to be babied for an extended time.

2. Boric Acid Soaks

Sig: 1 tablespoon of boric acid crystals to 1 quart of cool water. Soak hands for 15 minutes twice a day.

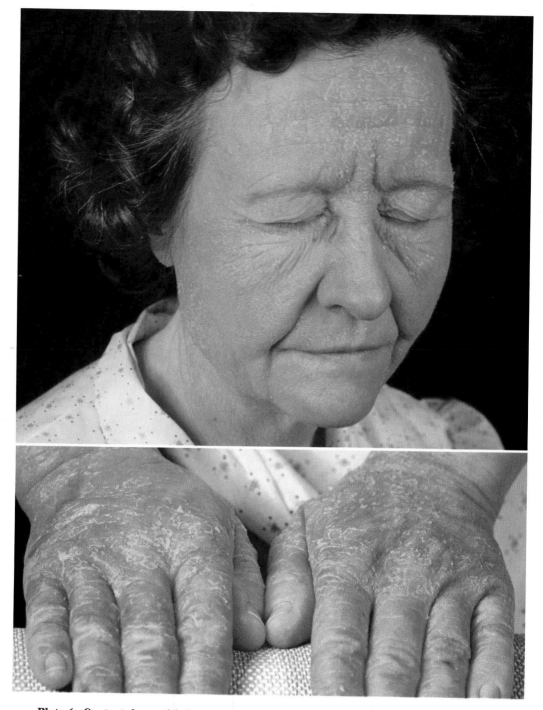

Plate 6. Contact dermatitis in a nurse due to chlorpromazine. The hands and the face were involved most severely. This eruption was aggravated following exposure to sunlight. (*K.U.M.C.*) (*Burroughs Wellcome & Company, Inc.*)

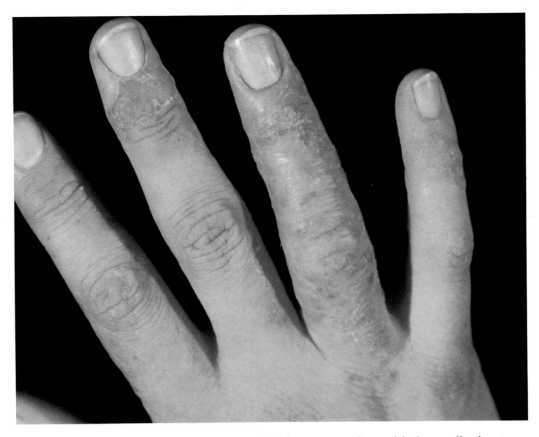

Plate 7. Contact dermatitis of the hand. This common dermatitis is usually due to continued exposure to soap and water. (*K.U.M.C.*) (*Burroughs Wellcome & Company, Inc.*)

3. Corticosteroid-antibiotic ointment (See p. 41.)   15.0

In place of a proprietary steroid ointment, hydrocortisone powder can be mixed with white petrolatum or water-washable bases. This cuts down the cost of the prescription. Example:

Hydrocortisone powder   0.5%-1%
White petrolatum or an antibiotic ointment q.s.   15.0
Sig: Apply sparingly locally q.i.d.

Housewives' eczema cannot usually be cured with a steroid salve alone without observing the other protective measures.

Treatment of Resistant, Chronic Cases

1. To the corticosteroid ointment add as indicated sulfur (3 to 5%), coal tar solution (3 to 10%), or an antipruritic agent such as menthol (0.25%) or camphor (2%).

2. Oral Corticosteroid Therapy. A short course of such therapy will often improve or cure a chronic dermatitis.

3. Superficial x-ray therapy administered by a competent dermatologist or radiologist is valuable for chronic persistent cases. Usually 3 or 4 treatments given at weekly or semiweekly intervals are effective. There is no danger from superficial x-ray radiation if it is given correctly and the total dosage is not excessive (see p. 47).

INDUSTRIAL DERMATOSES

Sixty-five percent of all the industrial diseases are dermatoses. The average case of occupational dermatitis is compensated for 10 weeks, resulting in a total cost of over $100,000,000 a year in the United States. The commonest cause of these skin problems is contact irritants, of which cutting oils are the worst offenders. Lack of adequate cleansing is a big contributing factor.

It is not possible to list the thousands of different chemicals used in the hundreds of varied industrial operations which have the potential of causing a primary irritant reaction or an allergic reaction on the skin surface. The most complete classic text on this entire subject of occupational dermatoses is that by Schwartz, Tulipan, and Birmingham, entitled *Occupational Diseases of the Skin* (ed. 3, Philadelphia, Lea and Febiger, 1956). A newer excellent book on this subject is by Adams, *Occupational Contact Dermatitis* (Philadelphia, J. B. Lippincott, 1969).

MANAGEMENT OF INDUSTRIAL DERMATITIS

A cutting-tool laborer presents himself with a pruritic red, vesicular dermatitis on his hands, forearms and face of 2 months duration.

1. Obtain a careful detailed history of his type of work, and any recent change such as use of new chemicals, new cleansing agents, exposure at home with hobbies, painting, etc. Question him concerning remission of the dermatitis on weekends, or while on vacation.

2. Question concerning the first-aid care given at the plant. Too often this care aggravates the dermatitis. Bland protective remedies should be substituted for potential sensitizers, such as sulfonamide and penicillin salves, antihistamine creams, benzocaine ointments, nitrofuran preparations, and strong antipruritic lotions and salves.

3. Treatment of the dermatitis with wet compresses, bland lotions, or salves is the same as for any contact dermatitis (see previous discussion). Unfortunately, many of the occupational dermatoses respond slowly to therapy. This is due in part to the fact that most patients continue to work and are re-exposed repeatedly to small amounts of the irritating chemicals, even though precautions are taken. Also, certain industrial chemicals, such as chromates, beryllium salts

and cutting oils, injure the skin in such a way as to prevent healing for months and years.

4. The legal complications with compensation boards, insurance companies, the industry and the injured patient can be discouraging, frustrating and time-consuming. However, most patients are not malingerers but they do expect and deserve proper care and compensation for their injury.

ATOPIC ECZEMA
(Plates 8 to 12)

Atopic eczema is a rather common, markedly pruritic, chronic skin condition that occurs in two clinical forms: *infantile* and *adult*.

Clinical Lesions. Infantile form—blisters, oozing and crusting with excoriation. Adolescent and adult forms—marked dryness, thickening (lichenification), excoriation and even scarring.

Distribution. Infantile form—on face, scalp, arms and legs, or generalized. Adolescent and adult form—on cubital and popliteal fossae and less commonly on dorsum of hands and feet, ears, or generalized.

Course. Varies from mild single episode to severe chronic, recurrent episodes resulting in the "psychoitchical" individual. The infantile form usually becomes milder or even disappears after the age of 3 or 4. At the age of puberty and the late teens flare-ups or new outbreaks can occur. Young housewives may have their first recurrence of atopic eczema since childhood due to their new job of dishwashing and baby care. Thirty percent of patients with atopic dermatitis eventually develop allergic asthma or hay fever.

Etiology. The following factors are important.

1. *Heredity* is the most important single factor. The family history is usually positive for one or more of the triad of allergic diseases, asthma, hay fever, or atopic eczema. Determination of this history in hand dermatitis cases is important because often it will enable you, on the patient's first visit, to prognosticate a more drawn-

out recovery than if the patient had a simple contact dermatitis.

2. *Dryness of the skin* is important. Most often atopic eczema is worse in the wintertime. The factor here is the decrease in home or office humidity that causes a drying of the skin. For this reason bathing and the use of soap and water should be reduced.

3. *Wool and lanolin* (wool fat) commonly irritate the skin of these patients. The wearing of wool clothes may be another reason for an increased incidence in the winter.

4. *Allergy to foods* is a factor often overstressed, particularly with the infantile form. The mother's history of certain foods causing trouble should be your guide for eliminating foods. The correctness of her belief can be tested by adding these incriminated foods to the diet, one new food every 48 hours, when the dermatitis is stable. Scratch tests and intracutaneous tests uncover very few dermatologic allergens.

5. *Emotional stress and nervousness* aggravate any existing condition such as itching, duodenal ulcers, or migraine headaches. Therefore, this "nervous" factor is important but not causative enough to label this disease *disseminated neurodermatitis.*

Differential Diagnosis

Dermatitis venenata (positive history usually of contactants, no family allergic history, distribution rather characteristic, p. 49).

Psoriasis (patches localized to extensor surfaces, mainly knees and elbows, p. p. 97).

Seborrheic dermatitis in infants (absence of family allergy history, lesions scaling and greasy, p. 87).

Localized neurodermatitis (single patches mainly, no family allergy history, p. 72).

General Management for Atopic Eczema: Inform the patient or family that this is usually a chronic problem, that this is an inherited allergy, that skin tests usually are not helpful, that you can give relief from the dermatitis and the itch but there is no "cure" except time. The forms shown in Fig. 4-1 are very useful to convey this type of information to the patient.

Treatment of Infantile Form: FIRST VISIT. Child aged 6 months with mild oozing, red, excoriated dermatitis on face, arms and legs.

1. Follow regular diet except for the avoidance of any foods which the mother believes aggravate the eruption.

2. Avoid exposure of baby to excessive bathing with soaps and to contact with wool and products containing lanolin.

3. Coal tar solution   120.0
    Sig: ½ tablespoon to the lukewarm bath water. Bathe only once or twice a week.

4. Hydrocortisone powder   1%
    White petrolatum q.s.   15.0
    Sig: Apply sparingly b.i.d. to affected areas.
(Proprietary corticosteroid-antibiotic preparations are listed in the Formulary, p. 41.)

5. Benadryl elixir   90.0
    Sig: 1 teaspoonful b.i.d.

SUBSEQUENT VISITS

1. Add coal tar solution (3% to 10%) to the above ointment.

SEVERE OR RESISTANT CASES

1. Restrict diet to milk only, and after 3 days add one different food every 24 hours. An offending food will cause a flare-up of the eczema in several hours.

2. Hydrocortisone liquid (Fluid Cortef)   90.0
    Sig: 1 teaspoonful (10 mg.) q.i.d. for 3 days, then 1 teaspoonful t.i.d. for 1 week. (Decrease the dose or discontinue as improvement warrants. Vary the dosage according to age of the child.)

3. Hospitalization with change of environment may be necessary for a severe case.

Treatment of Adult Form: FIRST VISIT. Young adult with dry, scaly lichenified patches in cubital and popliteal fossae:

1. Stress avoidance of excess soap and water for bathing, avoidance of lanolin

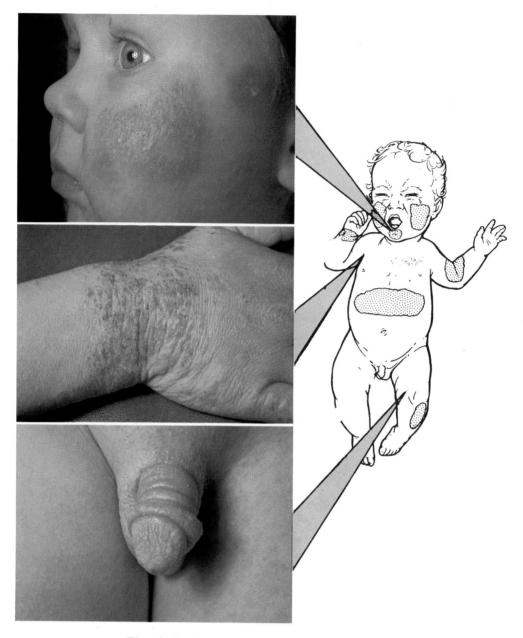

Plate 8. Atopic eczema (infant). (*Dome Chemicals*)

preparations locally, and contact with wool.

2. Menthol   ¼%
   Coal tar solution   5%
   Corticosteroid ointment (p. 39)
   q.s.   30.0
   Sig: Apply b.i.d. locally or p.r.n.
3. Phenergan tab., 12.5 mg.   #15
   Sig: 1 tab. h.s.

or Chlor-trimeton 12 mg.   #60
Sig: 1 b.i.d.

SUBSEQUENT VISITS

1. Gradually increase the concentration of the coal tar solution in the above salve up to 10%.

2. Nonspecific protein injections are of some value, such as: Piromen, beginning

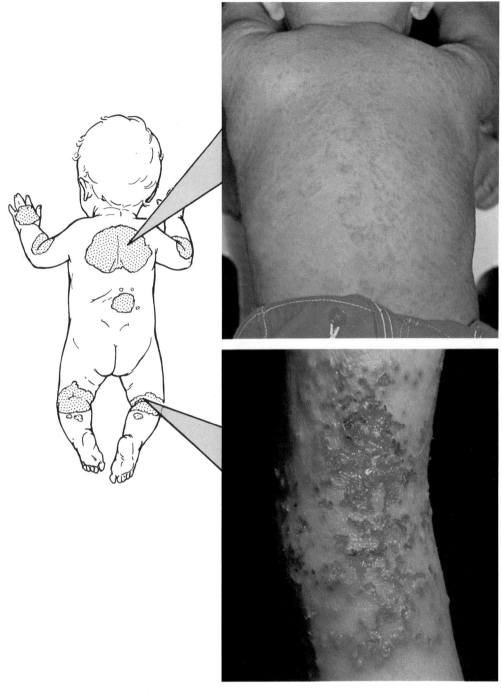

Plate 9. Atopic eczema (infant). (*Roche Laboratories*)

with 0.1 ml. of the 10 gamma per ml. dilution.

3. Unfiltered superficial x-ray therapy is often beneficial for chronic cases, given once a week for 4 to 6 treatments of 75 r each by a dermatologist or a radiologist.

4. Systemic ACTH or corticosteroid therapy may be indicated for severe and resistant cases.

5. *With every visit re-emphasize the fact of the chronicity of this disease and the ups and downs that do occur, particularly with seasons and stress.*

NUMMULAR ECZEMA
(Plate 13)

This is a moderately common distinctive eczematous eruption characterized by coin-shaped (nummular), papulovesicular patches mainly on the arms and the legs of young adults and elderly patients.

Primary Lesions. Coin-shaped patches of vesicles and papules usually on the extremities.

Secondary Lesions. Lichenification and bacterial infection.

Course. Very chronic, particularly in the older age group. Recurrences are common.

Subjective Complaints. Itching is usually quite severe.

Etiology. Nothing definite, but these factors are important:

1. History is usually positive for asthma, hay fever or atopic eczema, particularly in the young adult group.

2. Ingestion of iodides and bromides aggravates the disease.

3. Bacterial infection of the lesions is common.

4. In the older age group a history of a low-protein diet is common.

5. The low indoor humidity of wintertime causes dry skin which intensifies the itching, particularly in the elderly patients.

Differential Diagnosis

Atopic eczema (mainly in cubital and popliteal fossae, not coin-sized lesions, p. 56).

Psoriasis (not vesicular, see scalp and fingernail lesions, p. 97).

Contact dermatitis (will not see coin-sized lesions on both arms and legs, p. 49).

"Id" reaction, from stasis dermatitis of legs or a localized contact dermatitis (impossible to differentiate this clinically from nummular eczema but have history of previous primary dermatitis that suddenly became aggravated).

Treatment. FIRST VISIT in the winter of an elderly male with 5 to 8 distinct, coin-shaped, excoriated, vesicular, crusted lesions on the arms and the legs.

1. Instruct the patient to avoid excess bathing with soap and water.

2. Tell the patient to avoid these foods, which are rich in iodides and bromides: salted nuts, cheeses (except cottage cheese), sea foods, iodized salt (can use plain salt), tomatoes, melons and dark greens.

3. Increase the intake of protein-rich foods such as beef products, liver and gelatin.

4. Corticosteroid ointment   30.0
   Sig: Apply t.i.d. locally.

5. Benadryl, 50 mg.   #15
   Sig: 1 capsule h.s. for antipruritic and sedative effect.

TREATMENT OF RESISTANT CASES

1. Add coal tar solution, 3% to 10%, to the above salve.

2. A short course of oral corticosteroid therapy is effective, but relapses are common.

3. Depo-Testosterone (Upjohn), 50 mg. per ml.
   Sig: Give 1 ml. intramuscularly weekly for 3 to 4 weeks. Quite effective for resistant cases.

DRUG ERUPTIONS
(Plate 14)

It can be stated almost without exception that any drug systemically administered is capable of causing a skin eruption. *Any patient with a rather generalized skin eruption should be questioned concerning the use of oral or parenteral drugs.* To jog the memory of patients I often ask, "Do you take any medicine for any condition? What about medicated tooth paste, laxatives, vitamins, aspirin and tonics? Have you received any shots in the past month?" As stated in Chapter 4, this questioning also gives the doctor some general information regarding other ills of the patient which might influence the skin problem. An eruption due to allergy or primary irritation from *locally* applied drugs is a contact dermatitis.

Any of the larger dermatologic texts have extensive lists of common and uncommon drugs with their common and uncommon skin reactions. These books must be consulted for the rare reactions, but the following paragraphs will cover 95 percent of these idiosyncrasies.

Photosensitivity reactions from drugs are also covered in Chapter 26.

DRUGS AND THE DERMATOSES THEY CAUSE

Drug eruptions are usually not characteristic for any certain drug or group of drugs. However, the following drugs most commonly cause the associated skin lesions. Systemic drug reactions will not be stressed in this chapter.

Acetophenetidin (Phenacetin). In Empirin Compound, Phenaphen, A.S.A. Compound, A.P.C., BC, Nembudeine, Bromo Quinine, Super-Anahist and many other remedies. See urticaria and erythematous eruptions.

ACTH. See Cushing's syndrome, hyperpigmentation, acneiform eruptions, seborrheic-dermatitis-like eruptions and hirsutism.

Allopurinal (Zyloprim). (*See* erythema, maculopapular rash and severe bullae.)

Amantadine (*See* livedo reticularis)

Amphetamine (Benzedrine). Coldness of extremities and redness of neck and shoulders; it increases itching in neurodermatitis.

Ampicillin (*See* Antibiotics).

Antabuse. Redness of face and possible acne.

Antibiotics. Various agents have different reactions, but in general see monilial overgrowth in oral, genital and anal orifices resulting in pruritus ani, pruritus vulvae and generalized pruritus. Monilial skin lesions may spread out from these foci. Also commonly see urticaria, and erythema-multiforme-like eruptions, particularly from penicillin. Ampicillin not infrequently causes a generalized maculopapular rash. (*See* Streptomycin, *and* also Photosensitivity Reactions, p. 68.)

Anticoagulants. Bishydroxycoumarin (Dicumarol) and sodium warfarin (Coumadin) can cause severe hemorrhagic skin infarction and necrosis.

Antihistamines. In Corcidin, Super-Anahist and many other preparations. See urticaria, eczematous dermatitis and pityriasis-rosea-like rash.

Antitoxin. Get immediate reaction with skin manifestations of pruritus, urticaria and sweating; and delayed serum sickness reaction with urticaria, redness and purpura.

Apresoline. Causes systemic lupus-erythematosus-like reaction.

Arsenic. Inorganic arsenic (Fowler's solution, Asiatic pills) causes erythematous, scarlatiniform, vesicular, or urticarial rashes. Delayed reactions include palmar and plantar keratoses and eventual carcinomatous changes. Organic arsenic (Mapharsen, Neoarsphenamine, Tryparsamide) causes similar skin changes plus a severe form of exfoliative dermatitis. A mild erythema on the 9th day of therapy is not unusual. British Antilewisite (BAL) is effective therapy if given early for the skin reactions due to organic arsenicals.

Aspirin and Salicylates. Aspirin is found as an ingredient in a multitude of cold and antipain remedies. Pepto-Bismol contains salicylates. See urticaria, purpura and bullous lesions.

Atabrine. See universal yellow pigmentation, blue macules on face and mucosa, and lichen-planus-like eruption.

Atropine. Scarlet-fever-like rash.

Barbiturates. See urticarial, erythematous, bullous, or purpuric eruptions and fixed drug eruptions.

Bismuth. See bluish pigmentation of gums, and erythematous, papulosquamous and urtical skin eruptions.

Boric Acid. Accidental oral ingestion can cause exfoliative dermatitis and severe systemic reaction.

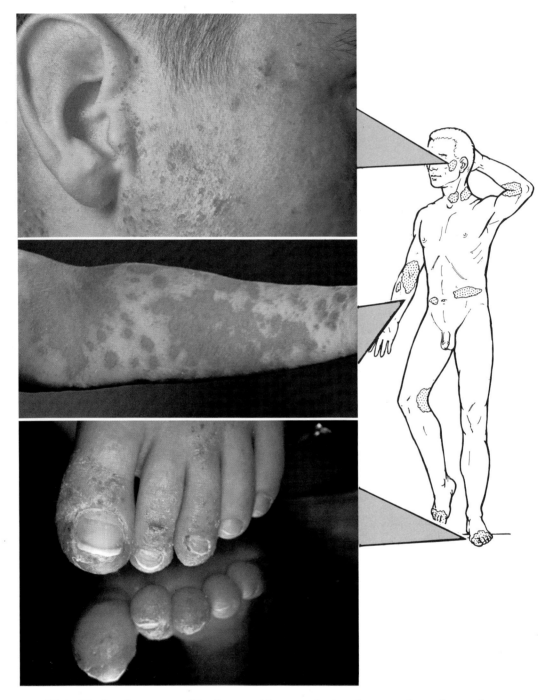

Plate 10. Atopic eczema. The bottom photograph, by the use of a mirror, demonstrates the under surface of the toes. (*Sandoz Pharmaceuticals*)

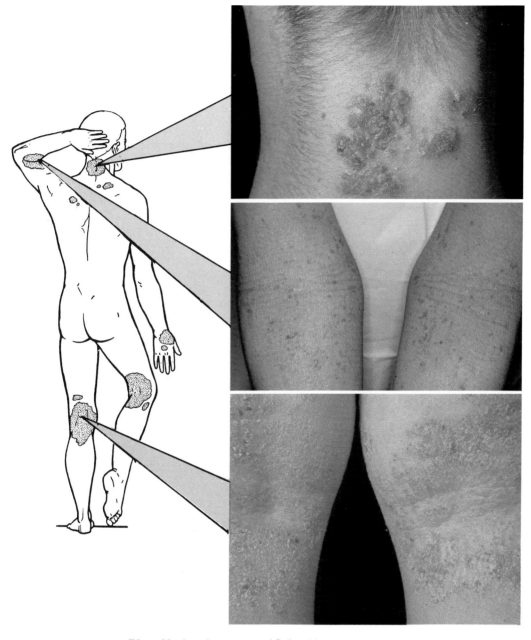

Plate 11. Atopic eczema. (*Geigy Pharmaceuticals*)

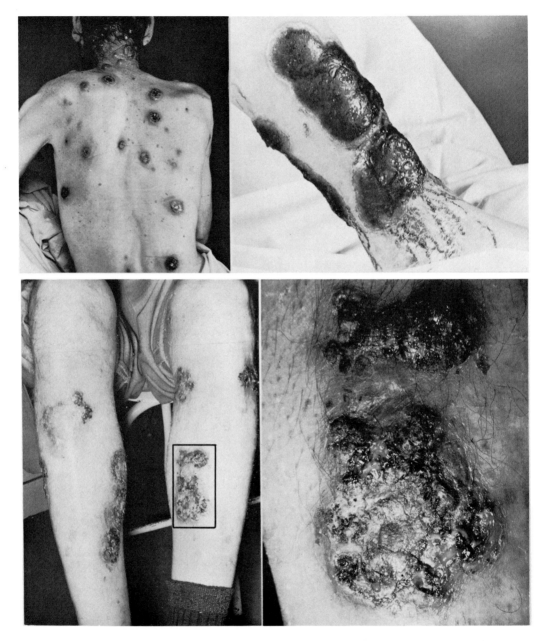

Fig. 7-3. Drug eruptions. (*Top*) From iodide, showing back and (on right) leg of same patient. (*Bottom*) From bromide, showing leg lesions and (on right) close-up.

Bromides. (*See* Iodides.) In Neurosine, Bromo Quinine, Bromo-Seltzer, Shut-eye and other drugs. Mainly see acnelike pustular lesions that can spread to form deep granulomatous pyodermas that heal with marked scarring. These must be differentiated from other granulomas (Fig. 7-3).

Butazolidin. Widespread erythematous, bullous eruptions.

Chloral Hydrate. Urticarial, papular, erythematous and purpuric eruptions.

Chloroquine. Erythematous or lichenoid eruptions with pruritus, and urticaria. (*Also see* p. 205.)

Chlorothiazide Diuretics. (*See* Photosensitivity Reactions, p. 68.)

Chlorpromazine (Thorazine). See maculopapular rash, increased sun sensitivity, purpura with agranulocytosis, and icterus from hepatitis. With long term therapy can develop slate gray to violet discoloration of skin.

Codeine and Morphine. Erythematous, urticarial, or vesicular eruption.

Contraceptive Drugs. Chloasmalike eruption, erythema nodosum and hives; aggravates some cases of acne.

Cortisone and Derivatives. Rarely see any cutaneous allergy.

Coumadin. (*See* Anticoagulants.)

Diasone. Red, maculopapular, vesicular eruption with agranulocytosis, occasionally like erythema nodosum.

Dicumarol. (*See* Anticoagulants.)

Diethylpropion Hydrochloride (Tenuate, Tepanil). Measleslike eruption.

Digitalis. Rarely, an erythematous, papular eruption is seen.

Digitoxin. Thrombocytopenic purpura.

Dilantin. Hypertrophy of gums, and erythema-multiforme-like eruption.

Doriden. (*See* Glutethimide.)

Estrogenic Substances and Stilbestrol. Edema of legs with cutaneous redness progressing to exfoliative dermatitis.

Glutethimide (Doriden). (*See* erythema, urticaria, purpura, or rarely exfoliative dermatitis.)

Gold. Eczematous dermatitis of hands, arms, legs, etc., or pityriasis-rosea-like eruption. Seborrheic-like eruption, urticaria, or purpura.

Insulin. See urticaria with serum sickness symptoms; also fat atrophy at injection site.

Iodides. (*See* Bromides.) Papular, pustural, ulcerative, or granulomatous lesions mainly on acne areas or legs (Fig 7-3). Administration of chloride hastens recovery.

Isoniazid. Erythematous and maculopapular generalized eruption, purpuric, bullous and nummular-eczema-like. Can aggravate acne.

Liver Extract. See urticaria, diffuse redness and itching.

Meclizine (Antivert). Urticaria.

Meprobamate. Small purpuric lesions and erythema-multiforme-like eruption.

Mercury. Erythema, pruritus, scarlatiniform eruption; also stomatitis.

Mesantoin. See macular rash and severe bullous eruption.

Methandrostenolone (Dianabol). Acnelike eruption.

Methyprylon (Noludar). (*See* fixed drug eruption).

Metronidazole (Flagyl). Urticaria and pruritus.

Morphine. (*See* Codeine.)

Noludar. (*See* Methyprylon.)

Para-aminosalicylic Acid. Scarlatiniform or morbilliform rash, fixed drug eruption and nummular-eczema-like rash.

Penicillin. (*See* Antibiotics.)

Phenacetin. (*See* Acetophenetidin.)

Phenolphthalein. Found in 4 Way Cold Tablets, Ex-Lax, Bromo Quinine, Phenolax, Petrogalar with Phenolphthalein, Agoral, Caroid and Bile Salts, Alophen and pink icing on cakes. See fixed drug eruption which consists of hyperpigmented or purplish, flat or slightly elevated, discrete, single or multiple patches.

Phenothiazine Group. (*See* Photosensitivity Reactions, p. 68.)

Psoralens. (*See* Photosensitivity Reactions, p. 68.)

Quinidine. See edema, purpura, scarlatiniform eruption that may go on to exfoliative dermatitis.

Quinine. See any kind of diffuse eruption.

Rauwolfia Alkaloids, Notably Reserpine. Urticaria, photosensitivity reactions, and petechial eruptions.

Salicylates. (*See* Aspirin.)

Silver. See diffuse bluish or grayish pigmentation of skin and gum margins due to a deposit of silver salts.

Stilbestrol. (*See* Estrogenic Substances.)

Streptomycin. Urticaria, erythematous, morbilliform and purpuric eruptions.

Sulfonamides. Urticaria, scarlatiniform eruption, erythema nodosum, eczematous flare of exudative dermatitis, erythema-multiforme-like bullous eruption or fixed eruption. (*Also see* Photosensitivity Reactions, p. 68.)

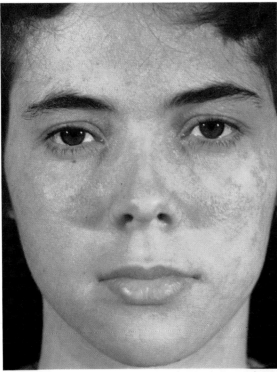

Plate 12. Atopic eczema. This case of facial atopic eczema resembled acute lupus erythematosus. The arm eruption is on another patient and exemplifies the chronic lichenified form of atopic eczema. (*K.U.M.C.*) (*Dome Chemicals*)

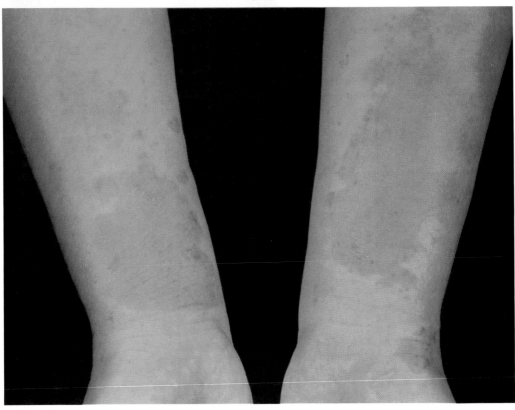

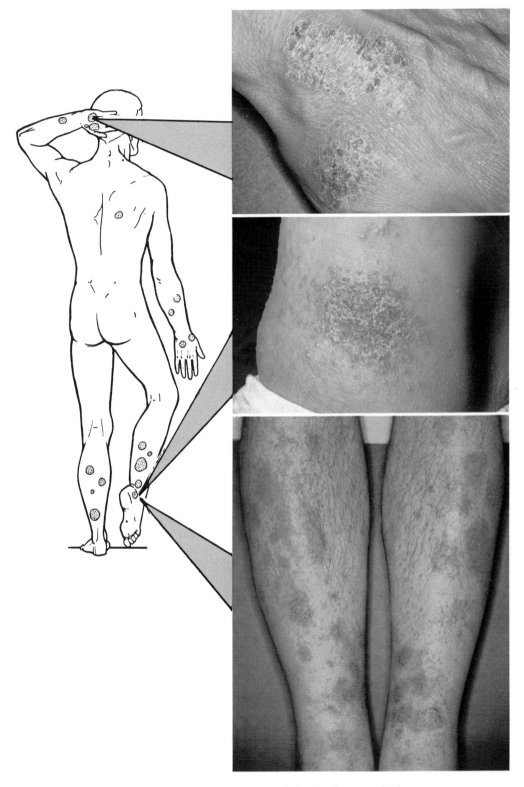

Plate 13. Nummular eczema. (*Schering Corporation*)

Sulfonylurea Hypoglycemics. (*See* Sulfonamides *and* Photosensitivity Reactions, p. 68.)

Testosterone and Related Drugs. Acnelike lesions and hypertrichosis.

Tridione. Acneiform eruption of face.

Triethylenemelamine (TEM). Pruritic maculopapular eruption.

Vitamins

Vitamin A. Due to long-term therapy with large doses, see scaly, rough, itchy skin with coarse, dry, scant hair growth and systemic changes.

Vitamin D. Rare skin lesions, but see headache, nausea, diarrhea, increased urination, sore gums and joints.

Vitamin B Group. See urticaria, pruritic redness and even anaphylactic reactions following I.M. or I.V. administration. Nicotinic acid quite regularly causes a red flush, pruritus and, less often, hives within 15 to 30 minutes after oral ingestion of 50 to 100 mg. The patient should be warned concerning this flush to eliminate unnecessary alarm.

Warfarin, sodium. (*See* Anticoagulants.)

DERMATOSES AND THE DRUGS THAT
CAUSE THEM

As stated above, drug eruptions are usually not characteristic for any particular chemical, but experience has shown that certain *clinical pictures* commonly follow absorption of certain drugs. (For description of these eruptions see the disease mentioned.)

Measleslike Eruption. Barbiturates, arsenic, sulfonamides, quinine and many others.

Scarlet-Fever-like Eruption or "Toxic Erythema." Arsenic, barbiturates, codeine, morphine, mercury, quinidine, salicylates, sulfonamides and others.

Pityriasis-Rosea-like Eruption. Bismuth, gold, barbiturates and antihistamines.

Eczematous Eruption. Quinine, procaine, antihistamines, gold, mercury, sulfonamides, penicillin and organic arsenic.

Nummular-Eczema-like Eruption. From combination of isoniazid and para-aminosalicylic acid.

Urticaria. Penicillin, salicylates, serums, sulfonamides, barbiturates, opium group, contraceptive drugs, and rauwolfia alkaloids.

Fixed Drug Eruption. (*See* the drug phenolphthalein, p. 65, for description.) Phenolphthalein, acetophenetidin, barbiturates, organic arsenic, gold, salicylates, sulfonamides and many others.

Erythema-Multiforme-like Eruption. Penicillin and other antibiotics, sulfonamides, phenolphthalein, barbiturates, Dilantin and meprobamate.

Erythema-Nodosum-like Eruption. Sulfonamides, iodides, bromides, salicylates, contraceptive drugs and Diasone.

Acnelike or Pustular Lesions. Bromides, iodides, Tridione, testosterone, methandrostenolone (Dianabol), and ACTH.

Vesicular or Bullous Eruptions. Sulfonamides, penicillin, Butazolidin and Mesantoin.

Purpuric Eruptions. Barbiturates, salicylates, meprobamate, organic arsenic, sulfonamides, chlorothiazide diuretics, Dicumarol and long-term use of corticosteroids.

Exfoliative Dermatitis. See in course of any severe generalized drug eruption, particularly due to arsenic, penicillin, sulfonamides and barbiturates.

Lichen-Planus-like Eruption. Atabrine, arsenic and gold.

Seborrheic-Dermatitis-like Eruption. Gold and ACTH.

Photosensitivity Reaction. Several of the newer drugs and some of the older ones cause a dermatitis on exposure to sunlight. These skin reactions can be urticarial, erythematous, vesicular or plaquelike. The mechanism can be either phototoxic or photoallergic, but this distinction can be difficult to ascertain. Here is a rather complete list of photosensitizing drugs, but also consult Chapter 26.

Sulfonamides

Sulfonylurea Hypoglycemics

    Tolbutamide (Orinase)

    Chlorpropamide (Diabinese)

    Acetohexamide (Dymelor)

Antibiotics

    Demethylchlortetracycline (Declomycin)

    Griseofulvin (Fulvicin, Grifulvin)

    Tetracycline (degraded products)

Chlorothiazide Diuretics
  Chlorothiazide (Diuril)
  Hydrochlorothiazide (Hydro-Diuril, Esidrix, Oretic, etc.)
  Cyclothiazide (Anhydron)
  Methyclothiazide (Enduron)
Phenothiazines
  Chlorpromazine (Thorazine)
  Promazine (Sparine)
  Prochlorperazine (Compazine)
  Promethazine (Phenergan)
  Trimeprazine (Temaril)
  Mepazine (Pacatal)
Psoralens
  8-Methoxypsoralen (Oxsoralen)

Pigmentary Changes. Contraceptive drugs, atabrine, chloroquine, chlorpromazine, and silver salts.

Nail Changes. Demethylchlortetracycline (Declomycin) and tetracycline can cause distal detachment of nails (onycholysis) apparently due to a phototoxic reaction.

Whitening of Hair. Chloroquine and hydroxychloroquine can cause this in blond or red-haired individuals.

Alopecia. Amethopterin (Methotrexate), colchicine, heparin, dicumarol, and coumarin derivatives.

Keratoses and Epitheliomas. Arsenic and mercury.

Course of Drug Eruptions. This depends on many factors, including the type of drug, severity of the cutaneous reaction, systemic involvement, general health of the individual, and efficacy of corrective therapy. Most cases with bullae, purpura or exfoliative dermatitis have a serious prognosis and a protracted course.

Treatment

1. Eliminate the drug. This simple procedure is often delayed, with resulting serious consequences, because a careful history is not taken. *When confronted with any diffuse or puzzling eruption, routinely question the patient regarding ANY medication taken by ANY route.*

2. Further therapy depends on the seriousness of the eruption. Most barbiturate measleslike eruptions subside with no therapy. An itching drug eruption should be treated to relieve the itch (starch baths and a nonalcoholic calamine lotion or white shake lotion). Cases of exfoliative dermatitis or severe erythema-multiforme-like lesions require corticosteroid and other supportive therapy (see pp. 197 and 80).

BIBLIOGRAPHY

CONTACT DERMATITIS AND ATOPIC ECZEMA

Adams, R. M.: Occupational Contact Dermatitis. Philadelphia, J. B. Lippincott, 1969.
Baer, R. L. (ed.): Atopic Dermatitis. Philadelphia, J. B. Lippincott, 1955.
Fisher, A. A.: Contact Dermatitis. Philadelphia, Lea & Febiger, 1967.
Schwartz, L., Tulipan, L., and Birmingham, D. J.: Occupational Diseases of the Skin, ed. 3. Philadelphia, Lea & Febiger, 1957. A classic text.
Sulzberger, M. B.: Dermatologic Allergy. Springfield, Charles C Thomas, 1940. An American classic on the subject.

DRUG ERUPTIONS

Baer, R. L., and Harris, H.: Types of cutaneous reactions to drugs. JAMA, *202*:150, 1967.
Baer, R. L., and Witten, V. H.: Year Book of Dermatology, 1960-1961 Series. pp. 9-37. Chicago, Year Book Publishers, 1961.
Bereston, E. A.: Reactions to antituberculous drugs. J. Invest. Derm., *33*:427, 1959.
Physicians' Desk Reference to Pharmaceutical Specialties and Biologicals. Oradell, N. J., Medical Economics. (Published yearly.) Toxic reactions to specific drugs are listed but the list lacks completeness.
Sams, W. M.: Photosensitizing therapeutic agents. JAMA, *174*:2043, 1960.
Sutton, R. L., Jr.: Diseases of the Skin, ed. 11. St. Louis, C. V. Mosby, 1956. A very extensive older list of drugs and reactions to them.
Also consult the larger general dermatologic texts listed in Chapter 33.

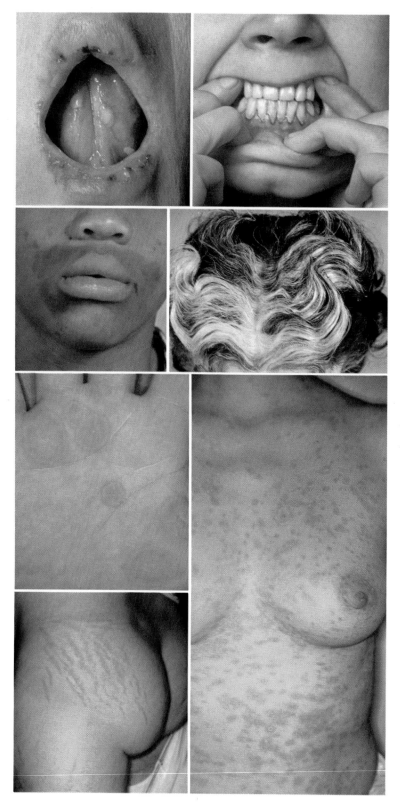

Plate 14. Drug Eruptions. (*Left*) Erosions of tongue and lips from sulfonamides. (*Right*) Bismuth line of gums.

(*Left*) Phenolphthalein fixed eruption of lips of a Negro boy. (*Right*) Whitening of scalp hair from chloroquine therapy for L. E.

(*Left, upper*) Erythema multiforme-like eruption of palm from oral antibiotic therapy. (*Left, lower*) Striae of buttocks of 30-year-old man following 9 months of corticosteroid therapy. (*Right*) Papulosquamous eruption of chest from phenolphthalein. (*E. R. Squibb*)

8

Pruritic Dermatoses

Pruritus or itching brings more patients to the doctor's office than any other skin disease symptom. Itchy skin is not easily cured or even alleviated. Many hundreds of proprietary over-the-counter and prescription drugs are touted as effective anti-itch remedies, but not one is 100 percent effective. However, many are partially effective, but it is unfortunate that the most effective locally applied chemicals frequently irritate or sensitize the skin.

Pruritus is a sympton of many of the common skin diseases such as contact dermatitis, atopic eczema, seborrheic dermatitis, hives, some drug eruptions and many other dermatoses. Relief of itching is of prime importance in treating these diseases.

In addition to the pruritus occurring as a symptom of many skin diseases, there are other clinical forms of pruritus that deserve special consideration. These special types include *generalized pruritus* of the winter, senile and essential varieties, and *localized pruritus* of the neurodermatitis type, of the ears, the anal area and the genitalia.

GENERALIZED PRURITUS

Diffuse itching of the body without perceptible skin disease usually is due to wintertime dry skin, senile skin or to unknown causes.

Winter pruritus or **pruritus hiemalis** is a common form of generalized pruritus, although most patients complain of itching confined mainly to their legs. Every autumn of the year a certain number of elderly patients, and occasionally young ones, will walk into the doctor's office complaining bitterly of the rather sudden onset of itching of their legs. These patients have dry skin due to the low humidity in their furnace-heated homes. Clinically, the skin shows excoriations and dry curled scaling plaques resembling a sun-baked muddy beach at low tide. The dry skin associated with winter itch is to be differentiated from *ichthyosis*, a congenital dermatosis of varying severity which is also worse in the wintertime.

Treatment of winter pruritus consists of (1) limiting general bathing to once a week; (2) sparing use of a bland soap such as Dove, Ivory, Oilatum or Basis Soap; (3) addition of an oil to the tub such as Lubath, Domol, Nivea, Mellobath or Alpha-Keri; (4) local application twice daily of white petrolatum, Nivea Skin Oil or Cream, Lowila Emollient, Keri Lotion,

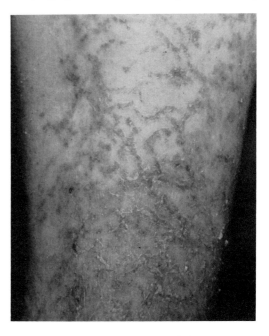

Fig. 8-1. Senile dry skin of the leg.

71

Nutraderm or Lubriderm; and (5) oral antihistamines which are sometimes effective such as Chlor-trimeton 4 mg. q.i.d., Temaril 2.5 mg. q.i.d., or Dimetane 4 mg. q.i.d. For some of the more severe localized areas of the itch, a corticosteroid ointment is indicated. (*See* p. 39).

Senile pruritus is a resistant form of generalized pruritus in the elderly patient (Fig. 8-1 and Chapter 30). It can occur at any time of the year and may or may not be associated with dry skin. This form of itch occurs most commonly on the scalp, the shoulders, the sacral areas and the legs. Clinically, some patients have no cutaneous signs of the itch, but others may have linear excoriations. *Scabies* should be ruled out, as well as the diseases mentioned under the next form of pruritus to be considered, essential pruritus.

Treatment is usually not very satisfactory. In addition to the agents mentioned previously in connection with winter pruritus, the injection of testosterone (Depo-Testosterone, 50 mg. intramuscularly) once a week for 2 to 4 weeks is often beneficial.

Essential pruritus is the rarest form of the generalized itching diseases. No age is exempt, but it occurs most frequently in the elderly patient. The itching is usually quite diffuse, with occasional "bites" in certain localized areas. All diffuse itching is worse at night, and no exception is made for this form of pruritus. Before a diagnosis of essential pruritus is made the following diseases must be ruled out by appropriate studies: *drug reaction, diabetes mellitus, uremia, lymphoblastoma* (mycosis fungoides, leukemia, or Hodgkin's disease), *liver disease,* or *intestinal parasites.* Treatment is the same as for senile and winter pruritus.

LOCALIZED PRURITIC DERMATOSES

Neurodermatitis
(Plates 15 and 16)

A few words must be said concerning the nomenclature of this disease. Other common terms for this condition include *lichen chronicus simplex* and *lichenified dermatitis*. There are pros and cons for all of the terms, but the term "neurodermatitis" has been selected because it is already being used rather universally, it stresses (perhaps too strongly) the emotional nervous habit of scratching, and it is simpler to use than the next best term, "lichen chronicus simplex."

Neurodermatitis is a common skin condition characterized by the occurrence of single or, less frequently, multiple patches of chronic, itching, thickened, scaly, dry skin in one or more of several classic locations (Plate 16). It is unrelated to atopic eczema, which unfortunately has the synonym "disseminated neurodermatitis," a term that should be abandoned.

Primary Lesions. This disease begins as a small, localized, pruritic patch of dermatitis that might have been an insect bite, a chigger bite, contact dermatitis, or other minor irritation which may or may not be remembered by the patient. Because of various etiologic factors mentioned below, a cycle of itching, scratching, more itching and more scratching supervenes, and the chronic dermatosis develops.

Secondary Lesions. These include excoriations, lichenification and, in severe cases, marked verrucous thickening of the skin with pigmentary changes. In these severe cases healing is bound to be followed by some scarring.

Distribution. This condition is seen most commonly at the hairline of the nape of the neck, on the wrists, the ankles, the ears (see external otitis), anal area (see pruritus ani), etc.

Course. Quite chronic and recurrent. The majority of cases respond quickly to correct treatment, but some can last for years and defy all forms of therapy.

Subjective Complaints. Intense itching, usually worse at night, even during sleep.

Etiology. The initial cause (a bite, stasis dermatitis, contact dermatitis, seborrheic dermatitis, tinea cruris, psoriasis) may be very evanescent, but it is generally agreed that the chronicity of the lesion is due to the nervous habit of scratching. It is a rare patient who will not volunteer the information or admit it if questioned that the itching is worse when he or she is upset, nervous, or tired. Why some people with a minor skin injury respond with the development of a lichenified patch of skin and others do not is due to the personality make-up of that individual.

Age Group. It is very common to see neurodermatitis of the posterior neck in menopausal women. Other clinical types of neurodermatitis are seen at any age.

Family Incidence. Unrelated to allergies in patient or family, thus differing from atopic eczema.

Related to Employment. Recurrent exposure and contact to irritating agents at work can lead to neurodermatitis.

Differential Diagnosis

Psoriasis (several patches on the body in classic areas of distribution, family history of disease, see classic whitish scales, sharply circumscribed patch, p. 97).

Atopic eczema (allergic history in patient or family, multiple lesions, classically seen in cubital and popliteal areas and face, p. 56).

Contact dermatitis (acute onset, contact history positive, usually red, vesicular and oozing; may see acute contact dermatitis overlying neurodermatitis due to overzealous therapy, p. 49).

Lichen planus, hypertrophic form on anterior tibial area (also see lichen planus in mouth and on other body areas; biopsy usually characteristic, p. 107).

Seborrheic dermatitis of scalp (does not itch as much, is better in summer; a diffuse, scaly, greasy eruption, p. 87).

Treatment

A 45-year-old female patient with severely itching, scaly, red lichenified patch on back of the neck at the hairline.

1. Explain the condition to the patient and tell her that your medicine will be directed toward stopping the itching. If this can be done, and if she will cooperate by keeping her hands off the area, the disease will disappear. Emphasize this effect of scratching by stating that if both arms were broken, the eruption would be gone when the casts were removed. How-

ever, this is not a recommended form of therapy.

2. For severe bouts of intractable itching:

Ice cold boric acid packs

Sig: 1 tbsp. of boric acid crystals to 1 quart of ice cold water. Apply cloth wet with this solution for 15 minutes p.r.n.

3. A corticosteroid ointment   15.0

Sig: Apply q.i.d. or more often as itching requires.

The fluorinated corticosteriod creams (Synalar, Cordran, Celestone, see p. 39) can be used under an occlusive dressing of Saran Wrap or Jiffy Wrap on lesions on an extremity. The dressing can be left on overnight or for 24 hours at a time.

TREATMENT ON RETURN VISIT

1. Add menthol (0.25%) or coal tar solution (3 to 10%) to above ointment for greater antipruritic effect.

2. Intralesional Corticosteroid Therapy. This is a very effective and safe treatment. The technic is as follows. Use a 1-inch long #24 or #25 needle and a Luer-lock type syringe. Inject 5 or 10 mg. of triamcinolone parenteral solution (Kenalog 10 Parenteral or Aristocort Intralesional Suspension) intradermally or subcutaneously directly under the skin lesion. An equal amount of procaine or other local anaesthetic solution should be mixed with the solution in the syringe to reduce the mild discomfort of the injection. Do not inject all the solution in one area but spread it around as you advance the needle. The injection can be repeated every 2 or 3 weeks as necessary to eliminate the patch of dermatitis.

A minor complication of an atrophic depression at the injection site usually can be avoided if the concentration of triamcinolone in one area is kept low.

TREATMENT OF RESISTANT CASES

1. A tranquilizer   #50

Sig: 1 tablet q.i.d., a.c. and h.s.

2. Triamcinolone or methylprednisolone, 4 mg.   #24

Sig: 1 tablet q.i.d. for 3 days, then 1 b.i.d. for 4 days.

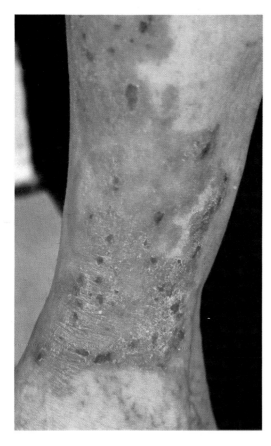

Plate 15. Neurodermatitis of the leg. This is a common location for neurodermatitis. Note the lichenification and the excoriations due to the marked pruritus. (*K.U.M.C.*) (*Duke Laboratories*)

3. X-ray therapy as given by a competent dermatologist or radiologist.

4. Dome Paste Boot. Apply in office for cases of neurodermatitis localized to arms and legs. This is a physical deterrent to scratching. Leave on for a week at a time.

5. Psychotherapy is of questionable value.

EXTERNAL OTITIS

External otitis is a descriptive term for a common and persistent dermatitis of the ears due to several causes. The agent most frequently blamed for this condition is "fungus," but pathogenic fungi are rarely found in the external ear. The true causes of external otitis, in order of frequency, are as follows: seborrheic dermatitis, neurodermatitis, contact dermatitis, atopic eczema, psoriasis, pseudomonas bacterial infection (which is usually secondary to other causes) and, lastly, fungal infection which also can be primary or secondary to other factors. For further information on the specific processes refer to each of the diseases mentioned.

Treatment. Primarily, this should be directed toward the specific cause, such as care of the scalp for seborrheic cases, or avoidance of jewelry for contact cases. However, when this is done, certain special technics and medicines must be used in addition to clear up this troublesome area.

An elderly woman comes in with an oozing, red, crusted, swollen left external ear with a wet canal but an intact drum. A considerable amount of seborrheic dermatitis of the scalp is confluent with the acutely inflamed ear area. The patient has had itching ear trouble off and on for 10 years, but in the past month it has become most severe.

1. Always inspect the canal and the drum with an otoscope. If excessive wax and debris are present in the canal, or if the drum is involved in the process, the patient should be treated for these problems or referred to an ear specialist. Salves should not be placed in the ear canal. An effective liquid to dry up the oozing canal is as follows:

Hydrocortisone powder	1%
Boric acid	2%
Burow's Solution, 1:10 strength, q.s.	15.0

Sig: 2 drops in ear t.i.d.

2. Boric acid solution wet packs

Sig: 1 tablespoon of boric acid to 1 quart of cool water. Apply wet cloths to external ear for 15 minutes 3 times a day.

3. A corticosteroid ointment   5.0

Sig: Apply locally to external ear t.i.d., not in canal.

SUBSEQUENT THERAPY. Several days later following decreased swelling, cessation of oozing and lessening of itching, institute the following changes in therapy:

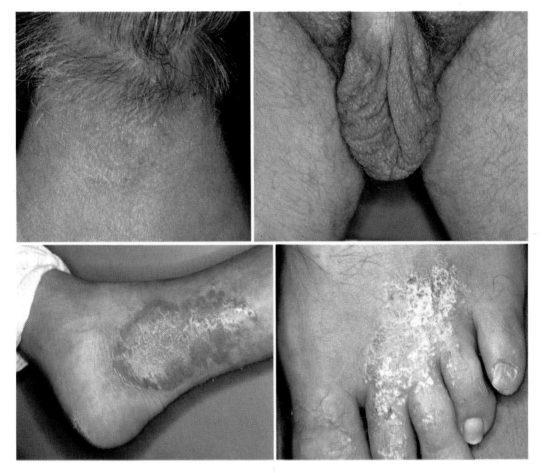

Plate 16. Neurodermatitis. (*Top, left*) In occipital area of scalp. (*Top, right*) Of scrotum, with marked lichenification and thickening of the skin. (*Bottom, left*) Of medial aspect of ankle, following lichen planus of this area. (*Bottom, right*) On dorsum of foot. (*Duke Laboratories*)

1. Decrease the boric acid soaks to once a day.
2. Sulfur, ppt.   5%
     A corticosteroid oint. q.s.   15.0
     Sig: Apply locally t.i.d. to ear.

For persistent cases, a short course of oral corticosteroid or antibiotic therapy often removes the fire so that local remedies will be effective. X-ray therapy, correctly administered, is also useful for chronic cases.

PRURITUS ANI

Itching of the anal area is a common malady that can vary in severity from mild to marked. The patient with this very annoying symptom is apt to resort to self-treatment and therefore delay the visit to the physician. Usually, he has overtreated the sensitive area, and the immediate problem of the physician is to quiet down the acute contact dermatitis. The original cause of the pruritus ani is often difficult to ascertain.

Primary Lesions. These can range from slight redness confined to a very small area to an extensive contact dermatitis with redness, vesicles and oozing of the entire buttock.

Secondary Lesions. Excoriations from the intense itching are very common and after a prolonged time they progress toward lichenification. A generalized papulovesicular id eruption can develop from an acute flare-up of this entity.

Course. The majority of cases of pruritus ani respond rapidly and completely to proper management, especially if the cause can be ascertained and eliminated. However, every physician will have his problem case who will continue to scratch and defy all therapy.

Etiology. The proper management of this socially unacceptable form of pruritus consists in searching for and eliminating the several factors that contribute to the persistence of this symptom-complex. These factors can be divided into general and specific etiologic factors.

1. GENERAL FACTORS

A. *Diet.* The following irritating foods should be removed from the diet: chocolate, nuts, cheeses and spicy foods. Coffee, because of its stimulating effect on any form of itching, should be limited to 1 cup a day. Rarely, certain other foods will be noted by the patient to aggravate the pruritus.

B. *Bathing.* Many patients have the misconception that the itching is due to uncleanliness. Therefore, they resort to excessive bathing and scrubbing of the anal area. This is harmful and irritating and must be stopped.

C. *Toilet Care.* Harsh toilet papers contribute greatly to the continuance of this condition. Cotton or a proprietary cleansing cloth called "Tucks" must be used for wiping. Mineral oil can be added to the cotton if necessary. Rarely, an allergy to the pastel tint in colored toilet tissues is a factor causing the pruritus.

D. *Scratching.* As with all of the diseases of this group, chronic scratching leads to a vicious circle. The chief aim of the physician is to give relief from this itching, but a gentle admonishment to the patient to keep his hands off is indicated. With the physician's help, the itch-and-scratch habit can be broken. The emotional and mental personality of the patient regulates the effectiveness of this suggestion.

2. SPECIFIC ETIOLOGIC FACTORS

A. *Oral Antibiotics.* Pruritus ani from this cause is being seen with increasing frequency. It may or may not be due to an overgrowth of monilial organisms. The physician who automatically questions his patients about recent drug ingestion will not miss this diagnosis.

B. *Neurodermatitis.* It is always a problem to know which comes first, the itching or the "nervousness." In most instances the itching comes first, but there is no denying that once pruritus ani has developed it is aggravated by emotional tensions and "nerves." However, it is a rare case that has a "deep-seated" psychological problem.

C. *Psoriasis* in this area is common. Usually, other skin surfaces are also involved.

D. *Atopic eczema* of this site in adults is rather unusual. A history of atopy in the patient or family is helpful in establishing this etiology.

E. *Fungal Infection.* Contrary to old beliefs, this cause is quite rare. Clinically, a raised, sharp, papulovesicular border is seen that commonly is confluent with tinea of the crural area. If a scraping or a culture reveals fungi, then stronger local therapy than usual is indicated for cure.

F. *Worm Infestation.* In children pinworms can usually be implicated. A diagnosis is made by finding eggs on morning anal smears or by seeing the small white worms when the child is sleeping. Worms are a rare cause of adult pruritus ani.

G. *Hemorrhoids.* In the lay person's mind this is undoubtedly the commonest cause. Actually, it is an unimportant primary factor but may be a contributing factor. Hemorrhoidectomy alone is rarely successful as a cure for pruritus ani.

H. *Cancer.* This is a very rare cause of anal itching, but a rectal or proctoscopic examination may be indicated.

Treatment. FIRST VISIT. A patient states that he has had anal itching for 4 months. It followed a 5-day course of an antibiotic for the flu. Many local remedies have been used; the latest, a supposed remedy for athlete's foot, aggravated the condition.

Examination reveals an oozing, macerated, red area around the anus.

1. Initial therapy should include removal of the general factors listed under "Etiology" and giving instructions as to diet, bathing, toilet care and scratching. Use the non-carbon paper pad (Fig. 4-1) for these instructions.

2. Boric acid wet packs.

Sig: 1 tablespoon of boric acid crystals to 1 quart of cool water. Apply wet cloths to the area b.i.d. while lying in bed for 20 minutes, or more often if necessary for severe itching. Ice cubes may be added to the solution for more anti-itching effect.

3. Nonalcoholic white shake lotion.
   (*See* p. 37)   60.0
   Sig: Apply to area b.i.d. (May burn slightly on first few applications.)

4. Benadryl, 50 mg.   #15
   Sig: 1 capsule h.s. (For itching and sedation.)

SECOND VISIT. After the acute contact dermatitis has subsided:

A corticosteroid ointment q.s.   15.0
Sig: Apply locally t.i.d.

SUBSEQUENT VISITS

1. As tolerated, add increasing strengths of sulfur, coal tar solution, or menthol (0.25%) or phenol (0.5%) to the above ointment or to any of the following:

Quotane ointment   15.0
Vioform ointment, with or without hydrocortisone   15.0
Sterosan ointment, with or without hydrocortisone   15.0

2. Intralesional corticosteroid injection therapy. Very effective. Usually the minor discomfort of the injection is quite well tolerated because of the patient's desire to "get cured." The technic is given under "Neurodermatitis" on page 73.

3. A short course of oral corticosteroid therapy may be indicated for resistant cases.

4. X-ray therapy is sometimes beneficial. It should be administered by a competent dermatologist or radiologist in a dose of 75 to 100 r weekly of unfiltered superficial radiation for a total dose of only 400 to 600 r.

GENITAL PRURITUS

Itching of the female vulva or the male scrotum can be treated in much the same way as pruritus ani if these special considerations are borne in mind.

Vulvar Pruritus. Etiologically, it is due to monilia or trichomonas infection; contact dermatitis from douche chemicals, contraceptive jellies and diaphragms; chronic cervicitis; neurodermatitis; menopausal or senile atrophic changes; or leukoplakia. Pruritus vulvae is frequently seen in patients with diabetes mellitus and during pregnancy. Treatment can be adapted from that for pruritus ani (p. 76) with the addition of a daily douche such as vinegar, 2 tablespoons to 1 quart of warm water.

Scrotal Pruritus. (Plate 16.) Etiologically, it is due to tinea infection; contact dermatitis from soaps, powders, clothing; or neurodermatitis. Treatment is similar to that given for pruritus ani (p. 76).

9

Vascular Dermatoses

Urticaria, erythema multiforme and its variants, and erythema nodosum are included under this heading because of their vascular reaction patterns. Stasis dermatitis is included because it is a dermatosis due to venous insufficiency in the legs.

URTICARIA

The commonly seen entity of urticaria or hives can be acute or chronic and due to known or unknown causes. The urticarial wheal results from liberation of histamine from damaged mast cells located around the smaller cutaneous blood vessels. There are many physical and chemical agents which can damage these mast cells and cause a sudden liberation of histamine.

Lesions can vary from pea-sized red papules to large circinate patterns with red borders and white centers that can cover an entire side of the trunk or the thigh. Vesicles and bullae are seen in severe cases along with hemorrhagic effusions. Edema of the glottis is a serious complication which can occur in the severe form of urticaria labeled *angioneurotic edema.*

Course. Acute cases may be mild or explosive but usually disappear with or without treatment in a few hours or days. The chronic form has remissions and exacerbations for months and years.

Etiology. Many cases of hives, particularly of the chronic type, after careful questioning and investigation are concluded to result from no apparent causative agent. Other cases, mainly the acute ones, have been found to result from the following factors or agents:

DRUGS. Penicillin is probably the commonest cause of acute hives, but any other drug, whether ingested, injected, inhaled or, rarely, applied on the skin, can cause the reaction. (*See* Drug Eruption, p. 60.)

FOODS are a common cause of acute hives. The main offenders are sea foods, strawberries, chocolate, nuts, cheeses, pork, eggs, wheat and milk. Chronic hives can be caused by traces of penicillin in milk products.

INSECT BITES AND STINGS. From mosquitos, fleas, spiders and contact with certain moths, leeches and jellyfish.

PHYSICAL AGENTS. Due to heat, cold, radiant energy and physical injury. *Dermographism* is a term applied to a localized urticarial wheal produced by scratching the skin of certain individuals (Fig. 9-1).

INHALANTS. Nasal sprays, insect sprays, dust, feathers, pollens and animal danders comprise a partial list of offenders.

INFECTIONS. A focus of infection is always considered sooner or later in chronic cases of hives, and in unusual instances it is causative. The sinuses, the teeth, the tonsils, the gallbladder and the genitourinary tract should be checked.

INTERNAL DISEASE. Urticaria has been seen with liver disease, intestinal parasites, cancer and rheumatic fever.

"NERVES." After all other causes of chronic urticaria have been ruled out there remain a substantial number of cases that appear to be related to nervous stress, worry or fatigue. These cases benefit most from the establishment of good rapport between the patient and the doctor.

Differential Diagnosis. *Hebra's erythema multiforme* (see systemic fever, malaise, and mouth lesions in children and young adults, p. 80).

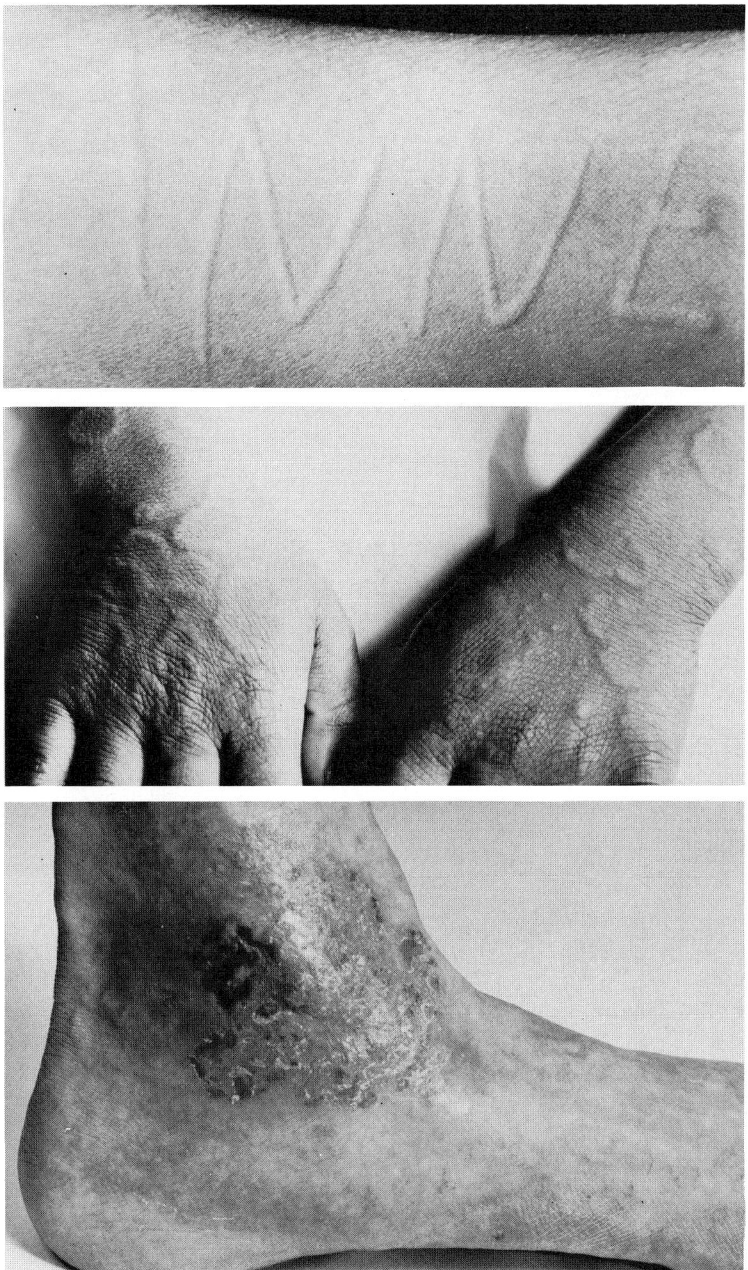

Fig. 9-1. Vascular dermatoses. (*Top*) Dermographism (arm).

(*Center*) Erythema multiforme in Negro boy.

(*Bottom*) Stasis dermatitis and ulcer of ankle.

Treatment

1. A case of *acute* hives due to penicillin injection one week previously for a "cold."

A. Colloidal bath

Sig: 1 cup of starch or oatmeal (Aveeno) to 6 to 8 inches of luke-warm water in the tub. Bathe for 15 minutes once or twice a day.

B. Camphor   1%
Alcoholic white shake lotion, q.s.   120.0
Sig: Apply b.i.d. locally for itching.

C. Atarax, 25 mg.   #30
Sig: 1 tablet t.i.d., a.c.

D. Benadryl, 50 mg.   #15
Sig: 1 capsule h.s.

2. *For a more severe case of acute hives:*

A. Benadryl injection. Give 2 ml. (20 mg.) subcutaneously, or

B. Epinephrine hydrochloride. Give 0.3 to 0.5 ml. of 1:1,000 solution subcutaneously, or

C. Acthar gel. Give 40 U. or 80 U. intramuscularly, or

D. Hydrocortisone tablets, 20 mg. (or newer related corticosteroid)   #20
Sig. 1 tablet q.i.d. for 3 days then 1 tablet t.i.d.

E. Penicillinase (Neutrapen). Give 800,000 U. intramuscularly if hives are known to be due to penicillin. This therapy occasionally causes severe constitutional reactions.

3. Treatment for patient with *chronic* hives of 6 months' duration. Cause undetermined after careful history and examination.

A. Atarax, 25 mg.   #60
Sig: 1-2 t.i.d. depending on drowsiness and effectiveness. Continue for weeks or months.

B. Diet. Suggest avoidance of chocolate, nuts, cheese and other milk products, sea foods, strawberries, pork, excess spicy foods, and excess of coffee or tea.

C. Staphylococcus Toxoid (Lederle), Dilution No. 1. Give 0.1 ml. subcutaneously and increase by 0.1 ml. twice or once a week up to 1.0 ml. (This is a mild form of nonspecific protein therapy that apparently is curative in some cases. Other agents that could be used are: Piromen, autohemotherapy, and crude liver injections.)

D. A mild sedative or tranquilizer such as meprobamate 400 mg. t.i.d. or phenobarbital 15 mg. t.i.d.

ERYTHEMA MULTIFORME

This term introduces a flurry of confusion in the mind of any student of medicine. It will be the purpose of this section to attempt to dispel that confusion. Erythema multiforme as originally described by Hebra is an uncommon distinct disease of unknown cause characterized by red iris-shaped or bulls-eye-like macules, papules, or bullae confined mainly to the extremities, the face and the lips, accompanied by mild fever, malaise and arthralgia, occurring usually in children and young adults in the spring and the fall, with a duration of 2 to 4 weeks, and frequently recurrent for several years (Fig. 9-1).

The only relationship between Hebra's erythema multiforme and the following diseases or syndromes is the clinical appearance of the eruption.

Stevens-Johnson syndrome is a very severe and oftentimes fatal variant of erythema multiforme. It is characterized by high fever, extensive purpura, bullae, and ulcers of the mucous membranes and, after 2 to 3 days, ulcers of the skin. Eye involvement can result in blindness.

Erythema Multiforme Bullosum. This is a severe, chronic, bullous disease of adults. (See p. 193.)

Erythema-Multiforme-like Drug Eruption. Frequently due to phenacetin, quinine, penicillin, mercury, arsenic, Butazolidin, barbiturates, Tridione, Dilantin, sulfonamides and antitoxins. (See p. 68.)

Erythema-Multiforme-like Eruption. This eruption is seen with rheumatic fever, pneumonia, meningitis, measles, herpes simplex, Coxsackie virus infection, pregnancy, cancer, following deep x-ray therapy, and as an allergic reaction to foods.

Erythema perstans group of diseases (Fig. 9-2). There are over a dozen clinical entities in this group with impossible-to-remember names. (See Dictionary-Index under "Erythema perstans.") All have varying sized erythematous patches, papules or plaques with a definite red border and a less active center forming circles, half circles, groups of circles, and linear bands. Multiple causes have been ascribed, including tickbites, allergic reactions, fungal, bacterial, viral and spirochetal infections, and internal cancer. The duration of and the response to therapy varies with each individual case.

Reiter's Syndrome. This is a triad of conjunctivitis, urethritis and, most important, arthritis, predominantly in males, which lasts approximately 6 months.

Behçet's syndrome consists of a triad of genital, oral and ophthalmic ulcerations seen most commonly in males; it can last for years with recurrences.

Differential Diagnosis of Hebra's Erythema Multiforme. *Urticaria* (clinically, it may resemble erythema multiforme, but hives are associated with only mild systemic symptoms; it can occur in any age group; iris lesions are unusual; usually it can be attributed to penicillin or other drug therapy; and it responds rapidly but often not completely to antihistamine therapy, p. 78).

Treatment. Child, aged 12, has bulls-eye-like lesions on hands, arms and feet, erosions of the lips and mucous membranes of the mouth, malaise and temperature of 101° orally. He had a similar eruption last spring.

1. Order bed rest and increased oral fluid intake.
2. Aspirin, 300 mg.   #30
   Sig: 2 tablets q.i.d.
3. Tetracycline capsules, 250 mg.   #20
   Sig: 1 capsule q.i.d.

For severe cases, such as the Stevens-Johnson form, intensive corticosteroid therapy with intravenous infusions, gamma globulin and other supportive measures will be indicated.

ERYTHEMA NODOSUM

Erythema nodosum is an uncommon reaction pattern seen mainly on the anterior tibial areas of the legs which appears as erythematous nodules in successive

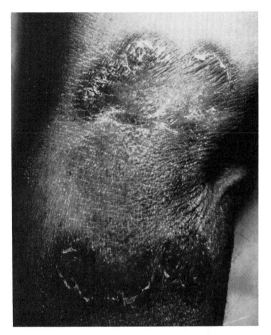

Fig. 9-2. Erythema perstans. Chronic lesions on elbow. (*Patient of Drs. L. Grayson and H. Shair.*)

crops preceded by fever, malaise and arthralgia (Fig. 9-3).

Primary Lesions. See bilateral red, tender, rather well-circumscribed nodules, mainly on the pretibial surface of the legs but also on the arms and the body. Later, the flat lesions may become raised, confluent and purpuric. Only a few lesions develop at one time.

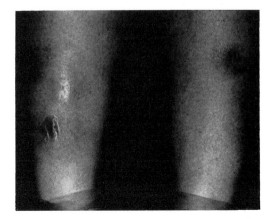

Fig. 9-3. Erythema nodosum of legs of pregnant woman.

Secondary Lesions. They never suppurate or form ulcers.

Course. The lesions last several weeks, but the duration can be affected by therapy directed to the cause if it is known. Relapses are related to the cause.

Etiology. Careful clinical and laboratory examination is necessary to determine the cause of this toxic reaction pattern. The following tests should be performed: complete blood count, sedimentation rate, urinalysis, serologic test for syphilis, chest roentgenogram, and specific skin tests as indicated. The causes of erythema nodosum are streptococcal infection (rheumatic fever, pharyngitis, scarlet fever, arthritis), fungal infection (coccidioidomycosis, *Trichophyton* infection), pregnancy, lymphogranuloma venereum, syphilis, chancroid, drugs (sulfonamides, contraceptive pills, iodides, bromides) and, rarely, tuberculosis.

Age and Sex Incidence. Predominantly in adolescent and young females.

Laboratory Findings. Histopathologic examination will reveal a nonspecific but characteristically localized inflammatory infiltrate in the subcutaneous tissue and in and around the veins.

Differential Diagnosis

Erythema induratum (this is a chronic tuberculid of young women that occurs on the posterior calf area and often suppurates; biopsy shows a tuberculoid infiltrate, usually with caseation).

Necrobiosis lipoidica diabeticorum (an uncommon cutaneous manifestation of diabetes mellitus characterized by well defined patches of reddish-yellow atrophic skin primarily on anterior areas of legs; can ulcerate; biopsy characteristic but usually not necessary or indicated because of possibility of poor healing; p. 213).

Periarteritis nodosa (a rare, fatal arteritis, most often in males; 25% of cases show painful subcutaneous nodules and purpura mainly of the lower extremities).

Nodular vasculitis (chronic painful nodules of the calves of middle-aged women which rarely ulcerate but recur commonly; biopsy is of value; it may be a variant of erythema nodosum).

Superficial thrombophlebitis migrans of Buerger's disease (an early venous change of Buerger's disease commonly seen in males, with painful nodules of the anterior tibial area; biopsy is of value).

Nodular panniculitis or *Weber-Christian disease* (mainly in obese middle-aged women; see tender, indurated, subcutaneous nodules, and plaques, usually on the thighs and the buttocks, each crop preceded by fever and malaise; leaves residual atrophy and hyperpigmentation).

For completeness, the following 5 very rare syndromes with inflammatory nodules of the legs are defined in the Dictionary-Index: *subcutaneous fat necrosis with pancreatic disease, migratory panniculitis, allergic granulomatosis, necrobiosis granulomatosis,* and *embolic nodules* from several sources.

Treatment

1. Treat the cause if possible.

2. Rest, local heat and aspirin are valuable. The eruption is self-limited if the cause can be eliminated.

3. Chronic cases can be disabling enough to warrant a short course of corticosteroid therapy.

STASIS DERMATITIS
(Plate 60)

This is a common condition due to impaired venous circulation in the legs of older patients. Almost all cases are associated with varicose veins, and since the tendency to develop varicosities is a familial characteristic, stasis dermatitis is also familial (Fig. 9-1.)

Primary Lesions. Early cases of stasis dermatitis begin as a red, scaly, pruritic patch that rapidly becomes vesicular and crusted, due to scratching and subsequent secondary infection. The bacterial infection is responsible for the spread of the patch and the chronicity of the eruption. Edema of the affected ankle area results in a further decrease in circulation and, consequently, more infection. The lesions may be unilateral or bilateral.

Secondary Lesions. Three secondary conditions can arise from untreated stasis dermatitis:

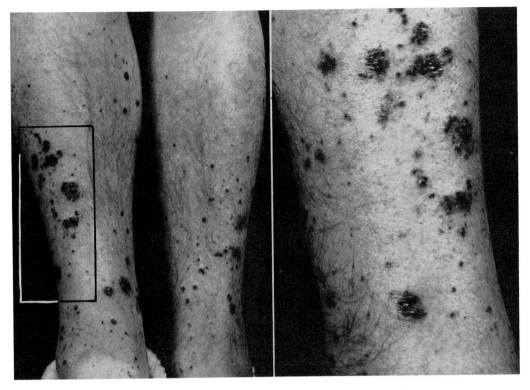

Fig. 9-4. Purpura of unknown cause on legs. (*K.U.M.C.*)

1. *Hyperpigmentation* is inevitable following the healing of either simple or severe stasis dermatitis of the legs. This increase in pigmentation is slow to disappear and in many elderly patients it never does.

2. *Stasis ulcers* (p. 126) can occur as the result of edema, deeper bacterial infection, or improper care of the primary dermatitis.

3. *Infectious eczematoid dermatitis* (p. 126) may develop on the legs, the arms and even the entire body, either slowly or as an explosive rapidly spreading eruption.

Course. The rapidity of healing depends on the age of the patient and other factors listed under "etiology." In elderly patients who have untreated varicose veins, stasis dermatitis can persist for years with remissions and exacerbations. If a patient in the 40-to-50 age group develops stasis dermatitis the prognosis is particularly bad for future recurrences and possible ulcers unless the varicosities are removed.

Etiology. Poor venous circulation due to the sluggish blood flow in tortuous dilated varicose veins is the primary cause. If the factors of obesity, lack of proper rest or care of the legs, pruritus, secondary infection, low protein diet and old age are added to the circulation problem, the result can be a chronic, disabling disease.

Differential Diagnosis

Contact dermatitis (history important, especially regarding nylon hose, new socks, contact with ragweed, high-top shoes, etc.; see no venous insufficiency, p. 49).

Neurodermatitis (thickened, dry, very pruritic patch; see no venous insufficiency, p. 72).

Treatment. Laborer, age 55, has scaly, reddish, slightly edematous, excoriated dermatitis on medial aspect of left ankle and leg of 6 weeks' duration.

1. Prescribe rest and elevation of the leg as much as possible by lying in bed. The foot of the bed should be elevated

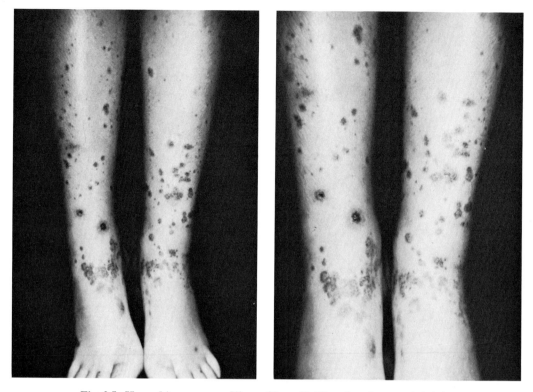

Fig. 9-5. Henoch's purpura. View of legs (*left*) and a close-up (*right*).

4 inches by placing 2 bricks under the legs. Sitting in a chair with the leg propped on a stool is of very little value.

  2. Boric acid wet packs

Sig: 1 tablespoon of boric acid crystals to 1 quart of warm water. Apply cloths wet with this solution for 30 minutes twice a day.

  3. An antibiotic-corticosteroid ointment q.s.   15.0

Sig: Apply to leg t.i.d.

  4. Surgical removal of varicose veins. This should be strongly recommended, particularly in younger patients, to prevent recurrences and eventual irreversible changes, including ulcers.

For the more *severe case* of stasis dermatitis with oozing, cellulitis, and 3-plus pitting edema, the following treatment should be ordered in addition:

  1. Hospitalization or enforced bed rest at home for the purpose of (A) applying the boric acid wet packs for longer periods of time, and (B) strict rest and elevation of the leg.

  2. A course of an oral antibiotic.

  3. Ace Elastic Bandage, 4 inches wide, No. 8.

After the patient is dismissed from the hospital and will be on his feet, give instructions for the correct application of this bandage to the leg before arising in the morning. This helps to reduce the edema that could cause a recrudescence of the dermatitis.

PURPURIC DERMATOSES

Purpuric lesions are caused by an extravasation of red blood cells into the skin or mucous membranes. The lesions can be distinguished from erythema and telangiectasia by the fact that purpuric lesions do not blanch under pressure applied by the finger or by diascopy (Fig. 9-4).

Petechiae are small superficial purpuric lesions. *Ecchymoses* or bruises are more extensive, round or irregularly shaped pur-

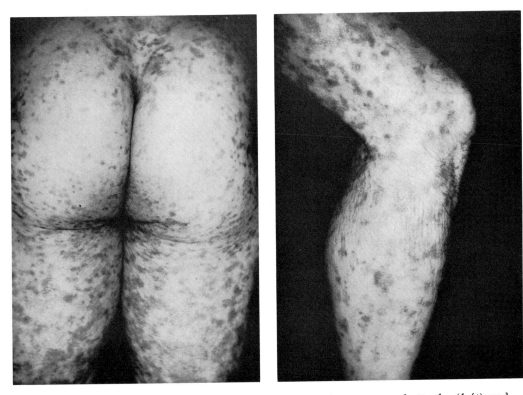

Fig. 9-6. Pigmented purpuric eruption of the Schamberg type on buttocks (*left*) and on thigh and leg (*right*).

puric lesions. *Hematomata* are large, deep, fluctuant, tumorlike hemorrhages into the skin.

The purpuras can be divided into the *thrombocytopenic* forms and the *nonthrombocytopenic* forms.

Thrombocytopenic purpura may be idiopathic or secondary to various chronic diseases or a drug sensitivity. The platelet count is below normal, the bleeding time is prolonged, and the clotting time is normal, but the clot does not retract normally. This form of purpura is rare.

Nonthrombocytopenic purpura is more commonly seen. *Henoch's purpura* (Fig. 9-5) is a form of nonthrombocytopenic purpura most commonly seen in children characterized by recurrent attacks of purpura accompanied by gastrointestinal pathology. It is thought to be related to *Schönlein's purpura*.

The ecchymoses or *senile purpura* seen in the elderly patients following minor injury are very common. Ecchymoses are also seen in patients who have been on long-term systemic corticosteroid therapy.

Another common purpuric eruption is that known as *stasis purpura*. These lesions are associated with vascular insufficiency of the legs and occur as the early sign of this change, or they are seen around areas of stasis dermatitis or stasis ulcers.

Quite frequently seen is a petechial *drug eruption* due to the chlorothiazide diuretics.

A less common group of cases are those seen in middle aged adults classified under the name of *pigmented purpuric eruptions*. Some cases of pigmented purpuric eruptions itch severely. The cause is unknown but the majority of cases have a positive tourniquet test but other bleeding tests are normal. Clinically these patients have grouped petechial lesions that begin on the legs and extend up to the thighs and occasionally up to the waist and on the arms.

Some clinicians are able to separate these pigmented purpuric eruptions into *purpura annularis telangiectodes* (*Majocchi*), *progressive pigmentary dermatosis* (*Schamberg*) and *pigmented purpuric lichenoid dermatitis* (*Gougerot-Blum*). Majocchi's disease commonly begins on the legs but slowly spreads to become generalized. Telangiectatic capillaries become confluent and produce annular or serpiginous lesions. The capillaries break down, causing purpuric lesions. Schamberg's disease (Fig. 9-6) is a slowly progressive pigmentary condition of the lower part of the legs which fades after a period of months. The Gougerot-Blum form is accompanied by severe itching; otherwise it resembles Schamberg's disease.

For these pigmented purpuric eruptions, therapy with Hesper-C Bitabs 3 times a day is occasionally effective, as is occlusive dressing therapy with a corticosteroid cream.

TELANGIECTASES

Telangiectases are abnormal dilated small blood vessels. Telangiectases are divided into *primary forms* where the causes are unknown, and *secondary forms* where they are related to some known disturbance.

The primary telangiectases include the simple and compound hemangiomas of infants (see p. 273) and the spider hemangiomas (see p. 275).

Secondary telangiectasia is very commonly seen on the fair-skinned individual as a result of aging and chronic sun exposure. X-ray therapy and burns can also cause dilated vessels.

BIBLIOGRAPHY

Fine, R. M., and Meltzer, H. D.: Chronic Erythema Nodosum. Arch. Derm., *100*:33, 1969.

Rook, A., Wilkinson, D. S., and Ebling, F. J. G.: Textbook of Dermatology, vol. 2. Philadelphia, Davis, 1968. An excellent section on "Disorders Affecting Blood Vessels."

Winkelman, R. K.: New inflammatory nodules of the legs. South. M. J., *57*:637, 1964.

10

Seborrheic Dermatitis, Acne and Rosacea

SEBORRHEIC DERMATITIS
(Plates 17 to 19)

Seborrheic dermatitis or dandruff is exceedingly common on the scalp but less common on the other areas of predilection: ears, face, sternal area, axillae and pubic area. It is well to consider seborrheic dermatitis as a "condition" of the skin and not as a "disease." It occurs as part of the "acne-seborrhea complex," most commonly seen in the brown-eyed brunette who has a family history of these conditions. Dandruff is spoken of as oily or dry, but it is all basically oily. If dandruff scales are pressed between two pieces of tissue paper, an oily residue is expressed, leaving its mark on the tissue.

Certain misconceptions that have arisen concerning this common dermatosis need to be corrected. Seborrheic dermatitis cannot be cured, but remissions for varying amounts of time do occur naturally or as the result of treatment. Seborrheic dermatitis does not cause permanent hair loss or baldness unless it becomes grossly infected. Seborrheic dermatitis is not infectious or contagious. The cause, contrary to magazine ads, is unknown.

Primary Lesions. Redness and scaling appear in varying degrees. The scale may be of the so-called "dry" type or of the "greasy" type (Plate 17).

Secondary Lesions. Rarely seen are excoriations from severe itching and secondary bacterial infection. Neurodermatitis with lichenification can follow a chronic itching and scratching habit.

Course. Exacerbations and remissions are common, depending on the season, treatment, and the age and general health of the individual. Since this is a condition of the skin and not a disease, a true cure is impossible.

Seasonal Incidence. This condition is worse in colder weather, presumably due to lower indoor humidity and lack of summer sunlight.

Differential Diagnosis

SCALP LESIONS

Psoriasis: sharply defined, whitish, dry, scaly patches; typical psoriasis lesions on elbows, knees, nails or elsewhere (p. 97).

Neurodermatitis: usually a single patch on the posterior scalp area or around the ears, intense itching, excoriation, and thickening of the skin (p. 72).

Tinea Capitis: usually in a child, see broken-off hairs with or without pustular reaction. Fluoresces under Wood's light. Culture is positive (p. 170).

Atopic Eczema: usually in infants or children, diffuse dry scaliness; eczema also on face, arms and legs (p. 56).

FACE LESIONS

Systemic Lupus Erythematosus: faint reddish, slightly scaly "butterfly" eruption, aggravated by sunlight, with fever, malaise, positive L. E. cell test (p. 205).

Chronic Discoid Lupus Erythematosus: sharply defined, red, scaly, atrophic areas with large follicular openings, resistant to local therapy (p. 204).

BODY LESIONS

Tinea Corporis (p. 170)
Psoriasis (p. 97)
Pityriasis Rosea (p. 104)
Tinea Versicolor (p. 107)

Treatment. Young man with recurrent, red, scaly lesions at border of scalp and

87

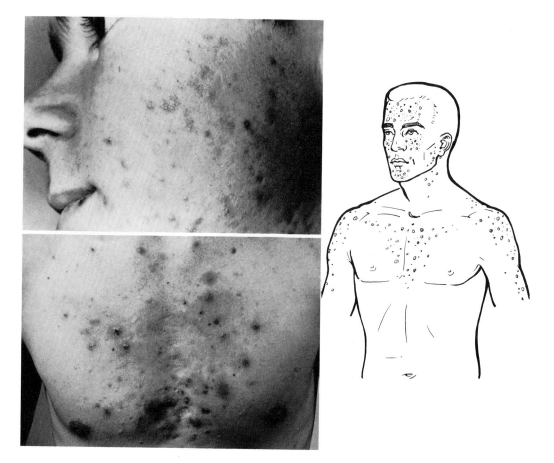

Fig. 10-1. Acne of face and chest.

forehead, and diffuse, mild, whitish scaling throughout scalp.

1. Management of cases of dandruff must include telling the patient what he has, that it is not contagious, that there is no true cure, that it will not cause baldness, and that there are seasonal variations. Therapy can be very effective but only for keeping the dandruff under control.

2. Shampooing. With the above information in mind, tell the patient that shampooing offers the best management. There are several shampoos available and the patient may have to experiment around to find the one most suitable to him. These can be suggested:

A. Selsun Suspension   120.0

Sig: Shampoo hair with 3 applications, leaving last application on for 5 minutes before rinsing off with hot water.

Repeat shampoo twice a week for 2 weeks, then weekly. Use no other soap. Refill prescription p.r.n.

The only major complaint about Selsun Suspension is that it often results in increased oiliness of the hair. It is nontoxic unless taken internally, and even then it would be regurgitated because of the soap base. Reports of hair loss following its use have not been substantiated.

B. Tar shampoos, such as Ionil T, Sebutone, X-Seb T, Vanseb-T, etc.

Sig: Shampoo as frequently as necessary to keep scaling and itching to a minimum.

Other effective shampoos are Head and Shoulders, Sebulex, Ionil, X-Seb, etc.

3. Pragmatar Ointment   15.0

Sig: Apply to scalp lesions nightly

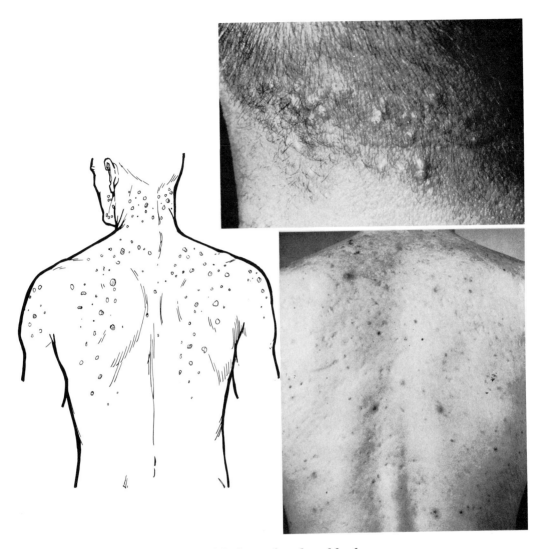

Fig. 10-2. Acne of neck and back.

for 1 to 2 weeks and to any recurrences not controlled by Selsun Suspension.

Pragmatar is also excellent for seborrheic dermatitis occurring on other locations of the body.

4. Vitamin B_{12}. For resistant cases give 500 mcg. subcutaneously once a week.

ACNE

Acne vulgaris is a very common skin condition of adolescents and young adults. It is characterized by any combination of comedones (blackheads), pustules, cysts and scarring of varying severity (Figs. 10-1 and 10-2).

Primary Lesions. Comedones, papules, pustules and, in severe cases, cysts.

Secondary Lesions. Pits and scars in severe cases. Excoriations of the papules are seen in some adolescents but most often they appear as part of the acne of women in their twenties and thirties.

Distribution. Face, neck and, less commonly, on the back, the chest and the arms.

Course. Begins at ages of 9 to 12 or later and lasts with new outbreaks for months or years. Subsides in the majority of cases by the age of 18 to 19, but occasional flare-ups may occur for years. The

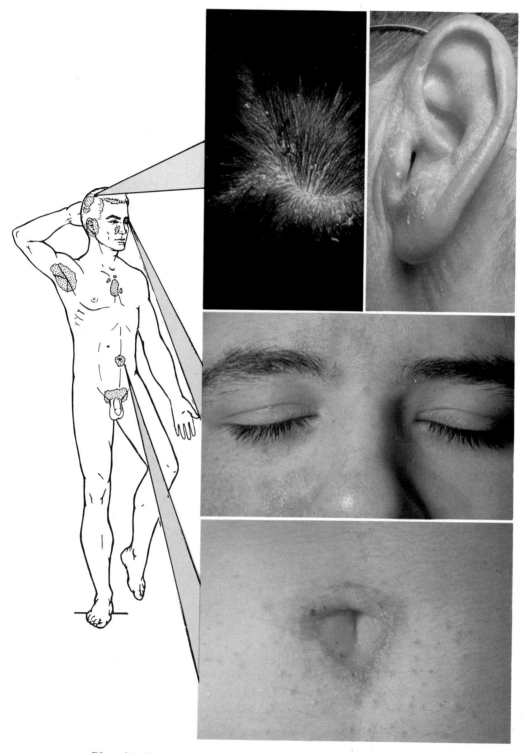

Plate 17. Seborrheic dermatitis. (*Owen Laboratories, Inc.*)

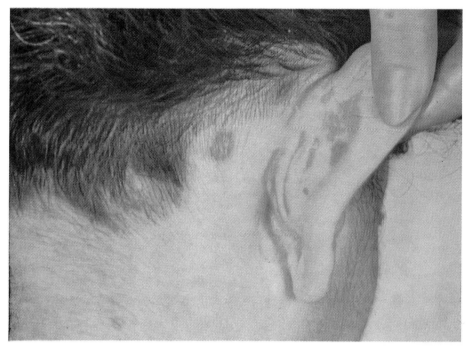

Plate 18. Seborrheic dermatitis behind the ear and at the border of the scalp. (*Smith, Kline & French Laboratories*)

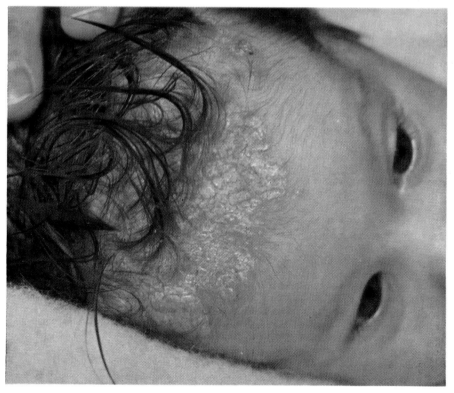

Plate 19. Seborrheic dermatitis of infancy. This is one of the causes of "cradle cap." (*Smith, Kline & French Laboratories*)

residual scarring varies with severity of the case and response to treatment.

Subjective Complaint. Tenderness of the large pustules, itching rarely. Emotional upset is common as a result of the unattractive appearance.

Etiology. These factors are important: heredity, hormonal balance, diet, cleanliness and general health.

Season. Most cases are better during the summer.

Contagiousness. None.

Differential Diagnosis

Drug Eruption: history of ingestion of iodides, bromides, Tridione, or testosterone and ACTH by injection (p. 60).

Contact Dermatitis from Industrial Oils (p. 55).

Adenoma Sebaceum: rare; see papular lesions; associated with epilepsy and mental deficiency (Fig. 292).

Treatment

FIRST VISIT of 14-year-old patient with moderate amount of facial blackheads and pustules:

1. Acne diet and instructions regarding skin care (see sheet that can be given to patient, "What You Should Know About Acne," p. 93) or the booklet "Acne and Other Complexion Problems," by Sauer, published by Lippincott). Stress the fact to the patient and the parent that not one factor but several factors (heredity, hormones, diet, cleanliness and general health) are important in clearing up acne.

2. Dial soap. The affected areas should be washed twice a day with a washcloth and this soap.

3. Sulfur, ppt.   6%
   Resorcinol   4%
   Colored alcoholic shake lotion
   (See in Formulary p. 37) q.s. 60.0
   Sig: Apply locally b.i.d. with fingers. (Boys may object to the powdery look and, if so, should use the lotion at night only.)

Proprietary substitutions for the above lotion include Resulin lotion (Almay), Liquimat (Texas), Komed lotion (Barnes-Hind), Acne-Aid Cream (Stiefel), Microsyn lotion (Syntex), Acno lotions (Cummins), and Rezamid lotion (Dermik).

4. Remove the blackheads with a comedone extractor in the office.

SUBSEQUENT VISITS. Ultraviolet therapy with increasing suberythema doses once or twice a week. Treat both sides of the face, back or chest as indicated.

TREATMENT FOR A CASE OF SCARRING ACNE

1. Tetracycline, or similar antibiotic, 250 mg.   #100
   Sig: 1 capsule q.i.d. for 3 days then 1 b.i.d. Following a good response, which may necessitate treatment for several weeks. This dose can be continued for weeks, months or years; or the dose can be lowered to 1 capsule a day for maintenance, depending, of course, on the extent of the involvement. Tetracycline should be taken ½ hour before meals or 2 hours after a meal.

2. Diethylstilbestrol (Enseals) 0.25 mg.   #30
   Sig: *Females:* 1 tablet a day for 10 days before and during the menstrual period. Take for 3 to 4 cycles. May temporarily alter the menstrual cycle. *Males:* 1 tablet a day. For very severe cystic acne the initial dose can be 1 mg. a day for 1 to 2 weeks, then decreased. A dose of 0.25 mg. a day can be safely continued for 1 to 2 months or until the breasts become tender.

3. X-ray Therapy. Seldom used now since the long-term therapy with oral antibiotics has proved to be so beneficial. X-ray therapy can be given after the age of 16 (younger in severe cases) and should be administered only by a dermatologist or a radiologist. The usual treatment consists of 75 r of unfiltered superficial x-ray given to both sides of the face (or to the back and the chest if needed) for 8 to 12 weekly treatments. The half-value layer of most superficial x-ray machines is 0.9 to 1.0 mm. of aluminum. Given in this manner, a total dose of 1,000 to 1,200 r is known to be safe. Further x-ray therapy should not be given to the area treated at *any time* in the future.

4. Other Treatments:
   A. Vitamin A (water-soluble natural Aqua-sol A or water-soluble synthetic Stabil A) 100,000 U.

Fig. 10-3. Residual scarring from severe facial acne.

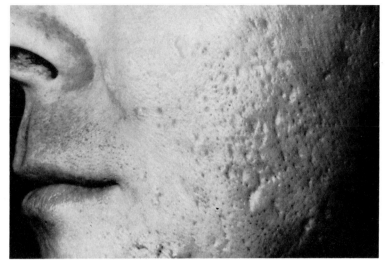

Sig: 1 capsule a day for 2 to 3 months.

B. Staphylococcus Toxoid (Lederle)

Sig: 0.1 ml. (Dilution 1) subcutaneously, increased by 0.1 ml. at weekly intervals, up to 1.0 ml.

C. Other cleansers include Fostex Cake and Cream (can also be used as a shampoo), piSec, Acnaveen Cream, etc.

D. Abrasive cleansers are somewhat effective in removing comedones. These include Brasivol, Pernox and Sastid.

E. Incision of fluctuant acne cysts. *Never* incise these widely, but if you feel the pus must be drained, do it through a very small incision.

5. The residual scarring of severe acne (Fig. 10-3) can be lessened by surgical dermabrasion, using a rapidly rotating wire brush or diamond fraise. This procedure is being done by many dermatologists and plastic surgeons.

What You Should Know About Acne*

Acne is a disorder in which the oil glands of the skin are overactive. It usually involves the face and, frequently, the chest and the back, for these areas are the richest in oil glands. When an oil gland opening becomes

* This information is from an instruction sheet given by the author to his acne patients. The author has also written a small booklet directed to the teenager, which the physician could give to his own acne patients, entitled "Acne and Other Complexion Problems," Philadelphia, Lippincott.

plugged, a blackhead is formed and irritates the skin in exactly the same way as any other foreign body, such as a sliver of wood. This irritation takes the form of red pimples or deep painful cysts. These infections destroy the tissues and, when healed, may result in permanent scars.

The tendency to develop acne may run in families, especially those in which one or both parents have an oily skin. Acne is aggravated by certain foods, improper care of the skin, lack of adequate sleep, and nervous tension. In girls, acne is usually worse before a menstrual period. Even in boys, acne flares on a cyclic basis. Any or all of these factors may exaggerate the tendency of the oily skin to develop acne. Therefore, the prevention of acne depends on your correcting not one but several of these factors.

Because acne is so common, is not contagious and does not cause loss of time from school or work, many people tend to ignore it or regard it as a necessary part of growing up. Actually, the old statement, "You'll be all right when you're married," has little or no significance. Marriage itself has no relationship to acne, except that ordinarily by the time a person is ready to get married, he or she usually is past the acne age and the acne would have cleared anyway.

REASONS FOR TREATING ACNE

There are at least two very important reasons for seeking medical care for acne. The first is to prevent the scarring mentioned previously. Once scarring has occurred, it is permanent in character. Then a patient must go through the rest of his life being embarrassed and annoyed by the scars, even though active pimples are no longer present. This scarring may vary from tiny little pits, which are frequently mistaken for "enlarged pores," to deep, large, disfiguring pockmarks.

The second reason for starting active treatment for acne, even without scarring, is that the condition may become the source of much psychological disturbance to a patient. Even though the acne may appear to others to be very mild and inconspicuous, it may seem very noticeable to the patient and lead to embarrassment, worry and nervousness.

TREATMENT MEASURES TO BE CARRIED OUT BY THE PATIENT

Cleansing Measures. Your face is to be washed twice a day with soap and a washcloth. The doctor may suggest a particular soap for use. Do not use any face cream, cold cream, cleansing cream, nourishing cream, or any other kind of grease on the face. This includes the avoidance of so-called pancake lotions which may contain oil, grease or wax. Acne is caused by excessive oiliness of the skin, and every effort will be made to make it dry. Use of greases and creams increases the oiliness. You may think your face is dry because of the flakes on it, but these are actually flakes of dried oil. Later, when the treatment begins to take effect, your skin will actually become dry, even to the point where it is chapped and tender, especially around the mouth and the sides of the chin. When this point is reached, you will be advised as to suitable corrective measures for this temporary dryness. If the skin becomes red and uncomfortable between office visits, the applied remedy may be discontinued for one or two nights.

Girls may use face powder, dry rouge (not cream rouge), lipstick, but no face creams. Boys with acne should shave as regularly as necessary, and should not use oils, greases, pomades or *hair tonics* except those which may be prescribed by the physician. Hair should be dressed only with water. Many cases of acne are associated with oily hair and dandruff and, for these cases, suitable local scalp applications and shampoos will be prescribed by the physician.

Plenty of rest is important. You should have at least 8 hours of sleep each night. Violent exercise should be avoided, since increased perspiration is usually accompanied by increased activity of the oil glands. Moderate suntanning is beneficial for acne, but a sunburn does more harm than good. When you go out in the sun, do not use oily or greasy suntan preparations.

Diet. These foods aggravate most cases of acne and should be restricted.

1. *Chocolate:* including chocolate candy, chocolate ice cream, chocolate cake, chocolate-covered nuts, chocolate sodas, cocoa and *cola* drinks. Hard candy (not chocolate) and soft drinks, other than the cola drinks, are all right in small or moderate amounts. Diet-type cola drinks can also be used.

2. *Nuts:* especially peanuts and peanut butter.

3. *Milk Products:* Avoid whole milk (homogenized) and 2 percent butterfat milk. You can drink 4 glasses of skim milk a day. Reduce the use of sweet and sour cream, whipped cream, butter, rich creamy cheeses and ice cream. Avoid sharp cheeses, but cottage and cheddar cheese are permitted.

4. *Avoid an excess of any sweets and fats,* especially French fried potatoes and fried fatty meats, such as hamburgers and tender steaks.

5. *Spicy Foods:* Reduce as much as possible the use of spicy sauces, Worcestershire, chili, catsup, pizza, spicy smoked meats and delicatessen products.

The following of this diet does not mean that you should starve yourself. Eat plenty of lean meats, fresh and cooked vegetables, fruits (and their juices) and all breads. Drink plenty of water (4 to 6 glasses) daily, especially on arising each morning.

Do not take any medicine internally without the knowledge of the physician.

MEDICAL TREATMENT OF ACNE

In addition to the prescribed treatment you will apply yourself, there are several aspects of the treatment of acne that must be carried out by the doctor or the nurse.

One important method of treatment is the proper removal of blackheads. *This is part of the doctor's job and should not be done by the patient.* Pimples which have pus in them and are ready to open should be opened by the doctor or the nurse. This is done with surgical instruments which are designed for the purpose and do not damage tissue or cause scars. Picking pimples by the patient can cause scarring and should be avoided completely. When the blackheads are removed and the pustules opened in the doctor's office, the skin heals faster, and scarring is minimized.

Ultraviolet light treatments and other medicines, including some taken internally (such as sulfa drugs, antibiotics or hormones) may be prescribed by the doctor. Vitamins, except vitamin A have no proven beneficial effect on acne.

Another method of treatment of severe and stubborn acne is x-ray therapy.

CONCLUSION

Do not become discouraged! Treatment is effective in at least 95 percent of all cases. It may be several weeks (4 to 6) before noticeable improvement appears. There may be occasional mild flare-ups, but, eventually, you will improve and you and your friends will notice the difference.

It is *very important* for you and your parents to realize that your doctor cannot shorten the length of time it takes for your oil glands to work normally. This maturing process of the skin can take several years in some persons. Therefore, after you improve, you will be dismissed from active medical care. But this does not mean that you stop using the lotion, the good cleansing measures, and the observation of the diet. If you develop a recurrence of your complexion trouble, then you must return to the physician for more active care. Don't foolishly think that because your complexion trouble returned the previous active medical care was not worthwhile. It was worthwhile, but it now needs to be resumed.

You can be sure that your doctor will do everything in his power to give you a clear healthy complexion. Your cooperation, patience and understanding will help.

ROSACEA

An uncommon pustular eruption of the butterfly area of the face in adults of the 40- to 50-year age group (Fig. 10-4).

Primary Lesions. Diffuse redness, papules, pustules, and later, dilated venules, mainly of the nose, the cheeks and the forehead.

Secondary Lesions. Severe long-standing cases eventuate in the bulbous greasy, hypertrophic nose characteristics of *rhinophyma*.

Course. The pustules are recurrent and difficult to heal. Rosacea keratitis of the eye is rare but can be very serious.

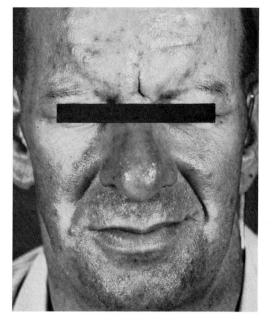

Fig. 10-4. Rosacea.

Etiology. Several factors influence the disease: (1) hereditary factor of oily skin and, usually, brunette complexion; (2) in some patients, no free hydrochloric acid in the stomach; (3) excess ingestion of alcoholic beverages, hot drinks and acne-producing foods.

Differential Diagnosis

Boils: usually only one large lesion; can be recurrent but may occur sporadically; an early case of rosacea may look like small boils (p. 120).

Iodide or Bromide Drug Eruption: clinically similar but drug eruption usually is more widespread; history positive for drug (p. 60).

Seborrheic Dermatitis: pustules uncommon; red and scaly; in scalp also (p. 87).

Roseacealike Tuberculid of Lewandowsky: rare; biopsy helpful.

Treatment

FIRST VISIT of a 44-year-old-male with redness and pustules on the butterfly area of the face.

1. Prescribe avoidance of these foods:

chocolate, nuts, cheese, cokes, iodized salt, seafood, alcohol, spices and very hot drinks.

2. Dial soap

Sig: Use as face cleanser with a washcloth twice a day.

3. Sulfur, ppt.   6%
   Resorcinol   4%
   Colored alcoholic shake
     lotion q.s.   60.0
   Sig: Apply to face h.s.

4. Tetracycline capsules (250 mg.) q.i.d. for 3 days then 1 b.i.b. for weeks as necessary for benefit.

SUBSEQUENT VISIT

1. Acidulin capsules (oral hydrochloric acid)   #50

   Sig: 1 capsule t.i.d., a.c.

2. X-ray therapy as given for acne by a dermatologist or a radiologist is indicated in severe cases.

11

Papulosquamous Dermatoses

This classic grouping of skin eruptions includes several specific entities that predominantly affect the chest and the back with clinically similar macular, papular, and scaly lesions (see Fig. 3-5). The commonest diseases in the group are psoriasis, pityriasis rosea, tinea versicolor, lichen planus, seborrheic dermatitis, secondary syphilis and drug eruptions. The last three conditions are considered elsewhere in the book. To be complete with regard to the differential diagnoses of this group, the following rarer diseases can also be included: parapsoriasis, lichen nitidus and pityriasis rubra pilaris.

PSORIASIS
(Plates 20 and 21)

Psoriasis is a common, chronically recurring, papulosquamous disease, characterized by varying sized whitish scaly patches seen most commonly on the elbows, the knees and the scalp (Figs. 11-1 and 11-2).

Primary Lesions. Erythematous, papulosquamous lesions vary in shapes and sizes from drop size to large circinate areas which can become generalized. The scale is usually thick and silvery and bleeds from minute points when it is removed by the fingernail (Auspitz's sign).

Secondary Lesions. Unusual, but can see excoriations, thickening (lichenification), or oozing.

Distribution. Most commonly on the scalp, the elbows and the knees but can involve any area of the body, including the nails.

Course. Notoriously chronic and recurrent. However, severe cases have been known to clear up and not recur.

Etiology. Unknown. Approximately 30 percent of patients with psoriasis have a family history of the disease.

There is an acute form of psoriasis called *guttate psoriasis* that very frequently develops following a streptococcal throat infection. The scaly lesions are the size of drops, hence guttate.

Subjective Complaints. Fortunately, only 30 percent of patients with psoriasis itch.

Season. Worse in winter usually, probably because of low winter indoor humidity and relative lack of sunlight.

Age Group. Any age but unusual in children.

Contagiousness. None.

Related to Employment. Psoriatic lesions can develop or flare up in areas of skin injury (Koebner phenomenon).

Laboratory Findings. Microscopic section is characteristic in typical cases.

Differential Diagnosis

Tinea Corporis: single lesion usually with healing in center; scraping and culture positive for fungi (p. 170).

Seborrheic Dermatitis: lesions more greasy; occur in hairy areas; scalp lesions are often impossible to differentiate from psoriasis (p. 87).

Pityriasis Rosea: "herald patch"; acute onset (p. 103).

Atopic Eczema: patches on flexural surfaces; allergic history (p. 56).

Secondary or Tertiary Syphilis: can be psoriasiform; blood serology positive; local therapy is of little value (p. 134).

Lichen Planus: lesions violaceous; small papules; very little scaling (p. 107).

A single lesion of psoriasis may resemble *neurodermatitis.*

Psoriasis of nails (Plate 51) is similar to *tinea of nails.*

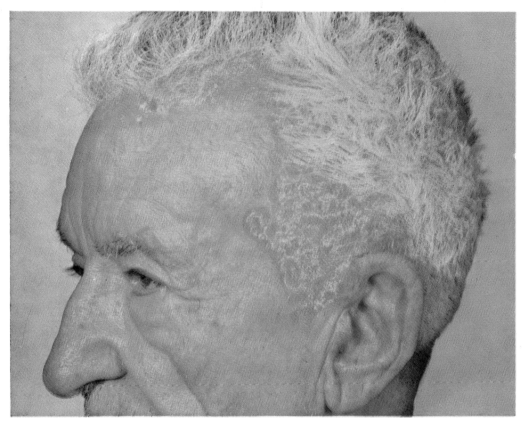

Plate 20. Psoriasis of the border of the scalp. Psoriasis in this location is often difficult to distinguish from seborrheic dermatitis. (*Smith, Kline & French Laboratories*)

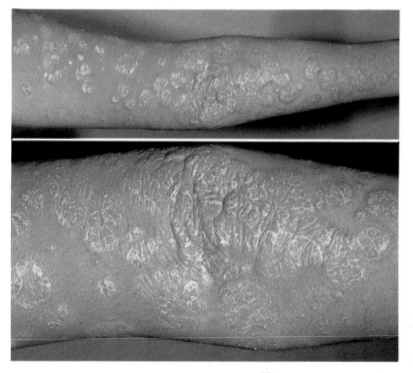

Plate 21. Psoriasis on elbows of a 17-year-old girl. (*Continued on facing page*).

98

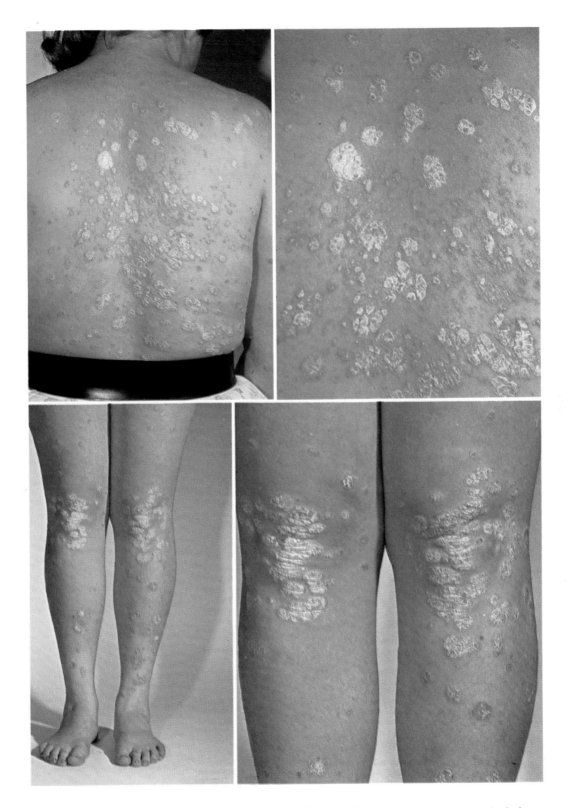

Plate 21 (*continued*). **Psoriasis of a 17-year-old girl.** Moderately extensive psoriasis in classic distribution on back and knees. (*K.U.M.C.*) (*Roche Laboratories*)

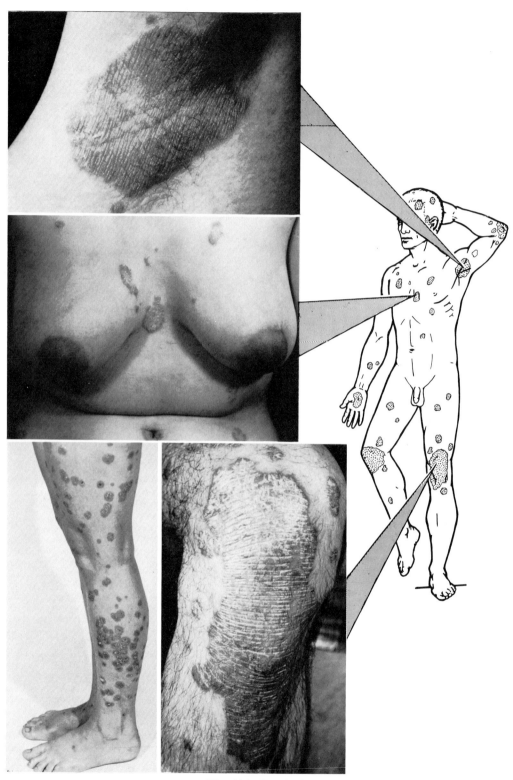

Fig. 11-1. Psoriasis.

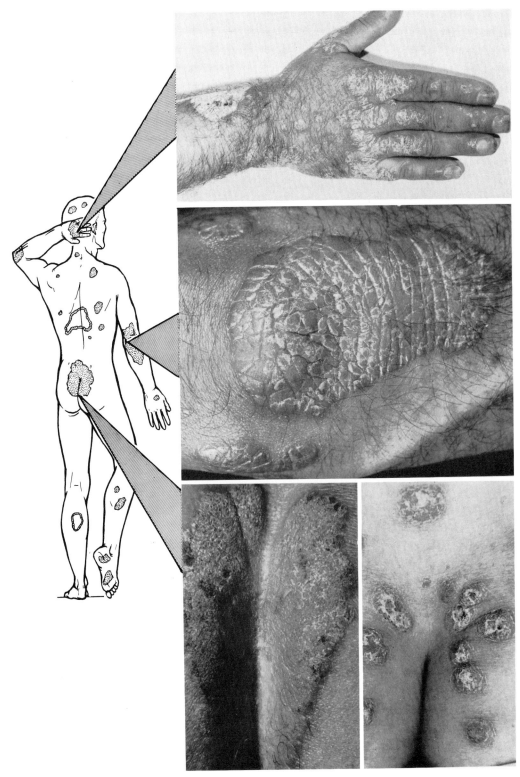

Fig. 11-2. Psoriasis.

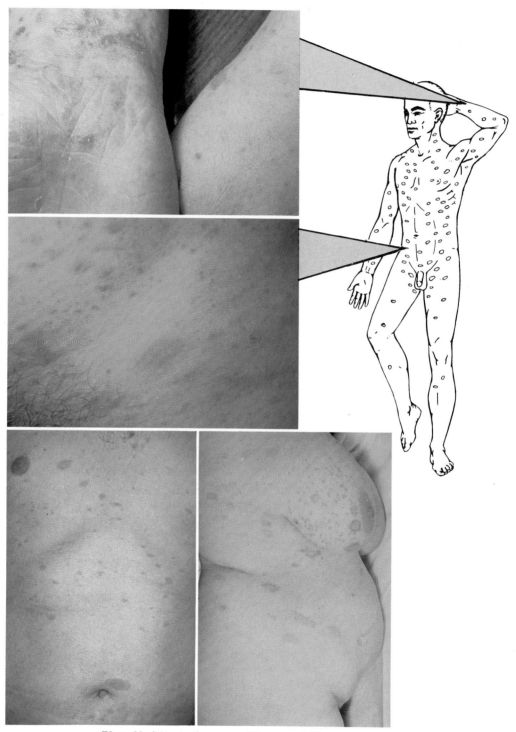

Plate 22. Pityriasis rosea. (*Westwood Pharmaceuticals*)

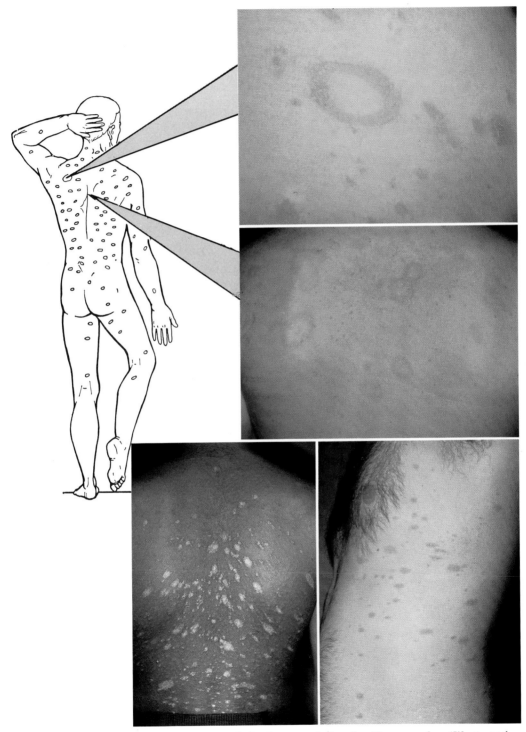

Plate 23. Pityriasis rosea. Bottom left photograph is of a Negro male. (*Westwood Pharmaceuticals*)

Treatment

It is most important in the management of patients with psoriasis that you be frank with them regarding the prognosis and "cure." Reassure them that it is not contagious, that the disease disappears in many cases, and that you can help them manage the disease. But be straightforward in saying that no doctor at this moment knows a "cure" for psoriasis. It might help the patient (or it might not) for you to say that psoriasis should not be considered a disease, but should be thought of as a hobby.

FIRST VISIT OF PATIENT WITH RED SCALY LESIONS ON SCALP AND ELBOWS ONLY

1. *For body lesions*
   Coal tar solution   5%
   Sulfur, ppt.   5%
   White petrolatum q.s.   30.0
   Sig: Apply locally b.i.d. to body lesions.
2. *For scalp lesions*
   Pragmatar ointment   15.0
   Sig: Apply to scalp lesions b.i.d. (Can use the ingredients of salve No. 1 in a water-washable base such as Unibase, Neobase, etc.).
3. Selsun Suspension   120.0
   Or a tar shampoo (See list in Formulary p. 35.)
   Sig: Shampoo scalp twice a week as long as salve is used in scalp. Use without any other soap. (Useful in relieving itching.)

SUBSEQUENT VISITS OF PATIENT WITH LOCALIZED CASE

1. For body lesions, gradually increase the strength of the medicines in the above salve (No. 1) to 10% and add salicyclic acid 4 to 10%.
2. Or stop above salve and use:
   Ammoniated mercury   5 to 10%
   White petrolatum q.s.   30.0
   (A salve containing both sulfur and ammoniated mercury will cause a black discoloration of the skin.)
3. Occlusive Dressing—Corticosteroid Therapy. For localized areas of psoriasis, especially on the extremities, Synalar, Cordran or Celestone cream can be applied at night and covered with an occlusive plastic dressing such as Saran wrap. This wrapping should be left on overnight, or for 24 hours. If the lesions of psoriasis are small, the cream can be covered with Blenderm Tape for occlusion.

For greater therapeutic effectiveness, on subsequent visits, coal tar solution (3 to 6%) can be incorporated in the cream.

4. Intralesional Corticosteroid Therapy. For localized patches of psoriasis, parenteral triamcinolone can be injected under the lesions. This is a very effective treatment for small lesions. The technic is given on page 73.

5. X-ray therapy can be given to localized areas by a dermatologist or a radiologist. If a lesion does not respond after 4 to 6 treatments of weekly doses of 75 r unfiltered, the lesion is not likely to respond to further x-ray therapy.

FIRST VISIT OF PATIENT WITH PSORIASIS ON 65 PERCENT OF THE BODY SURFACE

1. Coal tar solution (L.C.D.)   120.0
   Sig: 2 tablespoons to the bath tub with 6 to 8 inches of warm water. Soak for 15 minutes once a day. Soap may be used unless there is much itching.
2. Prescribe a mild body salve:
   Coal tar solution   3%
   White petrolatum q.s.   120.0
   Sig: Apply locally b.i.d.
   Later the concentration of the coal tar solution (L.C.D.) can be slowly increased.
3. Methischol or Lipotropic
   capsules   #100
   Sig: 2 capsules t.i.d., a.c.
   Given to correct a possible fat metabolism error.
4. Crude liver injection (2 mcg. of vitamin B_{12} per ml.)
   Sig: Give 2 ml. intramuscularly once or twice a week for 6 to 8 injections.
5. Ultraviolet therapy in increasing suberythema doses once or twice a week. This can be used following a daily thin application of a tar salve.
6. Methotrexate Therapy. In cases of severe psoriasis, dermatologists occasionally use this oral method of therapy with good results. Since methotrexate is a potent and dangerous drug, those wishing

to use it must consult recently published papers on the subject to become thoroughly familiar with the effects of the drug.

SUBSEQUENT VISITS OF PATIENT WITH RATHER GENERALIZED CASE

1. Increase the concentrations of medicines used locally or use:

Chrysarobin	0.1%
White petrolatum q.s.	30.0

Sig: Apply locally b.i.d. Avoid getting salve near the eyes.

The concentration of the chrysarobin can be increased cautiously, as necessary.

2. Low fat diet is thought by some to be helpful.

3. Systemic corticosteroids are of very little value except for triamcinolone (Aristocort or Kenacort). If conjunctive local therapy is not effective, relapses are the rule after corticosteroid therapy and may be difficult to handle. This is not a recommended form of therapy.

PITYRIASIS ROSEA
(Plates 22 to 24)

Pityriasis rosea is a moderately common papulosquamous eruption, mainly of the trunk of young adults, mildly pruritic, occurring most often in the spring and the fall.

Primary Lesions. Papulosquamous, oval erythematous discrete lesions. A larger "herald patch" resembling a patch of "ringworm" may precede the general rash by 2 to 10 days.

Secondary Lesions. Excoriations, rarely. The effects of overtreatment contact dermatitis are commonly seen.

Distribution. Chest and trunk mainly, along the lines of cleavage. In atypical cases the lesions are seen in the axillae and the groin only. Face lesions are rare in Caucasian adults but are rather commonly seen in children and Negroes.

Course. Following the development of the "herald patch," new generalized lesions continue to appear for 2 to 3 weeks. The entire rash commonly disappears within 6 weeks. Recurrences are rare.

Subjective Complaints. Itching varies from none to severe.

Etiology. Unknown.
Season. Spring and fall "epidemics" are common.
Age Group. Young adults mainly.
Contagiousness. None.

Differential Diagnosis

Tinea Versicolor: lesions tannish and irregularly shaped; fungi seen on scraping (p. 107).

Drug Eruption: no "herald patch"; positive drug history for bismuth or sulfa (p. 60).

Secondary Syphilis: no itching (99% true); history or presence of genital lesions; positive blood serology (p. 137).

Psoriasis: also usually on elbows, knees and scalp; lesions have whitish scale (p. 97).

Seborrheic Dermatitis: greasy, irregular scaly lesions on sternal and other hairy areas (p. 87).

Lichen Planus: lesions more papular, and violaceous colored; on mucous membranes of cheeks (p. 107).

Parapsoriasis: rare, very chronic.

If the pityriasis-rosea-like rash does not itch, obtain a blood serologic test for syphilis.

Treatment

FIRST VISIT

1. Reassure the patient that he does not have a "blood disease," that the eruption is not contagious, and that it would be rare to get it again. (Active treatment is preferred to saying, "Go home, it will disappear in six weeks." There are 3 reasons for this: (1) treatment *may* shorten the duration of the disease; (2) the usual itching must be alleviated; and (3) if you do not treat these patients they might go to someone else less qualified. If the eruption does not itch and the patient is reassured of the mild nature of the disease, then no treatment is necessary.)

2. Colloidal bath.

Sig: Use ½ box (small) of Linit or Argo starch, or 1 packet of Aveeno oatmeal preparation to the tub containing 6 to 8 inches of lukewarm water. Bathe for 10

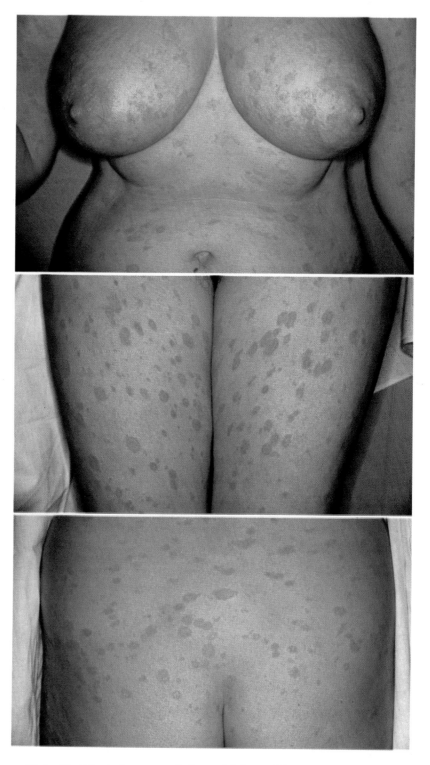

Plate 24. Pityriasis rosea of chest, thighs and buttocks of one patient. (*Syntex Laboratories, Inc.*)

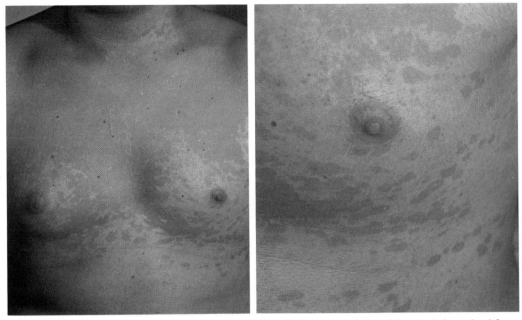

Plate 25. Tinea versicolor on the chest. The dark areas of the skin are infected with the fungus. (*K.U.M.C.*) (*Sandoz Pharmaceuticals*)

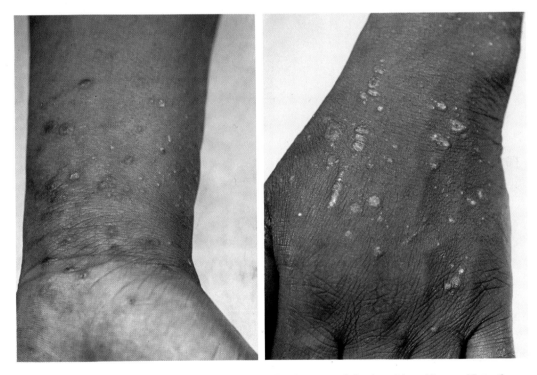

Plate 26. Lichen planus on the wrist and the dorsum of the hand in a Negro. Note the violaceous color of the papules and the linear Koebner phenomenon on the dorsum of the hand. (*E. R. Squibb*)

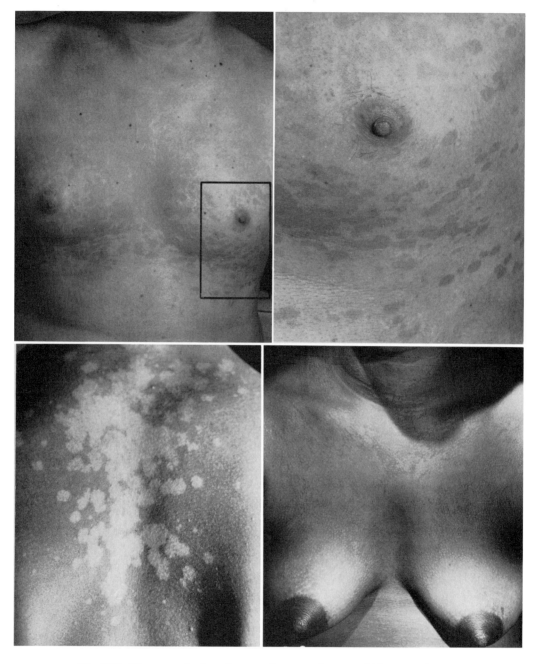

Fig. 11-3. Tinea versicolor. Lower photographs are of Negro patients.

to 15 minutes every day or every other day. Avoid soap as much as possible to reduce any itching.

3. Nonalcoholic white shake
   lotion q.s.   120.0
   (See Formulary p. 37.)
   Sig: Apply b.i.d. locally to affected areas.

4. If there is itching, prescribe an antihistamine drug such as:
   Temaril tablets, 2.5 mg., or
   Periactin, 4 mg.   #30
   Sig: 1 tablet a.c. and h.s.

5. Ultraviolet therapy in increasing suberythema doses once or twice a week may be given. The entire body is treated with 2 front and 2 back exposures.

SUBSEQUENT VISITS

1. If the skin becomes too dry from the colloidal bath and the sulfur lotion, stop the lotion or alternate it with the following:
   Hydrocortisone   ½%
   White petrolatum q.s.   30.0
   Sig: Apply b.i.d. locally to dry areas.

2. Continue the ultraviolet treatments.

SEVERELY PRURITIC CASES (in addition to the above)
   Prednisolone, 5 mg. or other
   corticosteriod   #40
   Sig: 1 tablet q.i.d. for 3 days, then 1 t.i.d. for 4 days, then 1 b.i.d. for 1 to 2 weeks, as symptom of itching demands.

TINEA VERSICOLOR
(Plate 25)

This is a moderately common skin eruption with characteristics of tannish colored, irregularly shaped, scaly patches causing no discomfort, usually located on the upper chest and back. It is caused by a fungus. (See p. 159.)

Primary Lesions. Papulosquamous or maculosquamous, tan and irregularly shaped (Fig. 11-3).

Secondary Lesions. Relative depigmentation due to the fact that the involved skin does not tan when exposed to sunlight. This cosmetic defect, obvious in the summer, often brings the patient to the office.

Distribution. Upper part of chest, back, neck and arms. Rarely on face or generalized.

Course. The eruption can persist for years unnoticed. Correct treatment is readily effective but, if treatment is not thorough, the tinea can recur.

Etiology. A fungus, *Malassezia furfur.*

Contagiousness. Rare.

Laboratory Findings. A scraping of the scale placed on a microscopic slide, covered with a 20 percent solution of potassium hydroxide (see p. 11) and a cover slip will show the fungus. Under the low-power lens of the microscope very thin mycelial filaments are seen. Diagnostic grapelike clusters of spores are seen best with the high-power lens. This fungus does not grow on routine culture media.

Differential Diagnosis

Pityriasis Rosea: acute onset; lesions oval-shaped with definite border (p. 103).

Seborrheic Dermatitis: greasy scales in hairy areas mainly (p. 87).

Mild Psoriasis: see thicker scaly lesions on trunk and elsewhere (p. 97).

Secondary Syphilis: more widely distributed and rarely only scaly (p. 134).

Treatment

1. Selsun Suspension   120.0
   Sig: Bathe and dry completely. Then apply medicine as a lotion to all the involved areas, usually from neck down to pubic area. Let it dry. Bathe again in 24 hours and wash off the medicine. Repeat procedure again at weekly intervals for 4 treatments. Recurrences are rare.

2. Depigmented spots may remain after the tinea is cured and, if desired, these can be tanned by gradual exposure to sunlight or ultraviolet light.

LICHEN PLANUS
(Plates 1 and 26)

Lichen planus is an uncommon, chronic, pruritic disease characterized by violaceous flat-topped papules which are usually seen on the wrists and the legs. Mucous membrane lesions on the cheeks or lips are whitish. (Figs. 11-4 to 11-6)

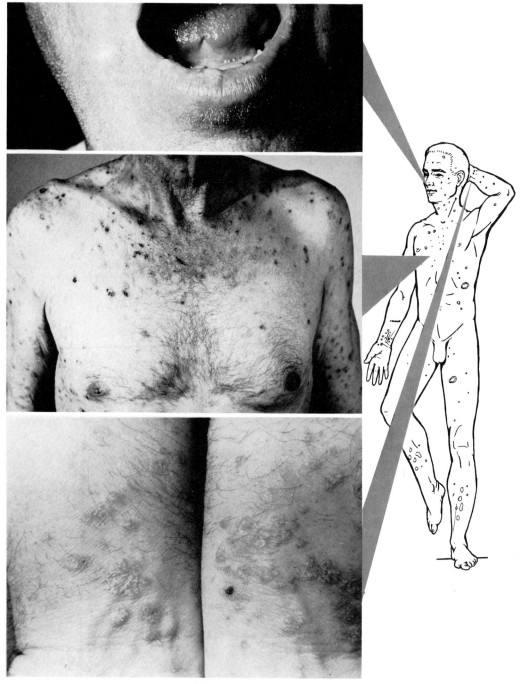

Fig. 11-4. Lichen planus.

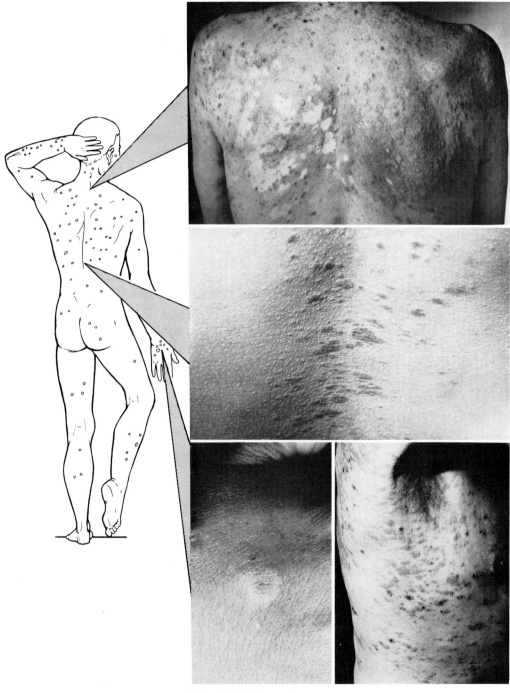

Fig. 11-5. Lichen planus.

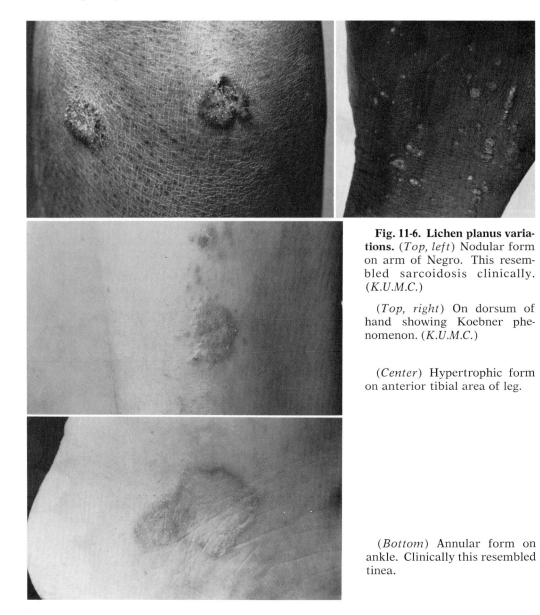

Fig. 11-6. Lichen planus variations. (*Top, left*) Nodular form on arm of Negro. This resembled sarcoidosis clinically. (*K.U.M.C.*)

(*Top, right*) On dorsum of hand showing Koebner phenomenon. (*K.U.M.C.*)

(*Center*) Hypertrophic form on anterior tibial area of leg.

(*Bottom*) Annular form on ankle. Clinically this resembled tinea.

Primary Lesions. Flat-topped, violaceous papules and papulosquamous lesions. Uncommonly, the lesions may assume a ring-shaped configuration. On the mucous membranes the lesions appear as a whitish lacy network.

Secondary Lesions. Excoriations and, on the legs, thick scaly lichenified patches.

Distribution. Most commonly on the flexural aspects of the wrists and the ankles, the penis and the oral mucous membranes, but can be anywhere on the body or become generalized.

Course. Rather sudden outbreak with chronic course averaging 9 months' duration. Some cases last several years. No effect on the general health except for itching. Recurrences are moderately common.

Etiology. Unknown. Rather frequently associated with nervous or emotional upsets.

Subjective Complaints. Itching varies from mild to severe.

Contagiousness. None.

Related to Employment. As in psoriasis, the lichen planus lesions can develop in scratches or skin injuries (Koebner phenomenon).

Laboratory Findings. Microscopic section is quite characteristic.

Differential Diagnosis

Secondary Syphilis: no itching; blood serology positive (p. 134).

Drug Eruption: history of taking atabrine, arsenic or gold (p. 60).

Psoriasis: lesions more scaly, whitish, on knees and elbows (p. 97).

Pityriasis Rosea: "herald patch," on trunk mainly (p. 103).

Lichen planus on leg may resemble *neurodermatitis* (usually one patch only, intensely pruritic, no mucous membrane lesions, p. 107).

Treatment

FIRST VISIT of case with generalized papular eruption and moderate itching.

1. Assure the patient that the disease is not contagious, is not a blood disease and is chronic but not serious.

2. Avoid excess bathing with soap.

3. Menthol ¼%
   Alcoholic white shake
      lotion q.s. 120.0
   Sig: Apply locally b.i.d.

4. Antihistamine tablet #50
   Sig: 1 tablet t.i.d. for itching (warn of drowsiness at onset of therapy).

SUBSEQUENT VISITS

1. Add phenol 0.5%, camphor 2%, or coal tar solution 5% to the lotion prescribed on the first visit.

2. Meprobamate, 400 mg. #40
   Sig: 1 tablet q.i.d. (For relief of tension and itching.)

3. Occlusive dressing—corticosteroid therapy. This is effective for localized cases. For technics, see page 102.

4. It is important in some resistant cases to rule out a focus of infection in teeth, tonsils, gallbladder, genitourinary system, etc.

5. Corticosteroids orally are of definite value for temporarily relieving the acute cases that have severe itching or a generalized eruption.

6. If necessary, have the patient consult a dermatologist to corroborate your diagnosis, reassure the patient and suggest further therapy.

12

Dermatologic Bacteriology

Bacteria exist on the skin as normal non-pathogenic resident flora, or as pathogenic organisms. The pathogenic bacteria cause primary, secondary and systemic infections. For clinical purposes it is justifiable to divide the problem of bacterial infection into these 3 classifications.

CLASSIFICATIONS

1. **Primary Bacterial Infections**
   A. Impetigo
   B. Ecthyma
   C. Folliculitis
      a. Superficial folliculitis
      b. Folliculitis of the scalp
         Superficial—acne necrotica miliaris
         Deep—folliculitis decalvans
      c. Folliculitis of the beard
      d. Stye
   D. Furuncle
   E. Carbuncle
   F. Sweat gland infections
   G. Erysipelas
2. **Secondary Bacterial Infections**
   A. Cutaneous diseases with secondary infection
   B. Infected ulcers
   C. Infectious eczematoid dermatitis
   D. Bacterial intertigo
3. **Systemic Bacterial Infections**
   A. Scarlet fever
   B. Granuloma inguinale
   C. Chancroid
   D. Myocobacterial infections
      a. Tuberculosis of the skin
      b. Leprosy
   E. Sarcoidosis

PRIMARY BACTERIAL INFECTIONS (PYODERMAS)

The commonest causative agents of the primary skin infections are the coagulase-positive micrococci (staphylocci) and the beta hemolytic streptococci. Superficial or deep bacterial lesions can be produced by these organisms.

In managing the pyodermas certain *general principles of treatment* must be initiated.

1. *Improve the Bathing Habits.* More frequent bathing and the use of a bactericidal soap, such as Dial soap, is indicated. Any pustules or crusts should be removed during the bathing to facilitate penetration of the local medications.

2. *General Isolation Procedures.* Clothing and bedding should be changed frequently and cleaned. The patient should have a separate towel and wash cloth.

3. *Diet.* For patients with persistent or chronic bacterial infections these foods should be restricted: chocolate, nuts, cokes and cheeses (see Acne Instruction Sheet, p. 93). The patient should be questioned regarding ingestion of drugs which can cause lesions that mimic pyodermas, such as iodides and bromides.

4. *Diabetes.* Rule out diabetes by history and laboratory examination in chronic skin infections, particularly recurrent boils.

IMPETIGO
(Plates 1G, 27 and 32)

Impetigo is a very common superficial bacterial infection seen most often in children. This is the "infantigo" every mother respects.

Plate 27. Impetigo of the face. The honey-colored crusts are very typical. (*From the late Abner Kurtin: Folia Dermatologica, No. 2, Geigy Pharmaceuticals*)

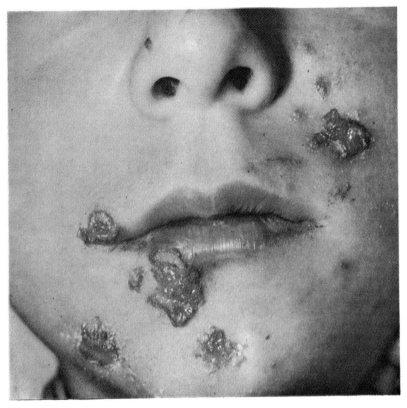

Primary Lesions. They vary from small vesicles to large bullae that rupture and discharge a honey-colored serous liquid. New lesions can develop rapidly in a matter of hours.

Secondary Lesions. Crusts form from the discharge and appear to be lightly stuck on the skin surface. When removed, a superficial erosion remains which may be the only evidence of the disease. In debilitated infants the bullae may coalesce to form an exfoliative type of infection called *Ritter's disease* or *pemphigus neonatorum*.

Distribution. Most commonly on the face but may be anywhere.

Contagiousness. It is not unusual to see brothers or sisters of the patient and, rarely, the parents similarly infected.

Differential Diagnosis

Contact Dermatitis Due to Poison Ivy: see linear blisters, does not spread as rapidly, itches (p. 49).

Tinea of Smooth Skin: fewer lesions, spread slowly, small vesicles in annular configuration which is an unusual form for impetigo, fungi found on scraping (p. 170).

Treatment

1. Outline the general principles of treatment. Emphasize the removal of the crusts once or twice a day during the bathing with Dial soap.

2. Sulfur, ppt.   4%
Neo-polycin or other antibiotic
ointment q.s.   15.0
Sig: Apply t.i.d. locally. (The addition of sulfur enhances the effectiveness of the antibiotic preparation.)

Advise the mother to continue the local treatment for 3 days after the lesions apparently have disappeared.

3. Systemic antibiotic therapy. Some physicians feel that every patient with impetigo should be treated with systemic antibiotic therapy to heal these lesions

and also to prevent chronic glomerulone-phritis.

ECTHYMA
(Plate 32)

Ecthyma is another superficial bacterial infection but it is seen less commonly than impetigo and is deeper than impetigo. It is usually caused by beta hemolytic streptococci and occurs on the buttocks and the thighs of children.

Primary Lesion. Vesicle or vesicopustule that rapidly changes into the secondary lesion.

Secondary Lesion. This is a piled-up crust 1 to 3 cm. in diameter overlying a superficial erosion or ulcer. In neglected cases scarring can occur as a result of extension of the infection into the corium.

Distribution. Most commonly seen on the posterior aspect of the thighs and the buttocks, from which areas it can spread. Ecthyma commonly follows the scratching of chigger bites.

Age Group. Mainly seen in children.

Contagiousness. Ecthyma is rarely found in other members of the family.

Differential Diagnosis

Psoriasis: unusual in children, see whitish firmly attached scaly lesion, also in scalp, on knees and elbows. (p. 97).

Impetigo: much smaller crusted lesions, not as deep (p. 114).

Treatment

1. Outline the general principles of treatment listed on p. 114. The crusts must be removed daily. Response to therapy is slower than with impetigo, but the treatment is the same for both conditions.

2. Systemic antibiotics. Commonly with extensive ecthyma in children, but only rarely with impetigo, there is a low-grade fever and evidence of bacterial infection in other organs, such as the kidney. If so, give penicillin by injection (600,000 units a day for 3 to 4 days) or one of the tetracycline syrups orally (125 mg. q.i.d. for 4 or more days).

FOLLICULITIS
(Plate 32)

This is a very common pyogenic infection of the hair follicles, usually caused by coagulase-positive staphylococci. Seldom does a patient consult the doctor for a single outbreak of folliculitis. The physician is consulted because of recurrent and chronic pustular lesions. The patient realizes that the present acute episode will clear up with the help of nature, but seeks the medicine and the advice that will prevent recurrences. For this reason the *general principles of treatment* listed on page 114, particularly the diet and the diabetes investigation, are important. Some physicians feel that a focus of infection in the teeth, the tonsils, the gallbladder or the genito-urinary tract should be ruled out when pyodermas are recurrent.

The folliculitis may invade only the superficial part of the hair follicle or it may extend down to the hair bulb. Many variously named clinical entities based upon the location and the chronicity of the lesions have been carried down through the years. A few of these entities bear presentation here, but the majority are defined in the Dictionary-Index.

Superficial Folliculitis

Most commonly seen on the arms, the face and the buttocks of children and adults with the "acne-seborrhea complex." The physician is rarely consulted for this minor problem; but if he is, a history of excessive use of hair oils, bath oils, or suntan oils, can often be obtained. These agents should be avoided.

Folliculitis of the Scalp

A *superficial form* has the appellation *acne necrotica miliaris.* This is an annoying, pruritic, chronic, recurrent folliculitis of the scalp in adults. The scratching of the crusted lesions occupies the patient's evening hours.

Treatment of superficial folliculitis of the scalp.

1. General principles

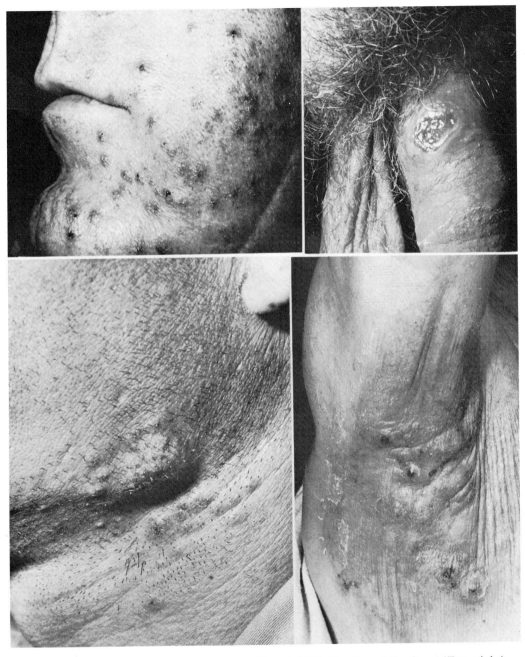

Fig. 12-1. Primary bacterial infections. (*Top, left*) Folliculitis of the face. (*Top, right*) Furuncle of the penis. (*Bottom, left*) Folliculitis of the face below ear. (*Bottom, right*) Chronic sweat gland infection of the axilla (hidradenitis suppurativa). (*K.C.G.H.*)

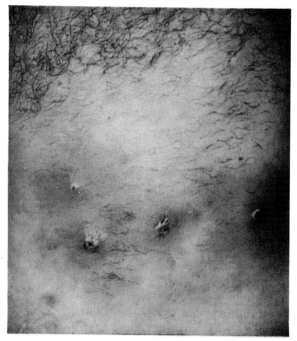

Plate 28. Multiple furuncles (boils) on the chest. (*From the late Abner Kurtin: Folia Dermatologica, No. 2, Geigy Pharmaceuticals*)

Plate 29. Carbuncle on the chin. Notice the multiple openings. (*From the late Abner Kurtin: Folia Dermatologica, No. 2, Geigy Pharmaceuticals*)

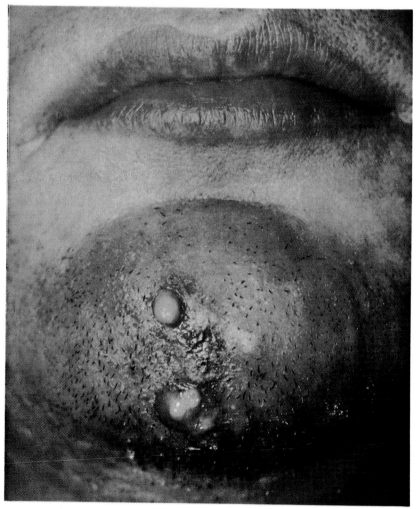

2. Selsun Suspension   120.0

Sig: Shampoo twice a week as directed on the label. Use no other shampoo or rinse.

3. Sulfur, ppt.   5%
   Coal tar solution   5%
   Antibiotic-corticosteroid   ointment
   q.s.   15.0

Sig: Apply to scalp h.s.

4. Staphylococcus toxoid (Lederle), Dilution 1

Give 0.1 ml. subcutaneously and increase by 0.1 ml. every 4 to 7 days until 1.0 ml. is given. This form of therapy works for some cases, apparently from a nonspecific protein action stimulating the adrenal cortex.

The *deep form* of scalp folliculitis is called *folliculitis decalvans.* This is a chronic, slowly progressive folliculitis with an active border and scarred atrophic center. The end-result after years of progression is patchy, scarred areas of alopecia, with eventual burning out of the infection.

Differential Diagnosis of deep form of folliculitis

Chronic Discoid Lupus Erythematosus: see redness, enlarged hair follicles (p. 204).

Alopecia Cicatrisata: rare, no evidence of infection (p. 226).

Tinea of the Scalp: it is important to culture the hair for fungi in any chronic infection of the scalp; *T. tonsurans* group can cause a similar clinical picture (p. 170).

Treatment of the deep form of scalp folliculitis is very disappointing. Follow the routine for the superficial form of folliculitis and give oral antibiotics.

Folliculitis of the Beard
(Plate 32)

This is the familiar "barber's itch" which in the days prior to antibiotics was very resistant to therapy. This bacterial infection of the hair follicles is spread rather rapidly by shaving, but after treatment is begun, shaving should be continued (Fig. 12-1 A and C).

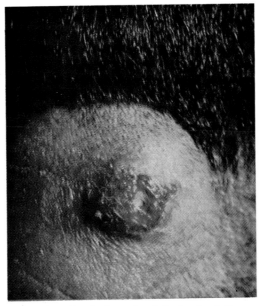

Plate 30. Carbuncle of the back of the neck. (*From J. Lamar Callaway: Folia Dermatologica, No. 4, Geigy Pharmaceuticals*)

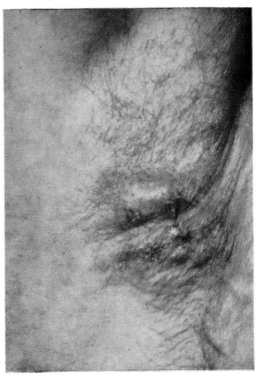

Plate 31. Sweat gland infection of the axilla (hidradenitis suppurativa). (*From the late Abner Kurtin: Folia Dermatologica, No. 2, Geigy Pharmaceuticals*)

Differential Diagnosis

Contact Dermatitis due to Shaving Lotions: history of new lotion applied, general redness of the area with some vesicles (p. 49).

Tinea of the Beard: very slowly spreading infection, hairs broken off, a deeper nodular type of inflammation is usually seen, culture of hair produces fungi (p. 174).

Ingrown Beard Hairs: see hair circling back into the skin with resultant chronic infection, a hereditary trait, especially in Negroes. Close shaving aggravates the condition. Local antibiotics rarely help, but locally applied depilatories do help.

Treatment of folliculitis of the beard

1. General principles, stressing the use of Dial soap for washing of the face.
2. Shaving instructions:

A. Change the razor blade daily or sterilize the head of the electric razor by placing it in 70% alcohol for 1 hour.

B. Apply the following salve very lightly to the face before shaving and again after shaving.

3. Neo-Polycin or other antibiotic ointment q.s.   15.0

Sig: Apply to face before shaving, after shaving and at bedtime.

For stubborn cases, add sulfur, 5%, or hydrocortisone, 1%, to ointment.

Stye (Hordeolum)

A stye is a deep folliculitis of the stiff eyelid hairs. A single lesion is treated with hotpacks of 1% boric acid solution and an ophthalmic antibiotic ointment. Recurrent lesions may be linked with the blepharitis of seborrheic dermatitis (dandruff). For this type, Selsun Suspension scalp shampoos are indicated.

FURUNCLE
(Plate 28)

A furuncle or boil is a more extensive infection of the hair follicle, usually due to the staphylococcus (Fig. 12-1B). A boil can occur in any individual at any age, but certain predisposing factors account for most outbreaks. An important factor is the "acne-seborrhea complex" (oily skin, dark complexion, and history of acne and dandruff). Other factors include poor hygiene, diet rich in sugars and fats, diabetes, local skin trauma from friction of clothing, and maceration in obese individuals. One boil usually does not bring the patient to the doctor, but recurrent boils do.

Differential Diagnosis

SINGLE LESION: *primary chancre-type diseases* (see list in Dictionary-Index)

MULTIPLE LESION: *Drug eruption from iodides or bromides* (p. 60).

Treatment. A young male has had recurrent boils for 6 months. He does not have diabetes, is not obese, is taking no drugs and bathes daily. He now has a large boil on his buttock.

1. Boric acid solution hot packs.

Sig: 1 tablespoon of boric acid crystals to 1 quart of hot water. Apply hot wet packs for 30 minutes twice a day.

2. Incision and drainage. This should be done only on "ripe" lesions where a necrotic white area appears at the top of the nodule. Drains are not necessary unless the lesion has extended deep enough to form a fluctuant *abscess*.

3. Penicillin injection   600,000 U.

Sig: Administer intramuscularly in hip daily for 2 to 4 days unless patient gives a history of penicillin sensitivity. (Other antibiotics could be substituted and used orally. Bacteriological culture and sensitivity studies are helpful in determining which antibiotic to use.)

4. To prevent recurrences:

A. General principles of treatment, stressing diet and use of Dial soap.

B. Rule out focus of infection in teeth, tonsils, genito-urinary tract, etc.

C. Staphylococcus Toxoid injections as outlined under folliculitis of the scalp (p. 119) may be of value.

D. Oral tetracycline therapy. Tetracycline, 250 mg. capsules, in a dose of 4 a day for 3 or 4 days, then 1 b.i.d. for weeks as for acne patients is very effective in breaking the cycle of recurrences.

CARBUNCLE
(Plates 29 and 30)

A carbuncle is an extensive infection of several adjoining hair follicles which drains with multiple openings onto the skin surface. Fatal cases were not unusual in the preantibiotic days. A common location for a carbuncle is the posterior neck region. Large, ugly, crisscross scars in this area in an older patient demonstrate the outdated treatment for this disease, namely, multiple, bold incisions. Since a carbuncle is in reality a multiple furuncle, the same etiologic factors apply. Recurrences are uncommon.

Treatment. The same as for a boil (p. 120) but with greater emphasis on systemic antibiotic therapy and physical rest.

SWEAT GLAND INFECTIONS
(Plate 31)

Primary *eccrine* sweat gland or duct infections are very rare. However prickly heat, a sweat retention disease, very frequently develops secondary bacterial infection.

Primary *apocrine* gland infection is rather common. Two types of infection exist:

Apocrinitis denotes infection of a single apocrine gland, usually in the axilla, and commonly associated with a change in deodorant. It responds to the therapy listed under furuncles (p. 120). In addition, a shake lotion containing a powdered antibiotic aids in keeping the area dry.

The second form of apocrine gland infection is *hidradenitis suppurativa* (Fig. 12-3D). This chronic, recurring, pyogenic infection is characterized by the development of multiple nodules, abscesses, draining sinuses and eventual hypertrophic bands of scars. The most common location is in the axillae, but it can also occur in the groin, the perianal and the suprapubic regions. It does not occur before puberty. Etiologically, there appears to be a hereditary tendency in these patients toward occlusion of the follicular orifice and subsequent retention of the secretory products. Two other diseases are related to hidradenitis suppurativa and may be present in the same patient: a severe form of acne called *acne conglobata* and *dissecting cellulitis of the scalp*.

Treatment of hidradenitis suppurativa: The management of these cases is difficult

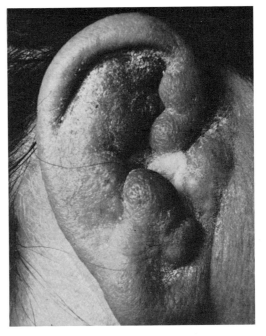

Fig. 12-2. Elephantiasis nostras of ear.
(Patient of Dr. M. Feldaker.)

and preferably should be in the hands of a dermatologist. In addition to the general principles mentioned above, one should use hot packs locally and an oral antibiotic for several weeks. Plastic surgery or a marsupialization operation is indicated in severe cases.

ERYSIPELAS
(Plate 33)

Erysipelas is an uncommon beta hemolytic streptococcus infection of the subcutaneous tissue that produces a characteristic type of cellulitis with fever and malaise. Recurrences are frequent.

Primary Lesion. A red, warm, raised, brawny, sharply bordered plaque that enlarges peripherally. Vesicles and bullae may form on the surface of the plaque. Usually a pre-existing skin wound or pyoderma will be found that initiated the acute infection. Multiple lesions of erysipelas are rare.

Distribution. Most commonly on the face and around the ears (following ear-piercing), but no area is exempt.

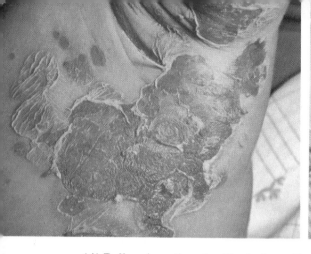
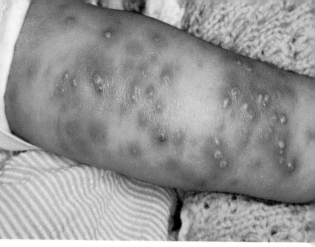

(A) Bullous impetigo of axillae in 1 yr. old   (B) Folliculitis of forearm in 7 mo. old baby

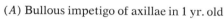

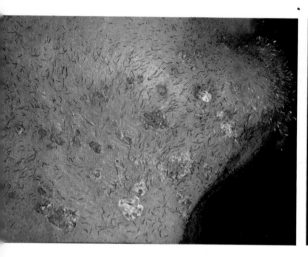
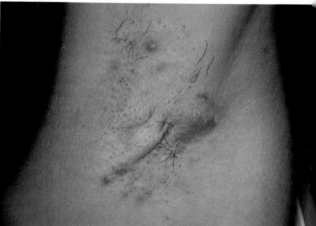

(C) Folliculitis of the beard area   (D) Hidradenitis suppurativa of axilla of 6 yrs. duration

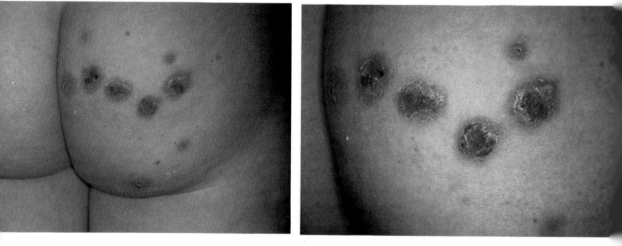

(E) Ecthyma of buttocks of 13 yr. old boy with (F) closeup of lesions

Plate 32. Primary Bacterial Infections. (*Burroughs Wellcome & Co., Inc.*)

122

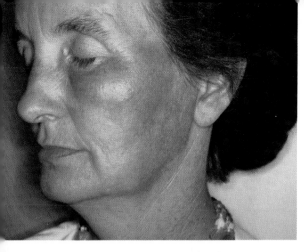 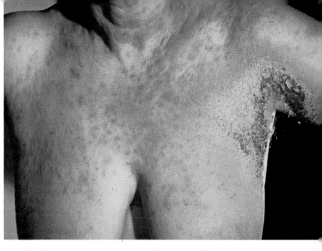

(A) Erysipelas of check   (B) Infectious eczematoid dermatitis
from axilla

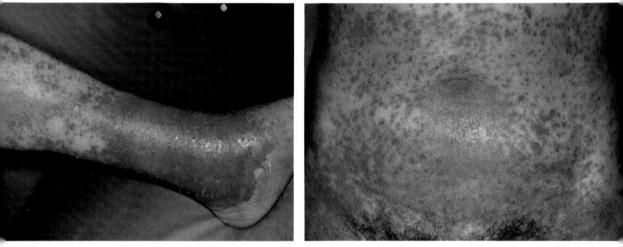

(C) Infectious eczematoid dermatitis from stasis dermatitis of legs with (D) spread to body

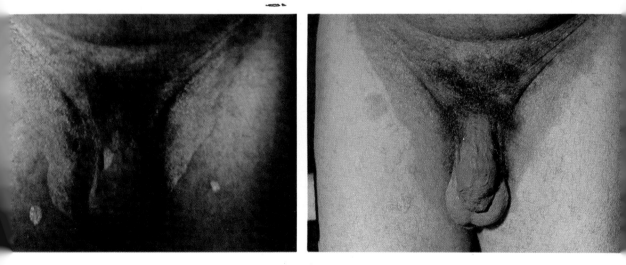

(E) Erythrasma of crural area with fluorescence under Wood's light and in natural light (F).

Plate 33. Bacterial Infections of Skin. (*Burroughs Wellcome & Co., Inc.*)

123

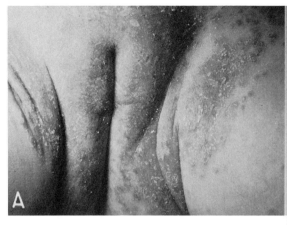

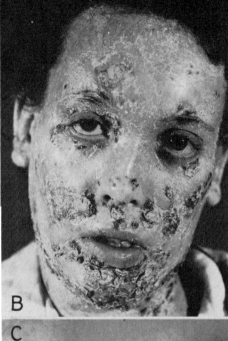

Fig. 12-3. Secondary bacterial infections.

(*A*) Bacterial intertrigo of infant.

(*B*) Atopic eczema with marked secondary bacterial infection.

(*C*) Infectious eczematoid dermatitis secondary to empyema sinus.

(*D*) Infectious eczematoid dermatitis secondary to external otitis.

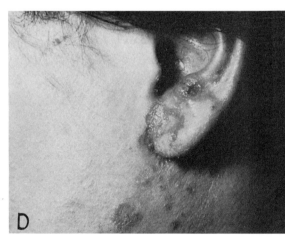

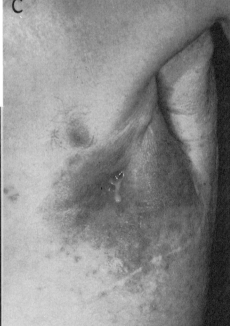

Course. Untreated cases last for 2 to 3 weeks, but when treated with antibiotics the response is rapid. Recurrences are common in the same location and may lead to *lymphedema* of that area which eventually can become irreversible. The lip, the cheek and the legs are particularly prone to this chronic change which is called *elephantiasis nostras* (Fig. 12-4).

Subjective Complaints. Fever and general malaise can precede the development of the skin lesion and persist until therapy is instituted. Pain at the site of the infection can be severe.

Differential Diagnosis

Cellulitis: lacks sharp border; recurrences are rare.

Contact Dermatitis: sharp border absent; fever and malaise absent; eruption is predominantly vesicular (p. 49).

Treatment

1. Bed rest, and therapy directed toward reducing the fever. If patient is hospitalized, semi-isolation procedures should be initiated.

2. Systemic antibiotic. Give appropriate antibiotic orally and/or by injection for 4 to 6 days.

3. Local cool wet dressing as necessary for comfort.

ERYTHRASMA
(Plate 33)

This is a rather uncommon bacterial infection of the skin that clinically resembles regular tinea or tinea versicolor. It affects the crural area, axillae and webs of the toes with flat, hyperpigmented, fine scaly patches. If the patient has not been using an antibacterial soap, these patches fluoresce a striking orange-red color under the Wood's light.

The causative agent is a diphtheroid organism called *Corynebacterium minutissimum.*

The treatment most effective is erythromycin 250 mg. q.i.d. for 5 to 7 days.

SECONDARY BACTERIAL INFECTIONS

Secondary infection develops as a complicating factor upon a pre-existing skin

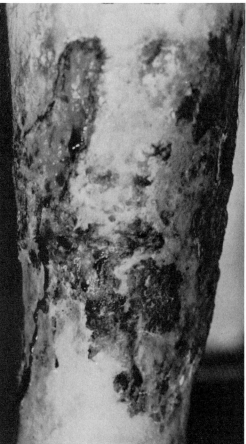

Fig. 12-4. Pyoderma gangrenosum of leg of patient with ulcerative colitis. (*K.C.G.H.*)

disease. The invasion of an injured skin surface with pathogenic streptococci or staphylococci is enhanced in skin conditions that are oozing and of long duration.

CUTANEOUS DISEASES WITH SECONDARY INFECTION

Failure in the treatment of many common skin diseases can be attributed to the physician's not recognizing the presence of secondary bacterial infection. Any type of skin lesion, such as hand dermatitis, poison ivy dermatitis, atopic eczema, chigger bites, fungus infection, traumatic abrasion, etc., can become secondarily infected (Fig. 12-3B).

The treatment is usually simple. Add an antibacterial agent to the treatment

you would ordinarily use for the dermatosis in question. For example, a secondary bacterial infection of contact dermatitis due to poison ivy would be treated by
the addition of an antibiotic, such as
chlortetracycline (Aureomycin) powder,
1% to 3%, to the antipruritic lotion or
salve.

INFECTED ULCERS
(Plate 60)

Ulcers are deep skin infections due to
injury or disease which invade the subcutaneous tissue and on healing leave
scars. Ulcers can be divided into primary
and secondary ulcers, but all become secondarily infected with bacteria.

Primary ulcers result from the following causes: gangrene due to pathogenic
streptococci, staphylococci and Clostrid-
ium species, syphilis, chancroid, tuberculosis, diphtheria, fungi, leprosy, anthrax,
cancer and lymphoblastomas.

Secondary ulcers can be related to the
following diseases: vascular (arterioscle-
rosis, thromboangiitis obliterans, Raynaud's phenomenon, phlebitis, thrombo-
sis) ; neurologic (spinal cord injury with
bedsores or decubiti, CNS syphilis, spina-
bifida, poliomyelitis, syringomyelia); diabetes; trauma; ulcerative colitis (Fig. 12-4);
allergic local anaphylaxis, and other conditions. Finally, there is a group of
secondary ulcers called *phagedenic ulcers,*
variously described under many different
names, that arise in diseased skin or on
the apparently normal skin of debilitated
individuals. These ulcers undermine the
skin in large areas, are notoriously chronic
and are resistant to therapy.

Treatment

1. For primary ulcers specific therapy
is indicated, if available. The response to
therapy is usually quite rapid.
2. For secondary ulcers appropriate
therapy should be directed toward the
primary disease. The response to therapy
is usually quite slow.
3. The basic rules of local therapy for
ulcers can be illustrated best by outlining
the management of a patient with a *stasis
leg ulcer* (see Stasis Dermatitis, p. 82).

A. Rest of the affected area. If rest
in bed is not feasible, then an Ace Elastic
Bandage, 4 inches wide, should be worn.
This bandage is applied over the local
medication and before getting out of bed
in the morning. A more permanent support is a modification of Unna's boot
(Dome-Paste Bandage or Gelocast). This
boot can be applied for a week or more
at a time, if secondary infection is under
control.

B. Elevation of the affected extremity. This should be carried out in bed
and can be accomplished by placing two
bricks, flat surface down, under both feet
of the bed. (Arteriosclerotic leg ulcers
should not be elevated.)

C. Boric acid wet packs
Sig: 1 tablespoon of boric acid
crystals to 1 quart of warm water. Apply
wet dressings of gauze or sheeting for 30
minutes 3 times a day.

D. If débridement is necessary, this
can be accomplished by enzymes, such as
Varidase jelly or Elase ointment, applied
twice a day and covered with gauze.

E. Gentian violet   1%
Distilled water, q.s.   15.0
Sig: Apply to ulcer b.i.d. with ap-
plicator.

A liquid is usually better tolerated
on ulcers than a salve. If the gentian violet
solution becomes too drying, the following salve can be used alternately for short
periods of time:

F. Neosporin or other antibiotic ointment, q.s.   15.0
Sig: Apply to ulcer and surrounding skin b.i.d.

G. Long-term tetracycline therapy.
Tetracycline capsules (250 mg.) 1 q.i.d. for
3 days then 1 b.i.d. for weeks is quite helpful for chronic pyogenic ulcers.

The best treatment for one ulcer, does
not necessarily work for another ulcer.
Many other local medications are available and valuable.

INFECTIOUS ECZEMATOID DERMATITIS
(Plate 33)   .

This term is more often used incor-
rectly than correctly. Infectious eczematoid dermatitis is an uncommon disease

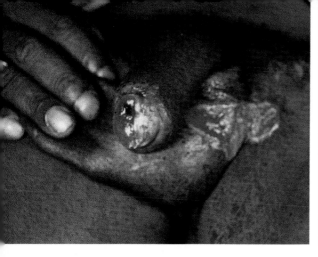

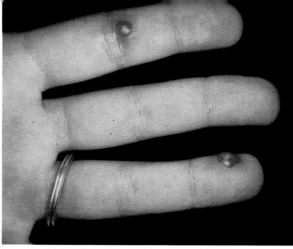

(A) Granuloma inguinale of penis and crural area

(B) Gonococcal septicemia with hemorrhagic vesicles

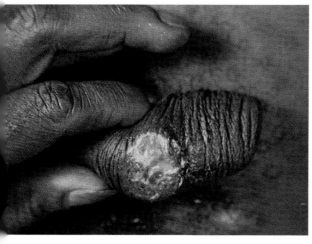

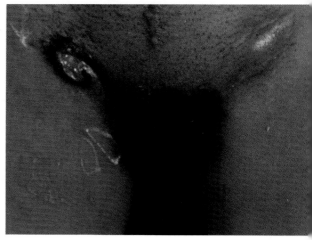

(C) Chancroid of penis

(D) Chancroid buboes in inguinal area

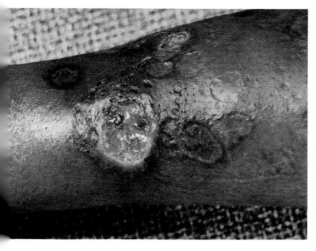

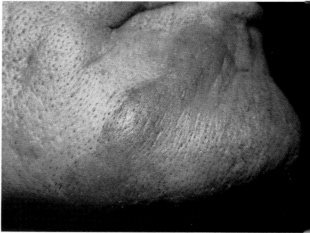

(E) Tuberculosis ulcer of leg

(F) Tuberculoid leprosy of the chin
(Drs. W. Schorr and F. Kerdel-Vegas)

Plate 34. Systemic Bacterial Infections. (*Derm-Arts Laboratories*)

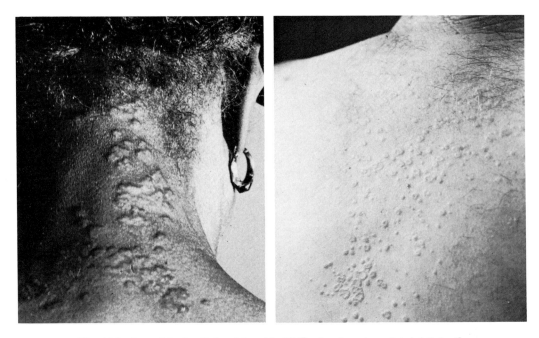

Fig. 12-5. Sarcoidosis of the skin. (*Left*) Back of neck and (*right*) back.

characterized by the development of an acute eruption around an infected exudative primary site, such as a draining ear, mastitis, a boil or a seeping ulcer (Fig. 12-5). Widespread eczematous lesions can develop at a distant site from the primary infection, presumably due to autoinoculation.

Primary Lesions. Vesicles and pustules in circumscribed plaques that spread peripherally from an infected central source. Central healing usually does not occur as with ringworm infection.

Secondary Lesions. Crusting, oozing and scaling predominate in widespread cases.

Distribution. Mild cases may be confined to a small area around the exudative primary infection, but widespread cases can cover the entire body, obscuring the initial cause.

Course. This depends on the extent of the eruption. Chronic cases respond poorly to therapy. Recurrences are common even after the primary source is healed.

Subjective Complaints. Itching is usually mild.

Etiology. Coagulase-positive staphylococci are frequently isolated.

Contagiousness. In spite of the strong autoinoculation factor, passage of the infective material to another individual rarely elicits a reaction.

Differential Diagnosis

Contact Dermatitis With Secondary Infection: no history or finding of primary exudative infection; history of contact with poison ivy, new clothes, cosmetics, or dishwater; responds faster to therapy (p. 49).

Nummular Eczema: no primary infected source, see coin-shaped lesions, on extremities, clinical differentiation of some cases can be difficult (p. 60).

Seborrheic Dermatitis: no primary infected source; see seborrhea-acne complex with greasy, scaly eruption in hairy areas (p. 87).

Treatment. Case of an 8-year-old boy with draining otitis media and pustular, crusted dermatitis on side of face, neck and scalp.

1. Treat the primary source, the ear infection in this case.

2. Boric acid wet packs.

Sig: 1 tablespoon of boric acid to 1

quart of warm water. Apply wet sheeting or gauze to area for 20 minutes t.i.d.
3. Antibiotic-corticosteroid cream
q.s.   15.0
Sig: Apply t.i.d. locally, after the wet packs are removed.

A widespread case might require hospitalization, potassium permanganate baths, oral antibiotics and corticosteroid therapy.

BACTERIAL INTERTRIGO
(Plate 57)

The occurrence of friction, heat and moisture in areas where two opposing skin surfaces contact each other will lead to a secondary bacterial or fungus infection. Bacterial intertrigo concerns us here (Fig. 12-3A).

Primary Lesion. Redness from friction and heat of opposing surfaces, and maceration from inability of the sweat to evaporate freely, leads to an eroded patch of dermatitis.

Secondary Lesion. The bacterial infection may become severe enough to result in fissures and cellulitis.

Distribution. Inframammary region, axillae, umbilicus, pubic, crural, genital and perianal areas, and between the toes.

Course. In certain individuals it tends to recur each summer.

Etiology. The factors of obesity, diabetes, prolonged contact with urine, feces and menstrual discharges predispose to the development of intertrigo.

Differential Diagnosis

Monilial Intertrigo: see scaling at border of erosion, presence of surrounding small satellite lesions; scraping and culture reveals *C. albicans* (p. 178).

Tinea: see scaly or papulovesicular border, scraping and culture positive for fungi (p. 168).

Seborrheic Dermatitis: greasy red scaly areas, also seen in scalp; bacterial intertrigo may coexist with seborrheic dermatitis (p. 87).

Treatment. Case of 2-month-old baby with red, pustular dermatitis in diaper area, axillae and folds of neck. (Also see Chapt. 29 on *Pediatric Dermatoses.*)

1. Bathe child once a day in lukewarm water with antibacterial soap. Dry affected areas thoroughly.
2. The diapers should be double-rinsed to remove all soap.
3. Change diapers as frequently as possible and apply a powder each time, such as:
Talc, unscented   45.0
Sig: Place in powder can.
4. Sulfur, ppt.   2%
Nonalcoholic white shake lotion
q.s.   90.0
Sig: Apply to affected areas t.i.d.

SYSTEMIC BACTERIAL INFECTIONS

SCARLET FEVER

Scarlet fever is a moderately common streptococcal infection characterized by a sore throat, high fever and a scarlet rash that avoids the circumoral area. The eruption develops after a day of rapidly rising fever, headache, sore throat and various other symptoms. The rash begins first on the neck and the chest but rapidly spreads over the entire body, except for the area around the mouth. Close examination of the pale scarlet eruption reveals it to be made up of diffuse pinhead size or larger macules. In untreated cases the rash reaches its peak on the 4th day, and scaling commences around the 7th day and continues for a week or two. The "strawberry tongue" is seen at the height of the eruption.

The presence of petechiae on the body is a grave prognostic sign. Complications are numerous and common in untreated cases. Nephritis, in mild or severe form, is a serious complication.

The Dick test is a seldom-used diagnostic test. A positive red reaction to the injected toxin supposedly indicates a susceptibility to scarlet fever due to lack of antitoxin.

Differential Diagnosis

Measles: see early rash on face and forehead, larger macular rash, running eyes, and cough (p. 157).

Drug Eruption: see lack of high fever and other constitutional signs; atropine and quinine can cause eruption clinically similar to scarlet fever (p. 60).

Treatment. Penicillin or a similar systemic antibiotic is the therapy of choice. Complications should be watched for and should be treated early.

GRANULOMA INGUINALE
(Plate 34)

Prior to the use of streptomycin this disease was one of the most chronic and resistant afflictions of man. Formerly, it was a rather common disease in the South, particularly among Negroes. Granuloma inguinale should be considered a venereal disease, although other factors may have to be present to initiate infection.

Primary Lesion. An irregularly shaped, bright-red, velvety appearing, flat ulcer with rolled border.

Secondary Lesions. Scarring may lead to complications similar to those seen with lymphogranuloma venereum. A squamous cell carcinoma can develop in old, chronic lesions.

Distribution. Genital lesions are most common on the penis, the scrotum, the labia, the cervix or the inguinal region.

Course. Without therapy, the granuloma grows slowly and persists for years, causing marked scarring and mutilation. Under modern therapy, healing is rather rapid, but recurrences are not unusual.

Etiology. Granuloma inguinale is due to *Calymmatobacterium granulomatis*, which can be cultured on special media.

Laboratory Findings. Scrapings of the lesion reveal Donovan bodies, which are dark-staining, intracytoplasmic, cigar-shaped bacilli, found in large macrophages. The material for the smear can be obtained best by snipping off a piece of the lesion with a small scissors and rubbing the tissue on several slides. Wright or Giemsa stains can be used.

Differential Diagnosis

Of a small lesion, consider *granuloma pyogenicum:* history of injury usually, short duration; rarely on genitalia; no Donovan bodies (p. 279).

Primary Syphilis: short duration, inguinal adenopathy, serology may be positive, find spirochetes (p. 134).

Chancroid: short duration, lesion small, not red and velvety, no Donovan bodies (see below).

Squamous Cell Carcinoma: more indurated lesion with nodules, may coexist with granuloma inguinale, biopsy specific.

Treatment. Dihydrostreptomycin, 4 Gm. daily for 1 to 2 weeks, or oxytetracycline (Terramycin) 1 to 2 Gm. a day for 2 to 4 weeks.

CHANCROID
(Plate 34)

Chancroid is a venereal disease with a very short incubation period of 1 to 5 days. It is caused by *Hemophilus ducreyi.*

Primary Lesion. A small, superficial or deep erosion with surrounding redness and edema. Multiple genital or distant lesions can be produced by autoinoculation.

Secondary Lesions. Deep, destructive ulcers form in chronic cases which may lead to gangrene. Marked regional adenopathy, usually unilateral, is common and eventually suppurates in untreated cases.

Course. Without therapy most cases heal within 1 to 2 weeks. In rare cases, severe, local destruction and draining lymph nodes (buboes) result. Early therapy is quite effective.

Laboratory Findings. The organisms arranged in "schools of fish" can often be demonstrated in smears of clean lesions. The Ducrey skin test is positive within 2 weeks after the appearance of the primary lesion and remains positive for life.

Differential Diagnosis

SYPHILIS *must be considered in any patient with a penile lesion. It can be ruled out only by darkfield examination or blood serology tests.*

Primary or Secondary Syphilis Genital Lesions: longer incubation period, more induration, *Treponema pallidum* found on darkfield examination, serology positive in late primary and secondary stage (p. 134).

Herpes Simplex Progenitalis: recurrent multiple blisters or erosions, mild inguinal adenopathy (p. 145).

Lymphogranuloma Venereum: rarely see primary lesion; Frei test positive (p. 156).

Granuloma Inguinale: chronic, red velvety plaque: Donovan bodies seen on tissue smear (p. 130).

Treatment. Triple sulfonamides, 2 to 4 Gm. daily for 7 days, or tetracycline 1 Gm. daily for 10 to 15 days. A fluctuant bubo should never be incised but aspirated with a large needle.

TUBERCULOSIS
(Plate 2B and 34)

Skin tuberculosis is rare in the United States. However, a text on dermatology would not be complete without some consideration of this infection. For this purpose the commonest tuberculous infection, lupus vulgaris, will be discussed. A classification of skin tuberculosis follows this section.

Lupus vulgaris is a chronic, granulomatous disease characterized by the development of nodules, ulcers and plaques arranged in any conceivable configuration. Scarring in the center of active lesions or at the edge in severe, untreated cases leads to atrophy and contraction resulting in mutilating changes.

Distribution. Facial involvement is most common.

Course. Often slow and progressive in spite of therapy.

Laboratory Findings. The histopathology shows typical tubercle formation with epithelioid cells, giant cells and a peripheral zone of lymphocytes. The organism, *Mycobacterium tuberculosis*, is not abundant in the lesions. The 48-hour tuberculin test is usually positive.

Differential Diagnosis. Other granulomas are to be ruled out by appropriate studies, such as *syphilis, leprosy, sarcoidosis, deep fungus disease* and *neoplasms.*

Treatment

1. Dihydrostreptomycin, 1 Gm. intramuscularly 2 or 3 times a week for several months. Can be given alone or with Isoniazid.

2. Isonicotinic acid hydrazid (Isoniazid), 150 to 300 mg. orally daily for adults for several months.

3. Para-aminosalicylic acid, 16 to 20 Gm. a day combined with Isoniazid or streptomycin.

CLASSIFICATION OF
CUTANEOUS TUBERCULOSIS

1. True cutaneous tuberculosis. (Lesions contain tubercle bacilli.)
   A. Primary tuberculosis. (No previous infection, individuals tuberculin-negative in initial stages.)
      (1) Primary inoculation tuberculosis. Tuberculosis chancre. (Exogenous implantation into skin producing the primary complex.)
      (2) Miliary tuberculosis of the skin. (Hematogenous dispersion.)
   B. Secondary tuberculosis. (Lesions develop in person already sensitive to tuberculin as result of prior tuberculous lesion. Tubercle bacilli difficult or impossible to demonstrate.)
      (1) Lupus vulgaris. Inoculation of tubercle bacilli into the skin from external or internal sources.
      (2) Tuberculosis verrucosa cutis. Inoculation of tubercle bacilli into the skin from external or internal sources.
      (3) Scrofuloderma. Extension to skin from underlying focus in bones or glands.
      (4) Tuberculosis cutis orificialis. Mucous membrane lesions and extension onto the skin near mucocutaneous junctions.
2. Tuberculids. (Allergic origin, no tubercle bacilli in lesions.)
   A. Papular forms.
      (1) Lupus miliaris disseminatus faciei. Purely papular.

(2) Papulonecrotic tuberculid. Papules with necrosis.

(3) Lichen scrofulosorum. Folliccular papules or lichenoid papules.

B. Granulomatous, ulceronodular forms.

(1) Erythema induratum. Nodules or plaques subsequently ulcerating. May be a nonspecific vasculitis.

LEPROSY
(Plate 34)

Leprosy is to be considered in the differential diagnosis of any skin granulomas. It is endemic in the southern part of the United States and in semitropical and tropical areas the world over.

Two definite types of leprosy are recognized: lepromatous and tuberculoid. In addition, there are cases that cannot presently be classified in either of these two categories but eventually develop either lepromatous or tuberculoid leprosy.

Lepromatous leprosy is the malignant form which represents minimal resistance to the disease with a negative lepromin reaction, characteristic histology, infiltrated cutaneous lesions with ill-defined borders, and progression to death from tuberculosis and secondary amyloidosis.

Tuberculoid leprosy is generally benign in its course because of considerable resistance to the disease on the part of the host. This is manifested by a positive lepromin test, histology not diagnostic, cutaneous lesions frequently erythematous with elevated borders, and minimal effect of the disease on the general health.

Early lesions of the lepromatous type include reddish macules with an indefinite border, nasal obstruction and nosebleeds. Erythema-nodosum-like lesions occur commonly. The tuberculoid type of leprosy is diagnosed early by the presence of an area of skin with impaired sensation, polyneuritis, and skin lesions with a sharp border and central atrophy.

Etiology. Due to *Mycobacterium leprae* (Hansen's bacillus).

Contagiousness. The source of infection is thought to be from patients with the lepromatous form. Infectiousness is of a low order.

Laboratory Findings. The bacilli are usually uncovered in the lepromatous type but seldom in the tuberculoid type. Smears should be obtained from the tissue exposed by a small incision made into the corium through an infiltrated lesion.

The lepromin reaction, a delayed reaction test similar to the tuberculin test, is of value in differentiating the lepromatous form from the tuberculoid form of leprosy, as stated above. False-positive reactions do occur.

Biologic false-positive tests for syphilis are common in patients with the lepromatous type of leprosy.

Differential Diagnosis. Consider any of the granulomatous diseases such as *syphilis, tuberculosis, sarcoidosis*, and *deep fungal infections*.

Treatment. The sulfones are more effective than any other form of therapy. Diaminodiphenyl sulfone (DDS) and Diasone are used predominantly.

GONORRHEA
(Plate 34)

Gonorrhea is considerably more prevalent than syphilis. Skin lesions with gonorrheal infection are rare (p. 143). But a statement is due here on the therapy of uncomplicated gonorrhea.

The therapy schedule suggested by the U. S. Public Health Service is 4.8 million units of aqueous procaine penicillin I.M. divided into 2 doses injected at 2 sites on the first visit. For penicillin sensitive individuals spectinomycin 2 to 4 Gm. I.M., or tetracycline orally in a dose of 9 Gm. given over 4 days can be prescribed.

RICKETTSIAL DISEASES

The commonest rickettsial disease in the United States is *Rocky Mountain spotted fever* which is spread by ticks of various types. The skin eruption occurs after 3 to 7 days of fever and other toxic signs, and is characterized by purpuric lesions on the extremities, mainly the wrists and the ankles, which then become generalized. The Weil-Felix test using Proteus

OX19 and OX2 is positive. The broad spectrum antibiotics are effective.

The typhus group of rickettsial diseases includes *epidemic* or *louse-borne typhus, Brill's disease* and *endemic murine* or *flea-borne typhus.* Less common forms include *scrub typhus* (tsutsugamushi disease), *trench fever* and *rickettsialpox.* The last-named rickettsial disease is produced by a mite bite. The mite ordinarily lives on rodents. Approximately 10 days after the bite a primary lesion develops in the form of a papule that becomes vesicular. After a few days fever and other toxic signs are accompanied by a generalized eruption that resembles chickenpox. The disease subsides without therapy.

SARCOIDOSIS

Sarcoidosis is a moderately common systemic granulomatous disease of unknown cause that affects skin, lungs, lymph nodes, liver, spleen, bones and eyes. Any one of these organs or all of them may be involved with sarcoid granulomas. Lymphadenopathy is the commonest single finding. Negroes are affected more commonly than Caucasians (Fig. 12-5). Only the skin manifestations of sarcoidosis will be discussed.

Primary Lesions. The superficial lesions consist of reddish papules, nodules and plaques which may be multiple or solitary, and of varying size and configuration. Annular forms of skin sarcoidosis are common. These superficial lesions usually involve the face, the shoulders and the arms. Subcutaneous nodular forms and telangiectatic lesions are more rare.

Secondary Lesions. Central healing can result in atrophy and scarring.

Course. Most cases of sarcoidosis run a chronic but benign course with remissions and exacerbations. Spontaneous "cure" is not unusual.

Etiology. The exact cause is unknown, but the clinicopathologic picture undoubtedly can be caused by several agents, including bacteria, fungi and certain inorganic agents.

Laboratory Findings. The histopathology is quite characteristic and consists of epithelioid cells surrounded by Langhans' giant cells. No acid-fast bacilli are found, and caseation necrosis is absent. The tuberculin skin test is negative, but the Kveim test using sarcoidal lymph node tissue is positive after several weeks. The total blood serum protein is high and ranges from 7.5 to 10.0 Gm. percent due mainly to an increase in the globulin fraction.

Differential Diagnosis. The other *granulomatous diseases,* particularly *secondary or tertiary syphilis,* can be ruled out by biopsy and other appropriate studies. *Silica granulomas* are histologically similar, but a history of such injury can usually be obtained.

Treatment. Time appears to cure or cause remission of most cases of sarcoidosis, but corticosteroids and calciferol are indicated for extensive cases.

BIBLIOGRAPHY

Dubos, R. J., and Hirsch, J. G.: Bacterial and Mycotic Infections of Man. ed. 4. Philadelphia, J. B. Lippincott, 1965.

13

Syphilology

The term "Syphilology" has been dropped from its long-term association with "Dermatology." The reason for this is simple: untreated syphilis is seen only rarely except in venereal disease clinics. When I was stationed at the West Virginia State Rapid Treatment Center from 1946 to 1948 our average admittance was 30 patients a day with venereal disease. Approximately one third of these patients had infectious syphilis. In 1949 the Center was closed because of the low patient census. As a result of this dramatic and rewarding decline in the incidence of syphilis, many responsible physicians feel that we prematurely lowered our guard. The incidence of reported syphilis has risen again to alarming heights. Because of this resurgence it is imperative for all physicians to have a basic understanding of this polymorphous disease.

In order to diagnose syphilis, the physician must have a high index of suspicion for it. Syphilis is the great imitator and can mimic many other conditions. Cutaneous lesions of syphilis occur in all 3 stages of the disease.

Under what circumstances will the present-day physician be called upon to diagnose, evaluate, or manage a patient with syphilis? (1) The cutaneous manifestations, such as a penile lesion or a rash that could be secondary syphilis, may bring a patient to the office. (2) A positive blood test found on a premarital examination or as part of a routine physical examination may be responsible for a patient's being seen by the physician. (3) Cardiac, central nervous system or other organ disease may be a reason for a patient's consulting a doctor.

To manage these patients properly a thorough knowledge of the natural *untreated* course of the disease is essential.

PRIMARY SYPHILIS

This first stage of acquired syphilis usually develops within 2 to 6 weeks (average 3 weeks) after exposure. The *primary chancre* most commonly occurs on the genitalia, but extragenital chancres are not rare and are often misdiagnosed (Plates 35 & 36). Without treatment the chancre heals within 1 to 4 weeks, depending on the location, the amount of secondary infection, and host resistance. The blood serologic test for syphilis (STS) may be negative in the early days of the chancre but eventually becomes positive. A spinal fluid examination during the primary stage reveals invasion of the spirochete in approximately 25 percent of cases. Clinically, the chancre may vary in appearance from a single small erosion to multiple indurated ulcers of the genitalia. Primary syphilis commonly goes unnoticed in the female. Bilateral or unilateral regional lymphadenopathy is common. Malaise and fever may be present.

Early Latent Stage

Latency, manifested by a positive serology and no other subjective or objective evidence of syphilis, may occur between the primary and the secondary stages.

SECONDARY SYPHILIS

Early secondary lesions (Fig. 13-1) may develop before the primary chancre has healed or after latency of a few weeks. **Late secondary lesions** (Figs. 13-2 and 13-3) are more rare and usually are seen

Plate 35. Primary syphilis with a chancre of the penis. This chancre is accompanied by marked edema of the penis. (*From the late J. E. Moore and The Upjohn Company*)

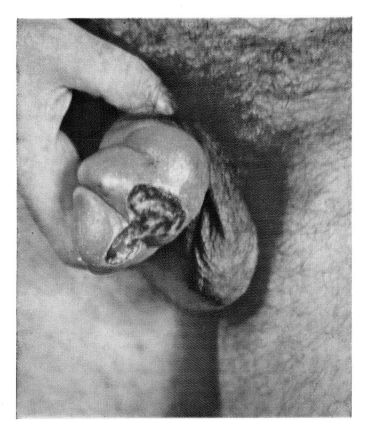

after the early secondary lesions have healed.

Both types of secondary lesions contain the spirochete, *Treponema pallidum*, which can be easily seen with the darkfield microscope. The STS is positive, and approximately 30 percent of the cases have abnormal spinal fluid findings.

Clinically, the early secondary rash can consist of macular, papular, pustular, squamous, or eroded lesions or combinations of any of these lesions. The entire body may be involved or only the palms and the soles, or the mouth, or the genitalia.

Condylomata lata is the name applied to the flat, moist, warty lesions teeming with spirochetes found in the groin and the axillae (Plate 37).

The late secondary lesions are nodular, squamous and ulcerative and are to be distinguished from the tertiary lesions only by the time interval after the onset of infection and by the finding of the spirochete in superficial smears of serum from the lesions. Annular and semiannular configurations of late secondary lesions are common.

Generalized lymphadenopathy, malaise, fever and arthralgia occur in many patients with secondary syphilis.

EARLY LATENT STAGE

Following the secondary stage, many patients with untreated syphilis have only a positive STS. After 4 years of infection the patient enters the late latent stage.

LATE LATENT STAGE

This time level of 4 years arbitrarily divides the early infectious stages from the later noninfectious stages which may or may not develop.

TERTIARY SYPHILIS

This late stage is manifested by subjective or objective involvement of any of the organs of the body, including the skin.

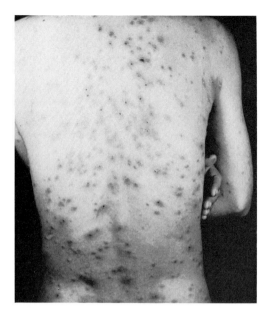

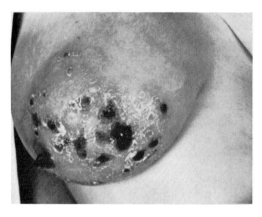

Tertiary changes may be precocious but most often develop 5 to 20 years after the onset of the primary stage. Clinically, the skin lesions are characterized by nodular and gummatous ulcerations (Fig. 13-4 and Plate 38). Solitary or multiple annular and nodular lesions are commonly seen. Subjective complaints are rare unless considerable secondary bacterial infection is present in a gumma. Scarring on healing is inevitable in the majority of the tertiary skin lesions. Larger texts should be consulted for the late changes seen in the central nervous system, the cardiovascular system, the bones (Fig. 13-5A), the eyes and the viscera. Approximately 15 percent of the patients who acquire syphilis and receive no treatment die of the disease.

LATE LATENT STAGE

Another latent period may occur after natural healing of some types of benign tertiary syphilis.

CONGENITAL SYPHILIS

This is syphilis acquired in utero from an infectious mother (Fig. 13-5B and Plate 57). The STS required of pregnant women by most states has lowered the incidence of this unfortunate disease. Stillbirths are not uncommon from mothers who are untreated. After the birth of a live infected child, the mortality rate depends on the duration of the infection, natural host re-

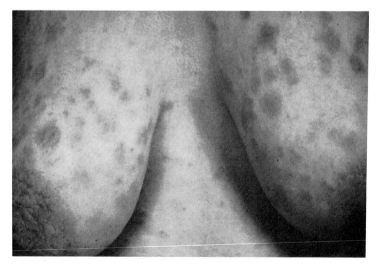

Fig. 13-1. Secondary syphilis.
(*Top*) Papulosquamous lesions on back.
(*Center*) Primary and secondary lesions on breast.
(*Bottom*) Macular lesions on breasts.

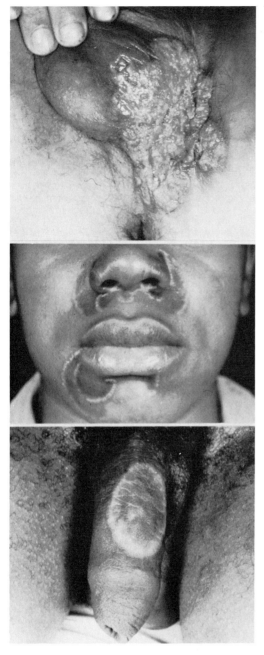

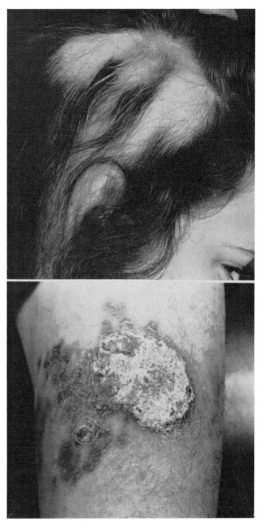

Fig. 13-3. Late secondary syphilis. (*Top*) Patchy alopecia of the scalp. (*Bottom*) Psoriatic-type lesions of the leg.

Fig. 13-2. Late secondary syphilis. (*Top*) Condyloma lata of crural area. (*Center*) Annular lesions on face. (*Bottom*) Annular lesion on penis.

sistance, and the rapidity of initiating correct treatment. Early and late lesions are seen in these children similar to those found in the adult cases of acquired syphilis.

LABORATORY FINDINGS

DARKFIELD EXAMINATION

The etiologic agent, *Treponema pallidum*, can be found in the serum from the primary or secondary lesions. However, a darkfield microscope is necessary, and very few doctor's offices or laboratories have this instrument. A considerable amount of experience is necessary to distinguish *T. pallidum* from other *Treponema*.

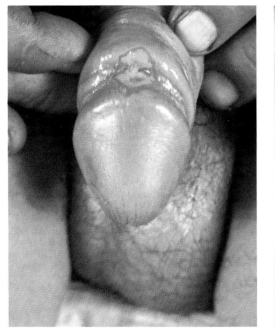

Penile chancre.

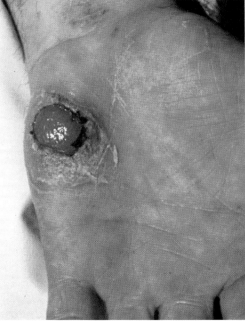

Chancre of the palm.

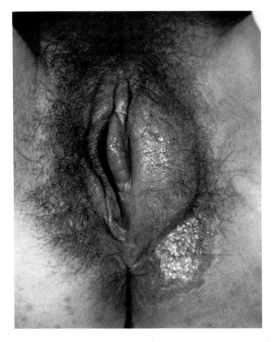

Vulvar chancre with edema of the
labia majora.

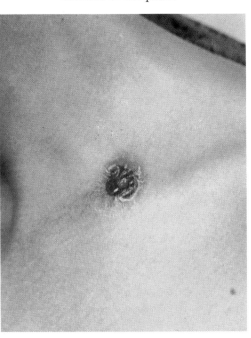

Chancre over the clavicle.

Plate 36. Primary Syphilis. (*The Upjohn Company*)

Plate 37. Secondary syphilis with condyloma lata of the vulva. (*From the late J. E. Moore and The Upjohn Company*)

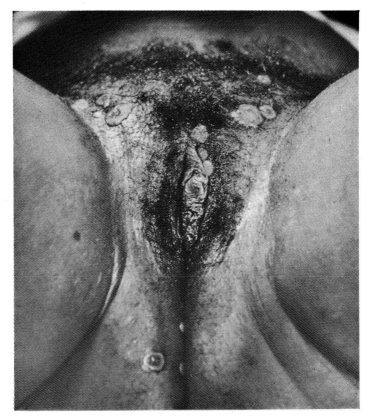

Serologic Test for Syphilis

A rather simple and readily available test is the serologic test for syphilis (STS), of which there are several modifications. The VDRL flocculation test is used most commonly. Fluorescent Treponemal Antibody Absorption test (FTA-ABS test) and modifications are more difficult to perform in the laboratory and therefore are used primarily when the VDRL test is "reactive."

When a report is received from the laboratory that the STS is positive (VDRL reactive), a second blood specimen should be submitted to obtain a *quantitative* report. In some laboratories this repeat test is not necessary, since a quantitative test is run routinely on all positive blood specimens. The use of the terms "2 plus" or "4 plus" is outdated and has been replaced by the more accurate measurement of the positivity by titers. A "4 plus" specimen may be positive in a dilution of 1:2, which is only weakly positive and might be a

biologic false-positive reaction, or it might be positive in a dilution of 1:32, which is strongly positive. In evaluating the response of the STS to treatment, remember that a change in titer from 1:2 to 1:4 to 1:16 to 1:32 to 1:64, or downward in the same gradations, is only a change in one tube in each instance. Thus a change from 1:2 to 1:4 is of the same magnitude as a change from 1:32 to 1:64. Quantitative tests enable the physician to (1) evaluate the efficacy of the treatment, (2) discover a relapse before it becomes infectious, (3) differentiate between a relapse and a reinfection, (4) establish a reaction as a sero-resistant (Wassermann-fast) type and (5) differentiate between true and biologic false-positive serologic reactions.

In most laboratories it is now routine to do a FTA-ABS test on all reactive VDRL tests. With rare exceptions, a positive FTA-ABS test means that the patient has or had syphilis and is not a biologic false-positive reactor.

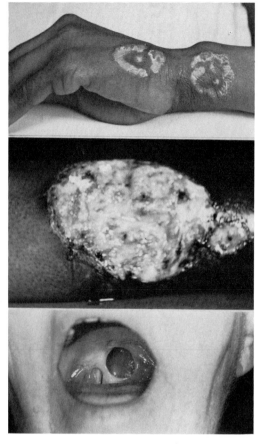

Fig. 13-4. Tertiary skin syphilis. (*Top*) Annular nodular lesions on arm of Negro. (*Center*) Gumma on leg of Negro. (*Bottom*) Perforation of soft palate due to healed gumma.

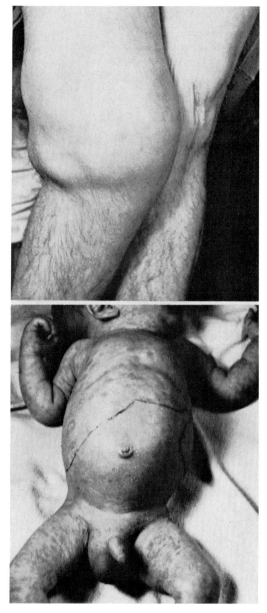

Fig. 13-5. Syphilis. (*Top*) Charcot knee joint of patient with tabes. (*Bottom*) Congenital syphilis. Note skin lesions and enlarged liver and spleen. (*See also* Plate 57.)

SPINAL FLUID TEST

As has been stated, the spinal fluid is frequently positive in the primary and the secondary stages of the disease. Invasion of the central nervous system is an early manifestation, even though the perceptible clinical effects are a late manifestation. The spinal fluid should be examined at least once during the course of the disease. The best routine is to perform a spinal fluid test before treatment is initiated and repeat the test as indicated. If the spinal fluid is negative in a patient who has had syphilis for 4 years, central nervous system syphilis will not occur, and future spinal fluid tests are not necessary. If the test is positive, repeat tests should be done every 6 months for 4 years.

The following 5 tests are run on the spinal fluid:

1. **Cell Count.** The finding of 9 or more lymphocytes or polymorphonuclear leukocytes is positive. The cell count is the most labile of the tests and becomes increased early in the infection and responds fastest to therapy. Therefore, it is a good index to activity of the disease. The cell count must be done within an hour after the fluid is withdrawn.

2. **Globulin or Pandy's Test.** This qualitative protein test is positive in most cases of central nervous system syphilis.

3. **Total Protein.** When measured in mg. percent, it normally should be below 40.

4. **Colloidal Gold.** Ten tubes are used, and in each tube the reactivity of the colloid varies from 0 to 5. A positive test shows reactivity from 2 to 5. Thus 0001111000 is negative and 0001233321 is positive.

5. **Complement-Fixation Test.** This is the most reliable test and should be done in dilutions of 1.0, 0.5, 0.25 and 0.1 ml. This test is the last to turn positive and the slowest to return to negativity. In some cases therapy causes a decrease in the titer, but slight positivity or "fastness" can remain for the lifetime of the patient.

DIFFERENTIAL DIAGNOSIS

Primary syphilis from chancroid, herpes simplex, fusospirochetal balanitis, granuloma inguinale, and any of the *primary chancre-type diseases* (see index).

Secondary syphilis from any of the papulosquamous diseases, fungal diseases, drug eruption and alopecia areata.

Tertiary skin syphilis from any of the granulomatous diseases, particularly tuberculosis, leprosy, sarcoidosis, deep mycoses and lymphoblastomas.

Congenital syphilis from atopic eczema, diseases with lymphadenopathy, hepatomegaly and splenomegaly.

A true-positive syphilitic serology is to be differentiated from a biologic false-positive reaction. This serologic differentiation is accomplished best by using the Fluorescent Treponemal Antibody Absorption test or its modifications along with a good history and a thorough examination of the patient. Many patients with biologic false-positive reactions develop one of the collagen diseases at a later date.

TREATMENT

A 22-year-old married male has a 1 cm. diameter sore on his glans penis of 5 days' duration. Three weeks previously he had extramarital intercourse and 10 days prior to this office visit he had marital intercourse.

FIRST VISIT

1. Perform a darkfield examination of the penile lesion. Treatment can be started if *Treponema pallidum* is found. If this examination is not available, then

2. Obtain a blood specimen for a serologic test for syphilis (STS).

3. While waiting for the STS report, advise the patient to soak the site in saline solution for 15 minutes twice a day. The solution is made by placing ¼ teaspoon of salt in a glass of water.

4. Advise against sexual intercourse until the reports are completed.

5. Explain to the patient the seriousness of treating him for syphilis if he does not have it. The "syphilitic" label is one he should not want if at all possible.

SECOND VISIT

Three days later. The lesion is larger, and the STS report is "VDRL nonreactive."

1. Obtain blood for a second STS.

2. Neosporin ointment   5.0
   Sig: Apply t.i.d. locally after soaking in saline solution.

3. Explain again why you are delaying therapy until a definite diagnosis is made.

THIRD VISIT

Three days later. The sore is smaller, but the STS report is "VDRL reactive." The diagnosis is now known to be "Primary Syphilis."

1. Reassure the patient that present-day therapy is highly successful, but he must follow your instructions closely.

2. His wife should be brought in for examination and a blood test. If the blood test is negative, it should be repeated weekly for 1 month. However, some syphilologists believe that therapy is indicated

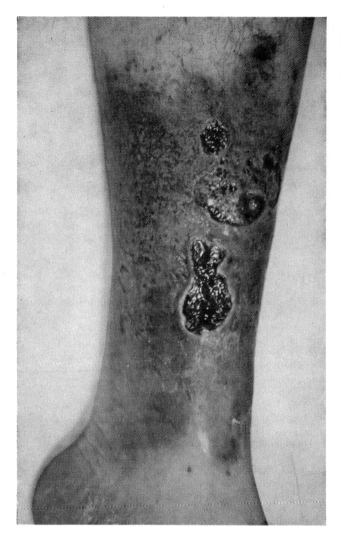

Plate 38. Tertiary syphilis with a gumma of the leg. This resembles a stasis ulcer. (*From the late J. E. Moore and The Upjohn Company*)

for the marital partner in the face of a negative STS if the husband has infectious syphilis and is being treated. A single injection of 2.4 million units of a long-acting type of penicillin is used. This will prevent "ping-pong" syphilis, which is a cycle of reinfection from one marital partner to another.

3. The patient's contact should be found. The patient knows her only as "Jane," and he cannot remember over which bar she presided. Report these findings to the local Health Department.

4. A spinal fluid specimen should be obtained. (The report was returned as normal for all 5 tests.)

5. Penicillin therapy should be begun. Here, two factors are important: (1) the dose must be adequate, and (2) the duration of effective therapy must be over a period of 10 to 14 days.

Dosage

Primary, Secondary, Early and Late Latent, and Benign Tertiary Syphilis: 600,000 or 1,200,000 units of a long-acting penicillin every 2 to 3 days for a total of 6,000,000 units.

For a proven primary or secondary case of syphilis, the U.S. Public Health Service states that one injection I.M. of 2,400,000 units of benzathine penicillin G is adequate.

Neurosyphilis or Cardiovascular Syphilis: A total of 9,000,000 units of a long-acting penicillin. For complicated cases, consult larger texts for therapy and care.

Congenital Syphilis: 100,000 units of penicillin per pound of body weight given twice weekly for 1 to 2 weeks. It is impractical to give doses smaller than 150,000 units in each dose. After the age of 6, or 60 pounds in weight, adult schedules should be used.

SYPHILIS PEARLS
GENERAL

1. Any patient treated for gonorrhea should have a serologic test for syphilis (STS) 4 to 6 weeks later.

2. 75 percent of the people who acquire syphilis suffer no serious manifestations of the disease.

3. Syphilis does not cause vesicular or bullous skin lesions, except in infants with congenital infection.

PRIMARY STAGE

1. Syphilis should be ruled in or out in the diagnosis of any penile or vulvar sores.

2. Multiple primary chancres are moderately common.

SECONDARY STAGE

1. The rash of secondary syphilis, except for the rare follicular form, does not itch.

2. Secondary syphilis should be ruled in or out in any patient with a generalized, nonpruritic rash. A high index of suspicion is necessary.

LATENT STAGE

The diagnosis of "latent syphilis" cannot be made for a particular patient unless spinal fluid tests have been done and are negative for syphilis.

TERTIARY STAGE

1. Tertiary syphilis should be considered in any patient with a chronic granuloma of the skin, particularly if it has an annular or circular configuration.

2. Invasion of the central nervous system occurs in the primary and the secondary stages of the disease. A spinal fluid test is indicated during these stages.

3. If the spinal fluid tests for syphilis are negative in a patient who has had syphilis for 4 years, central nervous system syphilis will not occur, and future spinal punctures are not necessary.

4. Twenty percent of patients with late asymptomatic neurosyphilis have a negative STS.

CONGENITAL SYPHILIS

An STS should be done on every pregnant woman to prevent congenital syphilis of the newborn.

SEROLOGY

1. The serologic test for syphilis may be negative in the early days of the primary chancre. The STS is always positive in the secondary stage.

2. A quantitative STS should be done on all syphilitic patients to evaluate the response to treatment or the development of relapse or reinfection. To label reactions as "2 plus" or "4 plus" is not now acceptable.

3. The finding of a low-titer STS in a patient not previously treated for syphilis calls for a careful evaluation to rule out a biologic false-positive reaction.

GONORRHEA
(Plate 34)

Untreated or inadequately treated infection due to *N. gonorrhoeae* can involve the skin through metastatic spread. *Primary cutaneous infection* with multiple erosions at the site of the purulent discharge is very rare.

Metastatic complications include a *bacteremia* where there is an intermittent high fever, arthralgia, and skin lesions. The skin lesions (Plate 34) are quite characteristic hemorrhagic vesicopustules most commonly seen on the fingers. Treatment with intravenous penicillin for 10 days in a total dose of 100 to 200 million units is indicated.

The rarer *septicemic form* with very high fever and meningitis or endocarditis may have purpuric skin lesions similar to those seen in *meningococcemia.*

BIBLIOGRAPHY

Stokes, J. H., Beerman, H., and Ingraham, N. R.: Modern Clinical Syphilology. ed. 3. Philadelphia, W. B. Saunders, 1945. A classic text.

Syphilis—A Synopsis. Washington, Public Health Service Publication No. 1660, 1968.

Termini, B. A., and Music, S. I.: The Natural History of Syphilis: A Review. Southern M. J. 65:241, 1972.

Youmans, J. B., (ed.): Syphilis and Other Venereal Diseases. Med. Clinics N. Am., Vol. 48, No. 3. Philadelphia, W. B. Saunders, 1964.

14

Dermatologic Virology

Virus diseases of the skin are exceedingly common. The various clinical entities are distinct, and, since we have no specific antiviral drug, the treatment varies for each entity. The following list contains the virus diseases that will be discussed. The exanthems of children will be covered in a cursory manner.

1. Herpes simplex
2. Kaposi's varicelliform eruption
3. Zoster
4. Chickenpox
5. Smallpox, vaccinia and cowpox
6. Warts
7. Molluscum contagiosum
8. Lymphogranuloma venereum
9. Exanthematous disease; measles, German measles, roseola and erythema infectiosum.

HERPES SIMPLEX
(Plate 39 A)

Herpes simplex (fever blister) is an acute, moderately painful, viral eruption of a single group of vesicles that commonly occurs around the mouth or the genitalia (Fig. 14-1). The commonest type of herpes simplex is the *recurrent form* seen in adults. An uncommon *primary form* of herpes simplex affects children and young adults. In this primary form, the vesicular lesions involve the mouth and the pharynx or vaginal and vulvar areas. High fever, regional lymphadenopathy and general malaise accompany the painful sores (Fig. 14-1 A).

The following discussion refers to the common *recurrent form* of herpes simplex.

Primary Lesions. A group of vesicles.

Secondary Lesions. Erosions and secondary bacterial infection.

Distribution. Lips, mouth, genital region of both males and females (herpes progenitalis), eye (marginal keratitis or corneal ulcer), or any body area.

Course. The vesicles last for 2 to 3 days before the tops come off. The residual erosions or crusted lesions last for another 5 to 7 days. Recurrences are common in the same area.

Etiology. Caused by a relatively large virus, *Herpesvirus hominis* (HVH). Certain precipitating factors are important in producing the recurrent eruptions. These factors, which include fever, common cold, sunlight, psychic influences, stomach upsets and trauma, apparently activate a dormant phase of the virus in the cells.

There are 2 antigenically and biologically different strains of the virus. Type 1 HVH is associated with most non-genital herpetic infections. Type 2 HVH occurs chiefly in association with genital infection and is probably venereally transmitted.

Contagiousness. This can occur through intimate contact. Kaposi's varicelliform eruption is a severe example (see p. 148).

Laboratory Findings. The virus may be easily isolated from the lesions, but this is not an office procedure. A biopsy is characteristic, and neutralizing antibodies in the blood show an increasing titer.

Differential Diagnosis

MOUTH LESIONS

Aphthous Stomatis: see only 1 or 2 painful eroded lesions; recurrent; not caused by herpes simplex virus.

BODY LESIONS

Zoster: see more than one group of vesicles, nerve segment distribution, not recurrent at same site; different virus (p. 149).

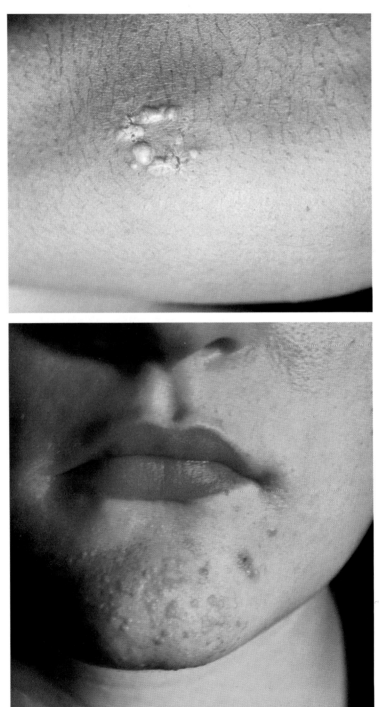

Plate 39. Dermatologic virology.
(*Top*) Herpes simplex on the forearm. (*K.U.M.C.*)

(*Bottom*) Flat warts on the chin. (*K.U.M.C.*) (*E. R. Squibb*)

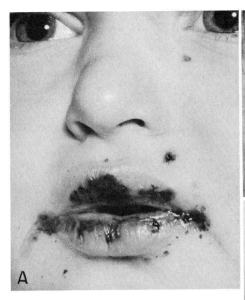

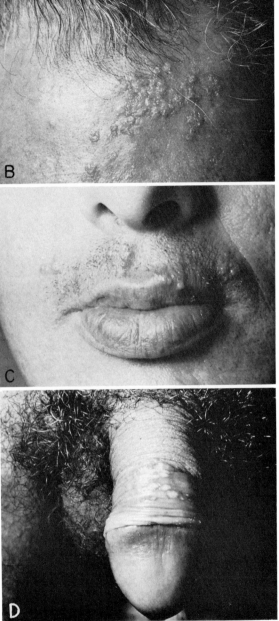

Fig. 14-1. Herpes simplex.

(*A*) Primary herpes simplex gingivostomatitis of 2-year-old boy. (*K.C.G.H.*)

(*B*) Recurrent herpes simplex on the forehead of an adult, initiated by a sunburn.

(*C*) Herpes simplex in a common location on the lips, concurrent with pneumonia.

(*D*) Herpes simplex on the penis.

Tinea of Body: early vesicular case can be clinically indistinguishable from herpes; later see central healing in tinea; fungus grown from scraping or culture (p. 170).

GENITAL LESIONS

Primary Syphilis: can be clinically similar to herpes simplex; history of illicit or extramarital intercourse; not recurrent usually; darkfield examination is definitely indicated and would be positive, but this test is rarely available (p. 134).

Treatment

Young woman with fever blisters on lower lip that have recurred every 2 or 3 months for the past 2 years.

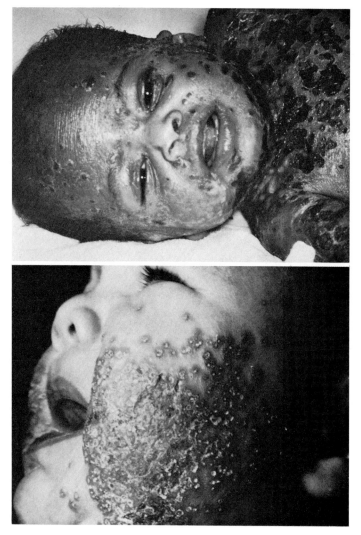

Fig. 14-2. Kaposi's varicelliform eruption. (*Top*) In a 6-month-old Negro girl with atopic eczema following accidental inoculation with the vaccinia virus. (*K.U.M.C.*)

(*Bottom*) In a child with atopic eczema inoculated with the herpes simplex virus.

1. Inform the patient that no specific treatment is available to shorten the natural course of the infection.

2. Neo-Polycin or other antibiotic ointment, q.s.   5.0
   Sig: Apply locally t.i.d.

This benefits by relieving the pain and the inflammation.

3. Therapeutic applications of dyes, such as neutral red, combined with exposure to incandescent light, are being studied now and may prove to be beneficial.

KAPOSI'S VARICELLIFORM ERUPTION

This viral disease is an uncommon but severe complication in children who have atopic eczema. It results from self-inoculation by scratching, due to the virus of either herpes simplex or vaccinia (Fig. 14-2). In the former type a history of exposure to fever blisters may or may not be obtained. With the vaccinia form a history of vaccination of the child or the sibling is commonly obtained. With either type, the child is acutely ill, has a high fever

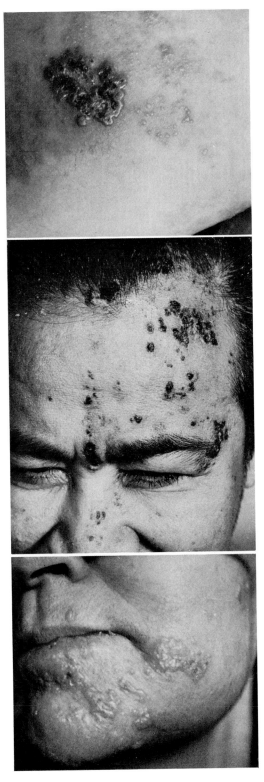

Fig. 14-3. Zoster. (*Top*) Grouped vesicles of zoster on the thigh of a 21-month-old child. (*Center*) Zoster of the ophthalmic branch of the trigeminal nerve. Note sharp mid-line demarcation on forehead. (*K.C.G.H.*) (*Bottom*) Zoster of the mandibular branch of the trigeminal nerve.

and has generalized umbilicated chickenpoxlike skin lesions. Supportive therapy consists of antibiotics systemically, intravenous infusions, and a nonalcoholic white shake lotion locally. Systemic corticosteroid therapy should not be given in the early stage of the disease but may be given later. Gamma globulin injections (2 to 4 ml. I.M. daily for 3 to 4 days) appear to be quite beneficial. For severe cases due to the vaccinia virus, vaccinia immune globulin is available from several centers in the United States through the American National Red Cross.

ZOSTER
(Plate 60)

Shingles is a common viral disease characterized by the appearance of several groups of vesicles distributed along a cutaneous nerve segment (Fig. 14-3). Zoster and chickenpox are thought to be caused by the same virus. Susceptible children who are exposed to cases of zoster often develop chickenpox. Less commonly, older individuals exposed to chickenpox may get zoster.

Primary Lesions. Multiple groups of vesicles or crusted lesions.

Secondary Lesions. Bacterial infection with pustules, rarely progressing to gangrenous ulcers and scarring.

Distribution. Unilateral eruption following a nerve distribution, frequently in the thoracic region, the face, the neck and less frequently the lumbosacral area and elsewhere. Eye involvement can be serious. Bilateral involvement of the body is rare but not fatal, contrary to the old wives' tale.

Course. New crops of vesicles can appear for 3 to 5 days. The vesicles then dry up and form crusts which take 3 weeks on the average to disappear. The general health is seldom affected except for low-grade fever and malaise. Recurrences are rare. The postheretic pain can persist for months in aged patients.

Subjective Complaints. Pain of a neuritic type can precede the eruption and, if in the abdominal area, can lead to erroneous diagnoses and surgical procedures. The common simple pain of young persons with shingles is readily treated and soon disappears. On the other hand, the severe true postherpetic pain of older patients can be very serious. In order to evaluate critically the therapeutic response to the many agents said to relieve this severe pain, *a nerve distribution pain should not be labeled as the true postherpetic type unless it has been present for over 30 days.* If this strict criterion is adhered to, many newly proclaimed treatments for such pain will be found to be of limited value.

Etiology. Caused by a virus similar to the one that causes chickenpox. Trauma is thought to play a role in development of some cases of shingles. "Nervousness" plays little if any role.

Contagiousness. The interrelationship between shingles and chickenpox has been referred to above.

Laboratory Findings. Isolation and identification of the virus is not an office procedure.

Differential Diagnosis

OF THE NEURITIC-TYPE PAIN THAT PRECEDES THE SKIN LESIONS: *appendicitis, ureteral colic, sciatica, migraine, etc.*

OF THE ERUPTION: *herpes simplex* (see single group of vesicles, recurrence history, p. 145); *blistered burn from hot application for neuritic pain* (very commonly the patient really has shingles and erroneously attributes the blisters as due to the hot application for the preceding herpetic pain).

Treatment

1. Forty-year-old female with multiple grouped vesicles on right cheek and forehead, causing moderately severe pain.

A. Reassure the patient that shingles, except in the elderly, is not a serious disease and advise her not to believe what her well-meaning friends will tell her about the disease.

B. Supply the name of an ophthalmologist to consult to rule in or out eye complications.

C. Chlortetracycline (Aureomycin) 500 mg.
Alcoholic white shake lotion q.s. 60.0
Sig: Apply locally to skin b.i.d. (The Aureomycin is added to help prevent secondary infection.)

D. Empirin or other analgesic tablets #50
Sig: 1 tablet q.i.d. for pain.

E. Meprobamate tablets, 400 mg. #30
Sig: 1 tablet q.i.d. (For the anxious apprehensive patient.)

2. Seventy-year-old male patient with *severe postherpetic pain* of 5 weeks' duration.

A. Reassure the patient that the majority of patients who have postherpetic pain lose it gradually day by day, week by week. It is extremely rare for the pain to remain persistent but, when this does happen, it can be disabling. Be optimistic, however. The following treatments can alleviate the neuritis.

B. Acthar Gel, 80 units. Inject subcutaneously in the hip area on the first visit and repeat in 2 days if necessary.

C. Hydrocortisone tablets, 20 mg. #20
Sig: 1 tablet t.i.d. for 4 days; then decrease dose slowly as symptoms subside.

D. Tuinal capsule, 50 mg. #10
Sig: 1 capsule h.s. for sleep.

E. For resistant cases, consult larger texts for additional therapy.

CHICKENPOX

This common viral disease of childhood is characterized by the development of tense vesicles first on the trunk and then spreading to a milder extent to the face and the extremities, appearance of new crops of vesicles for 3 to 5 days, and healing of the individual lesions in a week. The disease occurs 10 to 14 days after exposure to another child with chickenpox or to an adult with zoster. The clear vesicle becomes a pustule and then a crusted lesion before dropping off. Itching is more prominent during the healing stage.

Treatment

1. Usually nothing indicated, or
2. Menthol   0.25%
   Nonalcoholic white shake lotion q.s.   120.0
   Sig: Apply locally t.i.d. for itching.
3. Benadryl Hydrochloride elixir   60.0
   Sig: 1 tsp. t.i.d. for moderately severe itching.

SMALLPOX

Smallpox is an uncommon viral disease characterized by the development, after an incubation period of 1 to 3 weeks, of prodromal symptoms of high fever, chills and various aches. After 3 to 4 days a rash develops with lowering of the fever. The individual lesions are most extensive on the face and the extremities; they come out as a single shower and progress from papule to vesicle and in 5 to 10 days to pustule. With the occurrence of the pustule the fever goes up again with a high white blood cell count. Hemorrhagic lesions usually indicate a severe form of the disease.

Alastrim is a mild form of smallpox resulting from a less virulent strain of the virus.

Varioloid is a mild form of smallpox which occurs in vaccinated individuals. However, this strain of virus is very virulent and when transmitted to a nonvaccinated person often causes a fulminating disease.

Severe systemic complications of small pox include pneumonia, secondary bacterial skin infection and encephalitis.

Treatment

This consists of systemic antibiotics, parenteral infusions and locally applied white shake lotion containing an antibiotic.

Prophylactic treatment consists of vaccination. The best technic is by multiple puncture.

Never vaccinate a patient who has active atopic eczema; scratching of the vaccination can lead to development of Kaposi's varicelliform eruption (p. 148).

VACCINIA

Vaccinia is produced by the inoculation of the vaccinia virus into the skin of a person who has no immunity.

The *primary vaccination reaction* follows this timetable. The multiple puncture technic should be used. A red papule on a red base develops on the 4th day, becomes vesicular in 3 more days, pustular in 2 to 3 more days, and then gradually dries to form a crust which drops off within 3 to 4 weeks after the vaccination. A mild systemic reaction may occur during the pustular stage. The vaccination site should be kept dry and uncovered.

Generalized vaccinia is rare but can occur from auto-inoculation by scratching in atopic eczema patients (see Kaposi's varicelliform eruption, p. 148). A biologic false-positive serologic test for syphilis develops in approximately 20 percent of vaccinated persons. The test becomes negative within 2 to 4 months.

A *vaccinoid reaction* develops in a partially immune individual. A pustule with some surrounding redness occurs within 1 week.

An *immune reaction* consists of a papule that develops in 2 days which may or may not persist for 1 week.

An *absent reaction* indicates that the vaccine was inactivated by the procedure (alcohol used in cleaning the site, etc.), or that the vaccine was impotent.

A successful vaccination offers protection from smallpox within 3 weeks, and this immunity lasts for approximately 7 years.

COWPOX

Jenner used the cowpox virus to vaccinate humans against smallpox. For that reason, the vaccinia virus and the cowpox virus have been thought to be the same. Evidence now exists that proves these viruses to be different, presumably as a result of a change in the vaccinia virus through years of passage. The term "cow-

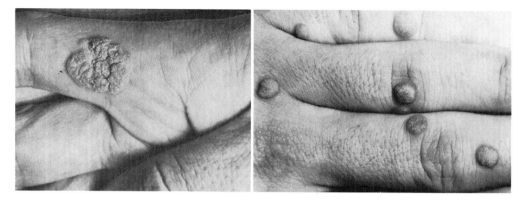

Fig. 14-4. Common warts on the hand.

pox" is now reserved for the viral disease of cows that occurs in Europe. Man can get the disease from infected teats and udders. A solitary nodule appears, usually on the hand, which eventually suppurates and then heals in 4 to 8 weeks.

WARTS (VERRUCAE)
(Plates 39 B and 51)

Warts or verrucae are very common small tumors of the skin. It is doubtful if any human escapes this viral infection. Warts have been played with for centuries, and cures have been attributed to burying a dead black cat in the graveyard at midnight and other such similar feats. The interesting fact is that these examples of psychotherapy do work. Physicians attempt the same type of therapy under more professional guise and are pleased but not surprised when such therapy is effective. Children, fortunately, are most amenable to this suggestion therapy. On the other hand, however, every physician is also familiar with the stubborn wart that has been literally blasted from its mooring in the skin but keeps recurring.

The various clinical types of warts relate to the appearance of the growth and to its location. The treatment varies somewhat for each type of wart and will be discussed separately for each type.

COMMON WART
(Fig. 14-4)

The appearance is a papillary growth, slightly raised above the skin surface, varying from pinhead size to large clusters of pea-sized tumors. These warts are seen most commonly on the hands. Rarely, they have to be differentiated from *seborrheic keratoses* (flatter, darker, velvety tumors of older adults, p. 259) and *pigmented verrucous nevi* (projections are not dry and rough to touch; longer duration; biopsy may be indicated. p. 278).

Treatment

1. Suggestion therapy can be attempted, particularly with children. One form of such therapy consists of the application by the doctor of a colored solution, such as podophyllum in alcohol, 25 percent solution. This has the added benefit of being a cell-destroying chemical.

2. Electrosurgery. Single warts in adults or older children are removed best by this method. The recurrence rate is minimal, and one treatment usually suffices. The technic is to cleanse the area, anesthetize the site with 1 percent procaine or other local anaesthetic, destroy the tumor with any form of electrosurgery (see p. 45), snip off or curette out the dead tissue, and desiccate the base. Recurrences can be attributed to failure to remove the dead tissue and to destroy the lesion adequately to its full depth. No dressing should be applied. The site will heal in 5 to 14 days with only minimal bacterial infection and scar formation. Warts around the nails have a high recurrence rate, and cure usually requires removal of part of the overlying nail.

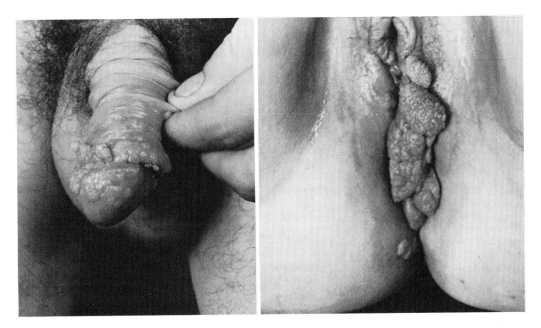

Fig. 14-5. Condyloma acuminata or moist warts. (*Left*) Of the penis. (*Right*) Of the vulva.

3. Liquid Nitrogen Therapy. If available, this freezing therapy is quite simple, effective, but moderately painful. (See p. 46.)

4. Salicylic acid   10%
   Flexible collodion q.s.   30.0

Sig: Apply to warts cautiously every night for 5 nights out of 7. The dead tissue can be removed with scissors.

This type of treatment is applicable to the case with 20 or more warts on one hand. The purpose is to remove as many warts as possible in this manner over a period of several weeks. Any remaining warts can be removed by electrosurgery.

5. Another form of treatment for multiple warts or for warts in children is as follows:

    Synalar Cream (0.025%) or
    Cordran Cream q.s.   15.0

Sig: Apply a very small quantity to each wart at night. Then cover the wart with Saran Wrap or Blenderm Tape and leave the occlusive dressing on all night or for 24 hours. Repeat nightly.

This treatment has the advantage of being painless and quite effective. Salicylic acid (2 to 4%) can be added to the cream for further benefit.

6. Vitamin A, 50,000 to 100,000
    Units   #50

Sig: 1 a day for no longer than 3 months. For the resistant case and for the one who says "Doctor, aren't there any pills I can take for these warts." Vitamin A is safe, and warts have disappeared after such a course of treatment.

FILIFORM WARTS

These are warts with long fingerlike projections from the skin that most commonly appear on the eyelids, the face and the neck. They are to be differentiated from *cutaneous horns* (seen in elderly patients with senile keratosis or prickle cell epithelioma at the base; has a hard keratin horn, p. 264), and *pedunculated fibromas* (on the neck and the axillae of middle-aged men and women, p. 260).

Treatment

1. Without anesthesia, snip off the wart with a small scissors and apply trichloracetic acid solution (saturated) cautiously

to the base. This is a fast and effective method, especially for children.

2. Electrosurgery. As above for common warts.

An annoying variant of this type of wart is the case with multiple small *filiform warts of the beard area*. Electrosurgery without anesthesia is well tolerated and effective for these warts. However, in order to achieve a permanent cure, the patient should be seen again in 3 to 4 weeks to remove the young warts that are in the process of enlarging. The physician's job is to keep ahead of these warts and eliminate the reinfection that occurs from shaving.

FLAT WARTS
(Plate 39 B)

These small flat tumors are often barely visible but can occur in clusters of 10 to 30 or more. They are commonly seen on the forehead and the dorsum of the hand and should be differentiated from small *seborrheic keratoses* or *nonpigmented nevi*.

Treatment

1. Suggestion therapy. This form of treatment is very effective for these warts in children. The following bland lotion has been used with excellent results:

Alcoholic white shake lotion q.s.
(See Formulary, p. 37)   60.0
Sig: Apply to warts b.i.d.

2. Electrosurgery or liquid nitrogen lightly.

Some adult cases can exhaust your therapeutic modalities only to have the warts disappear with time.

MOIST WARTS
(CONDYLOMATA ACUMINATA)
(Fig. 14-5)

These are quite characteristic single or multiple, soft, nonhorny masses that appear in the anogenital areas and, less commonly, between the toes and at the corners of the mouth. They are not always of a venereal nature.

Treatment

1. Podophyllum resin in alcohol (25% solution). Apply once to the warts cau-

tiously. Second or third treatments are rarely necessary. To prevent excessive irritation, the site should be bathed within 6 hours after the application.

PLANTAR WARTS
(Fig. 14-6)

(This is the layman's "planter's warts" which I am sure they believe are related to "Planter's Peanuts.") As the name signifies, this wart occurs on the sole of the foot, is flat, extends deep into the thick skin and, *on superficial trimming reveals small pinpoint-sized bleeding points.* Varying degrees of disability can be produced from the pressure type of pain. Single or multiple lesions can be present. The name *"mosaic"* is applied when the warts have coalesced into larger patches. One of the most vexing problems in dermatology is the patient with half of the sole of a foot covered with these warts.

Plantar warts are to be differentiated from a *callus* (no bleeding points visible on superficial trimming), and from *scar tissue from a previous treatment* (no bleeding points seen). *Never treat a plantar lesion as a wart until you have proved your diagnosis by trimming.*

Treatment

It would be impossible to list all of the forms of therapy that have proved to be curative for plantar warts or any other warts, but here are some favorite forms of therapy. I wager that if you start with number 1 and proceed down to number 6, either the warts will have left, or your patient will have gone to another doctor.

1. Electrosurgery. This is the simplest and most successful form of therapy for a single plantar wart. The procedure is the same as for common warts except that the downgrowth of the plantar wart is greater. The disadvantage of this type of treatment, as with any treatment except x-ray, is that healing takes from 3 to 4 weeks to be complete. Some bleeding is to be expected a few days after the surgery. Most patients do not complain of much pain during the healing stage.

2. Trichloracetic acid—tape technic. Useful for children and cases with multi-

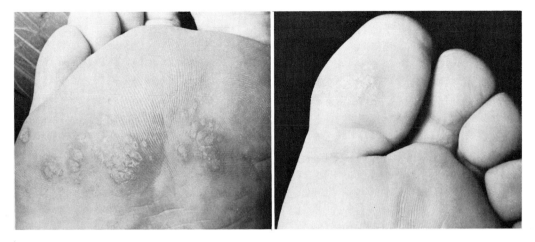

Fig. 14-6. Plantar warts. (*Left*) Such a large number of warts should be treated with a peeling local agent. (*Right*) These warts can be removed by electrosurgery.

ple plantar warts. The procedure is as follows: pare down the wart with a sharp knife, apply trichloracetic acid solution (saturated) to the wart, then cover the area with plain tape. Leave the tape on for 5 days without getting it wet. The physician then removes the tape and curettes out the dead wart tissue. Usually, more wart will remain, and the procedure is repeated until the wart is destroyed. This course of treatment may take from 3 to 6 weeks. After the first 2 visits the site may become tender and secondarily infected. If the disability and the infection are severe, therapy should be stopped temporarily and hot soaks instituted.

3. Fluorinated Corticosteroid—Occlusive Dressing Therapy. Have the patient apply a small amount of cream (Synalar Cream [0.025%], Cordran Cream or Celestone Cream) to the wart or warts at night and cover with Saran Wrap, Handi-Wrap or Blenderm Tape. Leave on for 12 to 24 to 48 hours and reapply. This form of treatment is painless.

4. Cantharidin Tincture (Cantharone, Ingram). Applied by the doctor to the pared wart. Use caution and do not get this vesicant on the surrounding normal skin. Cover with adhesive tape and leave on for 12 to 24 hours. This treatment can cause pain and infection, but it is quite

effective. The resulting blister can be trimmed off in 1 week and the medicine reapplied if necessary.

5. Liquid Nitrogen Therapy. This can be applied 2 ways. When applied for around 10 to 15 seconds, a blister will form in 24 hours and deep peeling of the wart will ensue. This can be quite painful but effective.

When applied lightly for around 5 to 8 seconds, the wart can be removed gradually on multiple visits with less pain and disability.

6. X-ray therapy. This painless form of therapy can be used for single warts. Only a dermatologist or a radiologist should administer this treatment. Once x-ray therapy is given in the usual dose, which varies with the size of the wart, the dose never should be repeated to that site. The cure rate is fairly high.

MOLLUSCUM CONTAGIOSUM
(Fig. 14-7)

This uncommon viral infection of the skin is characterized by the occurrence, usually in children, of one or multiple small skin tumors. These growths occasionally develop in the scratched areas of patients with atopic eczema.

Primary Lesion. An umbilicated, firm, waxy, skin-colored, raised papule varying

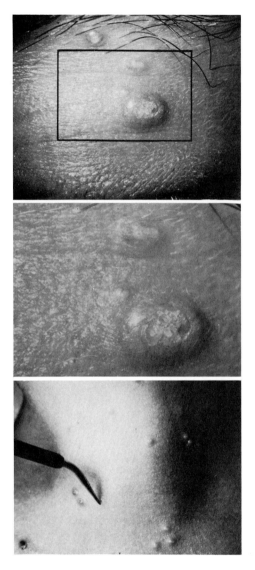

Fig. 14-7. Molluscum contagiosum.
(*Top*) Three molluscum contagiosum lesions on upper eyelid (*Drs. Calkins, Lemoine and Hyde*). (*Center*) Close-up of area marked in top photograph (*Drs. Calkins, Lemoine and Hyde*). (*Bottom*) Demonstrating the use of electrosurgery in treating multiple lesions on the neck and the shoulder.

in diameter from 2 mm. to 5 mm. and, rarely, larger.

Secondary Lesion. Inflamed from bacterial infection.

Distribution. Most commonly on trunk, face and arms but can occur anywhere.

Course. Onset of lesions is insidious, due to lack of symptoms. Trauma or infection of a lesion causes it to disappear. Recurrences are rare if lesions are removed adequately.

Contagiousness. Unusual.

Differential Diagnosis

Warts: no umbilication, not waxy (p. 152).

Keratoacanthoma: most commonly in older adults; larger lesion; biopsy characteristic (p. 271).

Basal Cell Epithelioma: in older adults; slow growing; biopsy characteristic (p. 267).

Treatment

A 6-year-old child has 10 small molluscum papules on his arms and upper trunk.

1. Curettement. Rapidly curette each lesion, apply pressure to stop bleeding, then apply bandage. A small amount of trichloracetic acid (saturated solution) on the broken pointed end of a swab stick helps to stop prolonged bleeding. Two or 3 visits may be necessary to treat recurrent lesions and new ones that have popped up.

2. Electrosurgery. Done lightly and rapidly, this is another effective method. It is not necessary to destroy the entire lesion as for a wart but only to induce some trauma and mild infection.

LYMPHOGRANULOMA VENEREUM

This uncommon veneral disease occurs mainly in Negroes and is characterized by a primary lesion on the genitals and secondary changes involving the draining lymph channels and glands (Fig. 14-8).

The primary erosion or blister is rarely seen, especially on the female. Within 10 to 30 days after exposure the inguinal nodes, particularly in the male, enlarge unilaterally. This inguinal mass may rupture if treatment is delayed. In the female the lymph drainage most commonly is toward the pelvic and the perirectal nodes, and their enlargement may be overlooked. Low-grade fever, malaise and generalized lymphadenopathy frequently occur during the adenitis stage. Scarlatinalike rashes and erythema nodosum lesions also may develop. The later manifestations of lymphogranuloma venereum occur as the result of scarring of the lymph channels and fibrosis of the nodes. These changes result in rectal stricture, swelling of the penis or the vulva, and ulceration.

Etiology. Lymphogranuloma venereum is caused by one of the chlamydozoaceae, *Miyagawanella lymphogranulomatosus*, which is related to the rickettsiae. Previously, the organism was classified as a "large" virus.

Diagnostic Skin Test. The Frei intradermal test is positive in any patient who has had the disease for 3 weeks. The test is performed by injecting 0.1 ml. of the antigen (Lygranum, Squibb) and 0.1 ml. of the control material intradermally. The reaction is of the delayed tuberculin-type. To be positive the papule should exceed 6 mm. in diameter within 48 hours (the surrounding zone of erythema is not important), and the control site should not exceed 3 mm.

Treatment. Sulfonamides, chlortetracycline (Aureomycin), and oxytetracycline (Terramycin) are effective in the early stages when continued for several weeks.

MEASLES

A very common childhood disease. The characteristic points are as follows. The incubation period averages 14 days before the appearance of the rash. The prodromal stage appears around the 9th day after exposure and consists of fever, conjunctivitis, running nose, Koplik spots and even a faint red rash. The Koplik spots measure from 1 to 3 mm. in diameter, are bluish-white on a red base and occur bilaterally on the mucous membrane around the parotid duct and on the lower lip. With increasing fever and cough the "morbilliform" rash appears, first behind the ears and on the forehead, then spreads over face, neck, trunk and extremities. The fever begins to fall as the rash comes out. The rash is a faint reddish, patchy eruption, occasionally papular. Scaling occurs in the end stage. Complications include

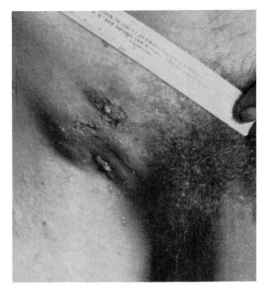

Fig. 14-8. Lymphogranuloma venereum, showing lymph node involvement. (*Dr. T. B. Hall*)

secondary bacterial infection and encephalitis.

Differential Diagnosis

German Measles: postauricular nodes, milder fever and rash, no Koplik spots (see below).

Scarlet Fever: circumoral pallor, rash brighter red and confluent (p. 129).

Drug Eruption: history of new drugs, usually no fever (p. 60).

Infectious Mononucleosis: rash similar, see characteristic blood picture, high titer of heterophile antibodies.

Treatment

Prophylactic. Measles virus vaccine, live, attenuated, can be administered.

Active. Supportive therapy for the cough, bed rest, and protection from bright light are measures for the active disease. The antibiotics have eliminated most of the bacterial complications. Corticosteroids are of value for the rare but serious complication of encephalitis.

GERMAN MEASLES

While this is a benign disease of children, it is serious if it develops in a pregnant woman during the first trimester, since it causes anomalies in a low percentage of newborns.

The incubation period is around 18 days and, as with measles, there may be a short prodromal stage of fever and malaise. The rash also resembles measles since it occurs first on the face and then spreads. However, the redness is less intense, and the rash disappears within 2 to 3 days. Enlargement of the cervical and the postauricular nodes is a characteristic finding. Serious complications are rare.

Differential Diagnosis

Measles: see Koplik spots; the fever and the rash are more severe; no postauricular nodes (p. 157).

Scarlet Fever: has high fever, perioral pallor; rash may be similar (p. 129).

Drug Eruption: get new drug history, usually no fever (p. 60).

Treatment

Prophylactic. Rubella virus vaccine, live, attenuated, can be administered.

Active. Active treatment is usually unnecessary. Gamma globulin given to a pregnant woman in the first trimester of pregnancy may prevent malformations in the fetus.

ROSEOLA

This is a common exanthem of children of 6 to 18 months of age. The incubation period is 10 days, but a contact history is rarely helpful. Characteristically, there is a high fever up to 105° for 4 to 5 days. With the appearance of the rash the fever and the malaise subside. The rash is mainly on the trunk as a faint red macular eruption. It fades in a few days. There are no severe complications.

Differential Diagnosis. Measles, German measles, scarlet fever, infectious mononucleosis and drug eruption.

Treatment. Not necessary except to reduce the high fever.

ERYTHEMA INFECTIOSUM

Also known as fifth disease, this exanthem occurs in epidemics and is thought to be caused by a virus.

It affects children primarily, but in a large epidemic many cases are seen in adults. In the Kansas City epidemic of the Spring of 1957 over 1,000 cases occurred, and this description is based on personal observation of that epidemic.

The incubation period varies from 1 to 7 weeks. In children the prodromal stage lasts from 2 to 4 days and is manifested by low-grade fever and occasionally joint pains. When the red macular rash develops it begins on the arms and the face and then spreads to the body. The rash in children is measleslike on the body, but on the face it looks as though the cheeks had been slapped. On the arms and the legs the rash is more red and confluent on the extensor surfaces. A low-grade fever persists for a few days after the onset of the rash, which lasts for approximately 1 week.

In adults the rash on the face—the "slap"—is less conspicuous, joint complaints are more common, and itching is present.

Etiology. A viral etiology has not been proved.

Differential Diagnosis

Drug Eruption (p. 60).

Measles (coryza, eruption begins on face and behind ears, p. 157).

Coxsackie and ECHO Virus Infections (Several distinct viruses have been isolated from these groups. The clinical picture varies somewhat for each virus and includes macules, papules and vesicles on the skin, and ulcers of the mouth. Most commonly seen in children in the summertime.)

Other Measleslike Eruptions

Treatment. Not necessary.

BIBLIOGRAPHY

Blank, H., and Rake, G.: Viral and Rickettsial Diseases of the Skin, Eye and Mucous Membranes of Man. Boston, Little, Brown & Co., 1955.

Horsfall, F. L., Jr., and Tamm, Igor: Viral and Rickettsial Infections of Man. ed. 4. Philadelphia, J. B. Lippincott, 1965.

Nahmias, A. J., Josey, W. E., and Naib, Z. M.: Infection with Herpesvirus Hominis Types 1 & 2. Progress in Dermatology, 4:7, 1969. (Published by the Dermatology Foundation)

15

Dermatologic Mycology

Fungi can be present as part of the normal flora of the skin or as abnormal inhabitants. We are concerned with the abnormal inhabitants or pathogenic fungi.

Pathogenic fungi have a predilection for certain body areas; most commonly it is the skin, but the lungs, the brain and other organs can be infected. Pathogenic fungi can invade the skin *superficially* and *deeply* and are thus divided into these two groups.

SUPERFICIAL FUNGAL INFECTIONS

The superficial fungi live on the dead horny layer of the skin and elaborate an enzyme that enables them to digest keratin, causing the superficial skin to scale and disintegrate, the nails to crumble, and the hairs to break off. The deeper reactions of vesicles, erythema and infiltration are presumably due to the fungi liberating an exotoxin. Fungi are also capable of eliciting an allergic or id reaction.

It will be necessary to define a few mycologic terms before proceeding further. When a skin scraping, a hair or a culture growth is examined with the microscope in a wet preparation (see p. 11 and Fig. 2-3) the two structural elements of the fungi will be seen: the spores and the hyphae.

Spores are the reproducing bodies of the fungi. Sexual and asexual forms occur. Spores are rarely seen in skin scrapings.

Hyphae are threadlike, branching filaments that grow out from the fungus spore. The hyphae are the identifying filaments seen in skin scrapings in potassium hydroxide (KOH) solution.

Mycelia are matted clumps of hyphae that grow on culture plates.

Culture media vary greatly in context, but modifications of Sabouraud's dextrose agar are used to grow the superficial fungi (Fig. 2-4). Sabouraud's agar and cornmeal agar are both used for the deep fungi. Hyphae and spores grow on the media, and identification of the species of fungi is established by the gross appearance of the mycelia, the color of the substrate, and the microscopic appearance of the spores and the hyphae when a sample of the growth is placed on a slide.

CLASSIFICATION

The latest classification divides the superficial fungi into three genera: *Microsporum, Epidermophyton* and *Trichophyton*. Only two of these species invade the hair: *Microsporum* and *Tricophyton*. As seen in a KOH preparation *Microsporum* causes an ectothrix infection of the hair shaft, whereas *Tricophyton* causes either an ectothrix or an endothrix infection. The ectothrix fungi cause the formation of an external spore sheath around the hair, whereas the endothrix fungi do not. The filaments of mycelia penetrate the hair in both types of infection.

Table 1 correlates the species of fungi with the clinical diseases. The organism causing tinea versicolor is not included in this table because it does not liberate a keratolytic enzyme.

ORAL GRISEOFULVIN THERAPY

Since the discovery of a specific systemic anti-fungal agent, griseofulvin, many physicians have felt that (1) griseofulvin was indicated for every fungus infection and (2) most skin diseases are due to a fungus, so they should treat the patient with griseofulvin and make a diagnosis later. Both of these assumptions are erroneous.

TABLE 15-1—RELATIONSHIP OF FUNGI TO BODY AREAS

	FEET AND HANDS	NAILS	GROIN	SMOOTH SKIN	SCALP	BEARD
Microsporum						
1. *M. audouini*	0	0	0	Mod. common	Common	0
2. *M. canis*	0	0	0	Common	Mod. common	Rare
3. *M. gypseum*	0	0	0	Rare	Rare	0
Epidermophyton						
E. floccosum	Mod. common	Rare	Common	Mod. common	0	0
Trichophyton						
1. Endothrix species						
a. *T. schoenleini*	0	Rare	0	Rare	(Favus) rare	0
b. *T. violaceum*	0	Rare	0	0	Rare	Rare
c. *T. tonsurans*	0	Rare	0	Rare	Mod. common	0
2. Ectothrix species						
a. *T. mentagrophytes*	Common	Mod. common	Common	Rare	Rare	Mod. common
b. *T. rubrum*	Common	Common	Mod. common	Rare	0	Rare
c. *T. verrucosum*	0	0	0	Rare	Rare	Rare

In general, the physician should be aware of the following facts:

1. Correct diagnosis of a fungal infection is necessary. Do not prescribe oral griseofulvin for your patient if you are not sure of the diagnosis. Griseofulvin is of no value in treating atopic eczema, contact dermatitis, psoriasis, monilial infections, pityriasis rosea, etc.

2. Treat with adequate dosage. Know (1) the correct daily dose for the particular type of fungal infection and (2) the correct duration of such dosage.

3. Generally speaking, oral griseofulvin therapy should not be used to treat tinea of the feet and tinea of the toenails. The recurrence rate after therapy is completed is very high, even after a year or more of "adequate" therapy.

4. Do not treat monilial infections with oral griseofulvin. Very commonly, monilial intertrigo of the groin or monilial paronychias are erroneously treated with griseofulvin. Griseofulvin is of no value in these conditions and, since it is a penicillin related drug, usually even aggravates the existing disease.

5. Tinea versicolor does not respond to oral griseofulvin therapy.

6. So-called "fungal infection of the ear" does not respond to oral griseofulvin therapy, since most external ear diseases are not caused by a fungus. (See External Otitis, p. 74).

CLINICAL CLASSIFICATIONS

Superficial fungal infections of the skin affect various sites of the body. The clinical lesions, the species of fungi, and the therapy vary for these different sites. Therefore, fungal diseases of the skin are classified, for clinical purposes, according to the location of the infection. These clinical types are as follows:

Tinea of the feet (Tinea pedis)
Tinea of the hands (Tinea manus)
Tinea of the nails (Onychomycosis)
Tinea of the groin (Tinea cruris)
Tinea of the smooth skin (Tinea corporis)
Tinea of the scalp (Tinea capitis)
Tinea of the beard (Tinea barbae)
Dermatophytid
Tinea versicolor (see p. 107)

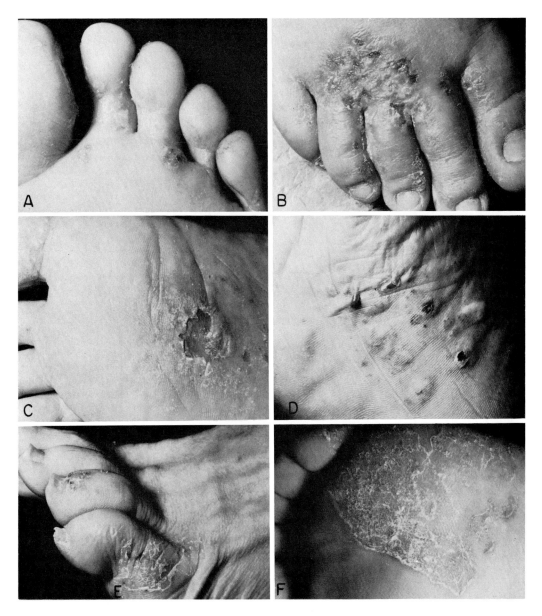

Fig. 15-1. Tinea of the foot. The top 4 photographs demonstrate acute infection, and the bottom 2 show chronic tinea infection.

Tinea of the external ear (see External Otitis, p. 74).

TINEA OF THE FEET
(Plate 40)

Tinea of the feet (athlete's foot, fungal infection of the feet, ringworm of the feet) is a very common skin infection. Many persons have the disease and are not even aware of it. The clinical appearance varies (Fig. 15-1).

Primary Lesions. Acute form: blisters on the soles and the sides of feet or between the toes. Chronic form: lesions are dry and scaly.

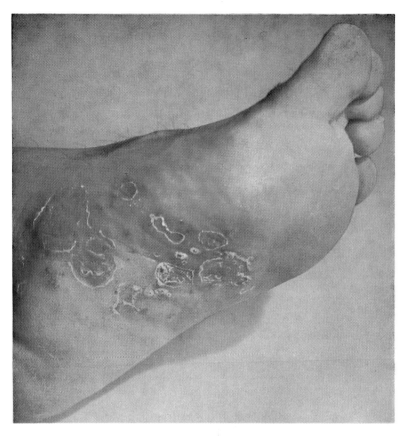

Plate 40. Tinea of the foot. This dry scaly form of fungus infection is usually due to *T. rubrum.* (*Smith, Kline & French Laboratories*)

Secondary Lesions. Bacterial infection of the blisters is very common; also see maceration and fissures.

Course. Recurrent acute infections can lead to a chronic infection. If the toenails become infected, a cure is highly improbable, since this focus is very difficult to eradicate.

The species of fungus influences the response to therapy. Most vesicular, acute fungal infections are due to *Trichophyton mentagrophytes* and respond readily to correct treatment. The chronic scaly type of infection is usually due to *T. rubrum* and is exceedingly difficult, if not impossible, to cure.

Contagiousness. Experiments have shown that there is a susceptibility factor necessary for infection. Males are much more susceptible than females, even when the latter are exposed.

Laboratory Findings. KOH-ink preparations of scrapings and cultures on Sabouraud's media serve to demonstrate the presence of fungi and the specific type. A KOH preparation is a very simple office procedure and should be resorted to when the diagnosis is uncertain or the response to therapy is slow (p. 11).

Differential Diagnosis

Contact dermatitis due to shoes, socks, gloves, foot powder (usually on dorsum of feet or hands; history of new shoes or new foot powder; fungi not found, p. 49).

Atopic eczema of feet, especially on

dorsum of toes in children (quite chronic; usually in winter; very pruritic; atopic family history; on dorsum of toes; fungi not found, p. 56 and Plate 58).

Psoriasis of soles and palms (rarely vesicular or pustular, thickened, well-circumscribed lesions; psoriasis elsewhere on body; fungi not found; p. 97).

Pustular Bacterid: pustular lesions only; chronic; resistant to local therapy; fungi not found.

Hyperhidrosis of Feet: can be severe and cause white, eroded maceration of the soles, accompanied by a foul odor.

Symmetric lividity of the soles. (Fig. 15-2) A rather common condition of the soles of the feet characterized by the presence of patches of macerated whitish sharply defined odoriferous skin associated with hyperhidrosis (see above).

Treatment

1. AN ACUTE VESICULAR, PUSTULAR FUNGAL INFECTION of 2 weeks' duration on the soles of the feet and between the toes in a 16-year-old boy. This clinical picture is usually due to the organism *T. mentagrophytes.*

A. Minimize the fear of the infectiousness of athlete's foot but emphasize normal cleanliness, including the wearing of slippers over bare feet, wiping the feet last after a bath (not the groin last), and changing socks daily (white socks are not necessary).

B. Débridement. The doctor or the patient should snip off the tops of the blister with small scissors. This enables the pus to drain out and allows the medication to reach the organisms. The edges of any blister should be kept trimmed, since the fungi spread under these edges. Follow this débridement by a foot soak.

C. Boric acid crystals

Sig: 1 tablespoon of boric acid crystals to 1 quart of warm water. Soak feet for 10 minutes twice a day. Dry skin carefully afterward.

D. Sulfur, ppt.   5%
   Neosporin or other antibiotic
   ointment q.s.   15.0

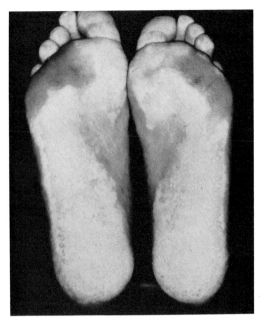

Fig. 15-2. Symmetric lividity of the soles. This is associated with hyperhidrosis.

Sig: Apply b.i.d. locally to feet after soaking. (The sulfur is antifungal, and the Neosporin is antibacterial for the secondary bacterial infection.)

E. Rest at home for 2 to 4 days may be advisable.

F. Place small pieces of cotton sheeting or cotton between the toes when wearing shoes.

SUBSEQUENT TREATMENT 5 days later. The secondary infection and blisters have decreased.

A. The soaks may be continued for another 3 days or stopped if no marked redness or infection is present.

B. Substitute the following salve for the first milder one:

Sulfur, ppt.   5%
Benzoic and salicylic acid oint.
(U.S.P.) q.s.   15.0

Sig: Apply small amount b.i.d. locally to feet. (Other antifungal ointments can be used as the base, such as Tinactin, Halotex, Desenex, Enzactin, Salundek and Verdefam.)

Tinactin soln (10 ml.) is quite effective. Apply a few drops on affected skin and rub in.

C. Boric Acid   2%
Sulfur   4%
Antifungal powder q.s. 45.0

Sig: Supply in powder can. Apply small amount to feet over the salve and to the shoes in the morning. (Antifungal powder bases include Desenex, Enzactin, Sopronal, Vioform, etc.)

D. Griseofulvin therapy. This form of oral treatment is not recommended for tinea of the feet because (1) response to griseofulvin is slow for these acute and rather disabling cases, (2) the recurrence rate is very high, and (3) the cost of oral therapy for 6 to 8 weeks is much greater than that of the more rapidly effective local therapy.

2. A CHRONIC, SCALY, THICKENED FUNGAL INFECTION of 4-years' duration that has in the past week developed a few small tense blisters on the sole of the feet. This type of clinical picture probably is due to the organism *T. rubrum*.

A. Tell the patient that you can clear up the acute flare-up (the blisters) but that it will be very difficult and time-consuming on his part to cure the chronic infection. If the toenails are found to be infected, the prognosis for cure is even poorer. (See "Tinea of the Nails," below.)

B. Debride and trim the blisters with manicure scissors.

C. Sulfur, ppt.   5%
Benzoic and salicylic acid oint.
(U.S.P.)   15.0

Sig: Apply locally to soles b.i.d. or
Tinactin soln.   10.0

Sig: rub in a few drops b.i.d.

D. Soaks in the following solution will soften the scales and aid in the penetration of the salve:

Sodium Thiosulfate (Hypo)
                               240.0

Sig: 2 tablespoons to 1 quart of warm water. Soak feet for 10 minutes once a day.

SUBSEQUENT VISIT OF RESISTANT CASE

A. 0.5% Anthralin ointment (Anthra-Derm, Dermik)   45.0

Sig: Apply to soles of feet h.s. Caution: Wash hands thoroughly afterward and do not touch eyes—an irritant.

B. Griseofulvin therapy. This type of oral therapy is not recommended for chronic tinea of the feet. But the patient may have heard or read about the "pill for athlete's feet," so it would be wise for you to discuss this with the patient. If you mention that you cannot guarantee a cure even after months of taking a large quantity of rather expensive pills, most patients will be content with keeping the chronic infection in an innocuous state with sporadic local therapy.

However, if after you have explained about the poor results and the expense of therapy the patient still wants to try oral therapy, use this dosage regime: Griseofulvin (Fulvicin U/F, 250 mg.; Grisactin, 250 mg.; Grifulvin, 250 mg.) q.i.d. for at least 6 weeks and preferably for 3 to 6 months.

TINEA OF THE HANDS
(Plate 41)

A primary fungal infection of the hand or hands is quite rare. In spite of this fact, the diagnosis of "fungal infection of the hand" is commonly applied to cases that in reality are contact dermatitis, atopic eczema, pustular bacterid or psoriasis. The best differential point is that tinea of the hand usually is seen only on one hand, not bilaterally. Since tinea of one hand is usually found with tinea of both feet, this is commonly called "one-hand, two-foot disease."

Primary Lesions. Acute: blisters on the palms and the fingers at the edge of red areas. Chronic: lesions are dry and scaly, and usually there is a single patch, not separate patches.

Secondary Lesions. Bacterial infection is rather unusual.

Course. A gradually progressive disease that spreads to fingernails. Usually nonsymptomatic.

Laboratory Findings. KOH-ink preparations will reveal mycelia, or cultures

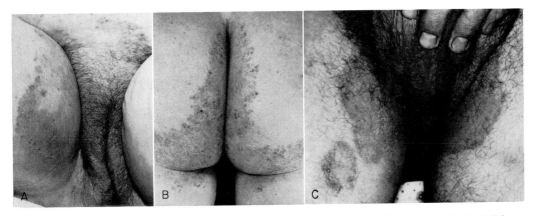

Fig. 15-3. Tinea of the groin area and the buttocks. (*A*) Fungal infection of the thigh and the pubic area in a female. (*B*) Fungal infection that has spread from the crural area to the buttocks. (*C*) Tinea of crural area of man. Note sharp border of lesions as compared with indefinite border of monilial intertrigo seen in Figure 15-7 & Plate 43.

on Sabouraud's media will grow the fungus (see p. 11).

Differential Diagnosis

Contact Dermatitis of Hands: due to soap, detergents and other irritants (usually bilateral, periodic, more vesicular and less frequently chronic; fungi not found; p. 49).

Atopic Eczema: history of atopy in patient or family; bilateral; periodic; fungi not found (see p. 56).

Psoriasis: see thick patch or patches in palms of menopausal women, usually bilateral; occasionally see psoriasis elsewhere; fungi not found (see p. 97).

Pustular Bacterid: pustular lesions only; periodic and chronic; resistant to local therapy; fungi not found.

Dyshidrosis of Palms: recurrent; seasonal incidence; mainly vesicular; not scaly; bilateral; related to atopic eczema; fungi not found.

Treatment

A man with scaly thickening of one palm of 8 years' duration. No fingernails involved. Itches slightly at times.

1. Griseofulvin therapy. Unless the cost is prohibitive, this oral therapy should be used for every case.

Griseofulvin, ultra-fine, (250 mg. or equivalent) q.i.d. for 3 months is usually curative. Rarely does the dose have to be higher or for a longer term.

TINEA OF THE NAILS
(Plate 41 and 51)

Tinea of the toenails is very common but tinea of the fingernails is uncommon. Tinea of the toenails is almost inevitable in patients who have recurrent attacks of tinea of the feet. Once developed, the infected nail serves as a resistant focus for future skin infection.

Primary Lesions. Begin as distal or lateral detachment of nail with subsequent thickening and deformity.

Secondary Lesions. Bacterial infection can result from the pressure of shoes on the deformed nail and surrounding skin.

Distribution. The infection usually begins in the 5th toenail and may remain there or spread to involve the other nails.

Course. *Tinea of the toenails can rarely be cured.* Aside from the deformity and an occasional mild flare-up of acute tinea, treatment is not necessary. Progression is slow, and spontaneous cures are rare.

Tinea of the fingernails can be cured, but the treatment usually takes months.

Etiology. Usually due to *T. rubrum* and, less importantly, to *T. mentagrophytes.*

Laboratory Findings. These organisms can be found in a KOH preparation of a scraping and occasionally can be grown

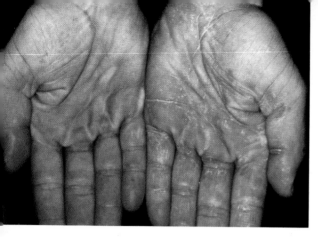

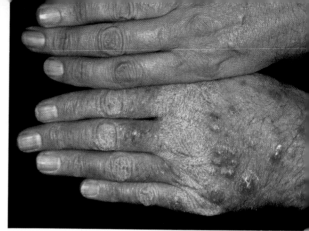

(A) Tinea of left palm only due to *T. mentagrophytes*

(B) Deep tinea of left hand, due to *T. mentagrophytes*

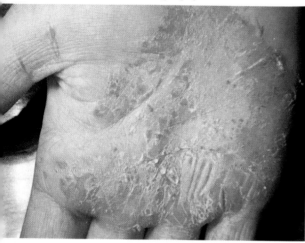

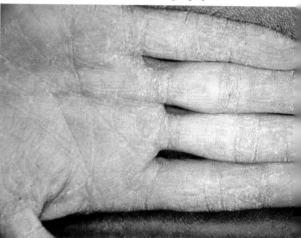

(C) Tinea of palm due to *T. rubrum*

(D) Tinea of palm of dry scaly type due to *T. rubrum*

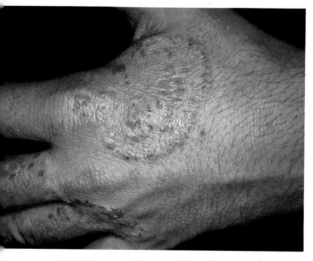

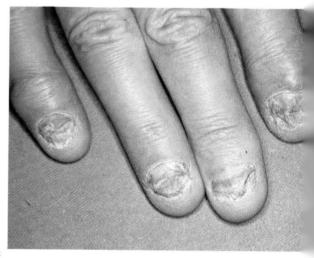

(E) Tinea on dorsum of hand due to *T. mentagrophytes* in a diabetic, age 15

(F) Tinea of fingernails due to *T. rubrum*

Plate 41. Tinea of the hand and fingernails. (Tinea of hand usually only affects *one* hand, but *both* feet. Thus, it is called "one hand, two foot syndrome.") (*Duke Laboratories, Inc.*)

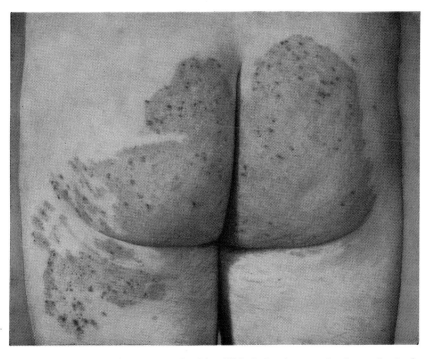

Plate 42. Tinea of the smooth skin. This infection on the buttocks had spread from the crural region. (*Smith, Kline & French Laboratories*)

on culture media. The material should be gathered from the debris under the nail plate.

Differential Diagnosis (See chapter on nail diseases, p. 228.)

Nail Injury: get history of such, although tinea infection often starts in an injured nail; absence of fungi.

Psoriasis of Fingernails: see pitting, red areas under nail with resulting detachment; psoriasis elsewhere usually; no fungi found (p. 97).

Psoriasis of Toenails: impossible to differentiate from tinea, since most psoriatic nails have some secondary fungal invasion.

Moniliasis of Fingernails: common in housewives; paronychial involvement common; monilia found (p. 175).

Green Nails: Another fingernail infection called "green nails" yields *C. albicans* and *Ps. aeruginosa* most commonly. Clinically, there is a distal detachment of the nail plate with underlying greenish-brown debris.

Treatment of Tinea of Fingernails. A young salesman has a fungal infection in 3 fingernails of 9 months' duration. The surrounding skin shows mild redness and scaling.

1. Griseofulvin therapy. This oral therapy is the treatment of choice.

Griseofulvin (250 mg. or equivalent) q.i.d for approximately 9 months. Therapy is stopped when there is no clinical evidence of infection (crumbling, thickening of nail plate, or subungual debris) and no cultural or KOH-ink mount evidence of fungi.

Treatment of Tinea of Toenails. A 45-year-old woman has 3 infected toenails on the right foot and 2 on the left foot. These are causing mild pain when she wears certain tight-fitting shoes. Scaliness of soles of feet is also evident.

1. Griseofulvin therapy. This oral therapy is *not* effective or indicated for tinea of the toenails. I have never seen a case that was cured. Apparently some derma-

tologists have cured cases after oral therapy was continued for several years or when oral griseofulvin was combined with evulsion of the toenails. Nonetheless, I do not recommend it. The only time such therapy for toenails is prescribed, in my practice, is when the patient understands the problem but still wants to attempt a a cure with at least 18 months of therapy.

2. Onycho-Phytex liquid, 15 ml. For the patient who wants to "do something," applications 2 to 4 times a day for months might help some mild cases. One can combine this therapy with débridement of the nails.

3. Debriding of thick nails by patient, dermatologist or chiropodist offers obvious relief from discomfort. This can be accomplished by filing or picking away with a broken piece of glass, a sharp knife, a razor blade or a motor-driven drill (see p. 337).

4. Surgical evulsion of the toenail is rarely curative. As stated above, this surgical approach can be combined with oral griseofulvin therapy with probable enhancement of the end-result.

TINEA OF THE GROIN
(Plate 42)

This is a common, itching, annoying fungal infection of the groin appearing usually in males and often concurrently with tinea of the feet (Fig. 15-3). Home remedies often result in a contact dermatitis that adds fuel to the fire.

Primary Lesions. Bilateral fan-shaped, red, scaly patches with a sharp, slightly raised border. Small vesicles may be seen in the active border.

Secondary Lesions. Oozing, crusting, edema and secondary bacterial infection. In chronic cases lichenification may be marked.

Distribution. Crural fold and extending to involve scrotum, penis, thighs, perianal area and buttocks.

Course. The type of fungus influences the course, but most acute cases respond rapidly to treatment. Other factors that affect the course and recurrences are obesity, hot weather, sweating, and chafing garments.

Etiology. Commonly due to the fungi of tinea of the feet, *T. rubrum*, and *T. mentagrophytes*, and also the fungus *E. floccosum*.

Infectiousness. Minimal, even between husband and wife.

Laboratory Findings. The organism is found in KOH preparations of scrapings and can be grown on culture. Take material from the active border (see p. 11).

Differential Diagnosis

Moniliasis: no sharp border; see fine scales, oozing, redness, satellite pustule-like lesions at edges; commoner in obese females; monilia found (p. 175 and Plate 43).

Contact Dermatitis: often coexistent but can be separate entity; new contactant history; no fungi found; no active border (p. 49).

Prickly Heat: pustular, papular; no active border, no fungi; may also be present with tinea (p. 320).

Neurodermatitis: unilateral usually; may have resulted from old chronic tinea; no fungi (p. 72).

Psoriasis: usually unilateral; may or may not have raised border; psoriasis elsewhere; no fungi (p. 97).

Erythrasma: faint redness, fine scaling with no elevated border, also seen in axilla and webs of toes; reddish fluorescence under Wood's light; due to a diphtheroid organism called *Corynebacterium minutissimum* (p. 125).

Treatment

Oozing, red dermatitis with sharp border in crural area of young man.

1. Since the infection usually comes from chronic tinea of the feet, to prevent recurrences advise the patient to dry the feet last and not the groin area last when taking a bath.

2. Griseofulvin oral therapy
   Griseofulvin (ultra-fine) 250 mg.
   Sig: 1 tablet q.i.d. for 6 to 8 weeks.

For mild cases or where the expense of oral griseofulvin therapy is a factor, the following local treatment is quite effective.

3. Vinegar wet packs

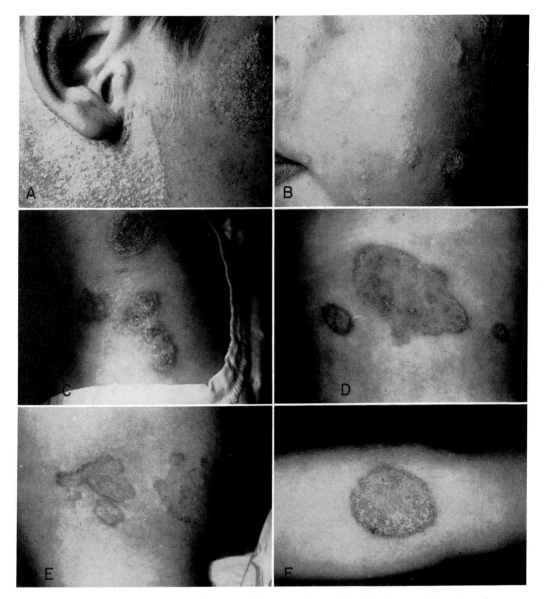

Fig. 15-4. Tinea of the smooth skin. (*See also* Plate 58) (*A*) Tinea of face in a farm boy. (*B*) Tinea of face due to *M. canis.* (*C*) Tinea of the side of neck. (*D*) Tinea of thigh due to *T. mentagrophytes.* (*E*) Tinea of buttocks due to *T. rubrum.* (*F*) Tinea of forearm due to *T. mentagrophytes.*

Sig: ½ cup of white vinegar to 1 quart of warm water. Wet the sheeting or thin toweling and apply to area for 15 minutes twice a day.

4. Sulfur, ppt.   5%
    Nonalcoholic white shake lotion
        (See Formulary p. 37) q.s.   90.0
    Sig: Apply locally t.i.d.

SUBSEQUENT VISIT, oozing gone.
1. Tinactin soln. 10 ml. or this cream:
    Sulfur ppt.   5%
    Hydrocortisone powder   1%
    Antifungal cream q.s.   15.0
    Sig: Apply locally t.i.d.
2. Apply a small amount of this solution in the office with a cotton swab:

| Chrysarobin | 3% |
| Chloroform q.s. | 15.0 |

This is very effective for resistant, dry, scaly patches. It stings after application. Caution patient to avoid touching the area with his fingers and then rubbing his eyes.

TINEA OF THE SMOOTH SKIN
(Plate 58)

The familiar ringworm of the skin is most common in children because of their intimacy with animals and other children (Fig. 15-4). The lay public believes that *most* skin conditions are "ringworm," and many physicians erroneously agree with them.

Primary Lesions. Round, oval, or semi-circular scaly patches with slightly raised border that commonly is vesicular. Rarely, deep ulcerated granulomatous lesions are due to superficial fungi.

Secondary Lesions. Bacterial infection, particularly at the advancing border, is common in association with certain fungi, such as *M. canis* and *T. mentagrophytes.*

Course. Infection is short-lived if treated correctly. Seldom recurs unless treatment is inadequate.

Etiology. Most commonly due to *M. canis* from kittens and puppies; to *M. audouini* from other children who usually also have scalp infection; and less commonly due to *E. floccosum* and *T. mentagrophytes* from groin and foot infections.

Infectiousness. Incidence is high.

Laboratory Findings. Same as for previously discussed fungal diseases.

Differential Diagnosis

Pityriasis Rosea: history of herald patch; sudden shower of oval lesions; fungi not found (p. 103).

Impetigo: vesicular, crusted; most commonly on face; no fungi found (p. 114).

Contact Dermatitis: no sharp border or central healing; may be coexistent with ringworm due to overtreatment (p. 49).

Treatment

A child has several 2- to 4-cm. sized scaly lesions on his arms of 1 week's duration. He has a new kitten which he holds and plays with.

1. Examine the scalp, preferably with a Wood's light, to rule out scalp infection.

2. Advise the mother regarding moderate isolation procedures in relation to the family and others.

3. Tinactin soln. 10 ml. or this cream:

| Sulfur ppt. | 5% |
| Antifungal salve q.s. | 15.0 |

Sig: Apply b.i.d. locally. (Antifungal bases that can be used include Tinactin, Desenex, Salundek, Enzactin, etc.)

SUBSEQUENT VISIT OF RESISTANT CASE OR A NEW WIDESPREAD CASE

Griseofulvin oral therapy.

Griseofulvin (ultra-fine) can be given in tablet or oral suspension form. The usual dose for children is 250 mg. b.i.d., but the pharmaceutical company's product information sheet should be consulted. Therapy should be maintained for 3 to 6 weeks or until lesions are gone. Occasionally a higher dose is needed in deeper forms of infection.

TINEA OF THE SCALP
(Plate 58)

Tinea of the scalp is the commonest cause of patchy hair loss in children (Fig. 15-5). Endemic cases are with us always, but epidemics, usually due to the human type, were, until the discovery of griseofulvin, the real therapeutic problem. Griseofulvin orally finds its greatest therapeutic usefulness and triumph in the management of tinea of the scalp. Before griseofulvin, children with the human type of scalp tinea had to be subjected to traumatic shampoos and salves for weeks or months, or they had to be epilated by x-ray. Often they were kept out of school for this entire period of therapy.

Tinea capitis infections can be divided into two clinical types: *noninflammatory* and *inflammatory.* The treatment, the cause and the course vary for these two types.

Noninflammatory Type

Primary Lesions. Grayish, scaly, round patches with broken-off hairs, causing balding areas. The size of the areas varies.

Fig. 15-5. Tinea of the scalp. (*See also* Plate 58)

(*A*) Due to *M. audouini.* Note absence of visible inflammation.

(*B*) Due to *T. tonsurans.* Wood's light examination revealed no fluorescence.

(*C*) Due to *T. mentagrophytes.* Note inflammation.

(*D*) Favus, due to *T. schoenleini,* of 11 years' duration.

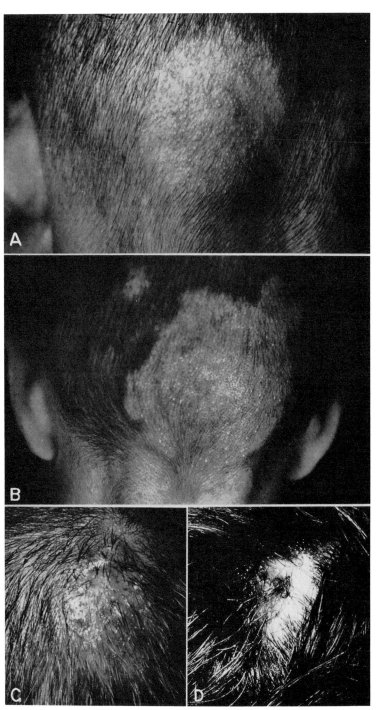

Secondary Lesions. Bacterial infection and id reactions are rare. A noninflammatory patch can become inflamed spontaneously or as the result of strong local treatment. Scarring almost never occurs.

Distribution. Commonest in posterior scalp region. Body ringworm from the scalp lesions is common, particularly on the neck and the shoulders. *Perform Wood's light examination of scalp on any child with ringworm of the smooth skin.*

Course. The incubation period in and on the hair is short, but clinical evidence of the infection cannot be expected under 3 weeks after inoculation. Parents often do not notice the infection for another 3 weeks to several months, particularly in girls. Spontaneous cures are rare in 2 to 6 months but after that time occur with greater frequency. Some cases last for years if untreated. Recurrence of the infection after the cure of a previous episode is rare but not impossible, since adequate immunity does not develop.

Age Group. Infection of the noninflammatory type is commonest between the ages of 3 and 8 and is rare after the age of puberty. This adult resistance to infection is attributed in part to the higher content of fungistatic fatty acids in the sebum after puberty. This research laboratory finding had great therapeutic significance, and the direct outgrowth was the development of Desenex, Timofax, Salundek and other fatty acid ointments and powders.

Etiology. The noninflammatory type of scalp ringworm is caused most commonly by *M. audouini*, occasionally by *M. canis*

and rarely by *T. tonsurans*. *M. audouini* and *T. tonsurans* are anthropophilic fungi (human-to-human passage only), whereas *M. canis* is a zoophilic fungus (animals are the original source, mainly kittens and puppies).

Contagiousness. High incidence in children. The case can be a part of a large urban epidemic.

Laboratory Findings. *Wood's light examination of the scalp hairs* is an important diagnostic test. The Wood's light is a specially filtered ultraviolet light. The hairs infected with *M. audouini* and *M. canis* fluoresce with a bright yellow-green color (Plate 58). Over 90 percent of the tinea capitis in the United States and Canada is due to these fungi, so very few cases will be missed by this light. *The bright fluorescence of fungus-infected hairs is not to be confused with the white or dull yellow color emitted by lint particles or sulfur-laden scales.* An inexpensive but excellent Wood's light is described on page 337.

Microscopic examination of the infected hairs in 20 percent potassium hydroxide solution shows an ectothrix arrangement of the spores when due to the *Microsporum* species, and endothrix spores when due to *T. tonsurans*. Culture is necesary for species identification but is not practical in most offices. The cultural characteristics of the various fungi can be found in many larger dermatologic or mycologic texts and will not be presented here.

Differential Diagnosis

	Wood's Light	Scales	Redness	Hair Loss	Remarks
Tinea capitis	+	Dry or crusted	Uncommon	Yes	Back of scalp, child
Alopecia areata (p. 224)	−	None	No	Yes	Exclamation point hairs at edges
Seborrheic derm. (p. 87)	−	Greasy	Yes	No	Diffuse scaling
Psoriasis (p. 97)	−	Thick and dry	Yes	No	Look at elbows, knees and nails
Trichotillomania (p. 225)	−	None	No	Yes	Psychoneurotic child
Pyoderma (p. 114) (with or without lice)	−	Crusted	Yes	Occasional	Poor hygiene

Prophylactic Treatment

1. Infected individuals may attend school, provided that (a) the child wears a cotton stockinette cap at all times (no swapping allowed), and (b) a note must be presented from the physician every 3 weeks, stating that the child is under a doctor's care. Infected children should be restricted from theaters, churches, and other public places. Consult your own Health Department for specific rulings.

2. Inspection of all susceptible school children with a Wood's light by school nurse every 4 weeks during an epidemic.

3. Wash hair after every haircut at a barber shop.

4. Provide parent-and-teacher education on methods of spread of disease, particularly during an epidemic.

5. Suggest provision for individual storage of clothing, particularly caps, in school and home.

Active Treatment

1. Griseofulvin oral therapy. The ultra-fine types of griseofulvin (Fulvicin U/F, Grifulvin V, and Grisactin) can be administered in tablet form or liquid suspension (not all brands available in liquid form). The usual dose for a child age 4 to 8 is 250 mg. b.i.d., but some require a larger dose. The duration of therapy is usually 6 to 8 weeks. But both dose and duration have to be individualized and based on clinical, Wood's light or culture response.

2. Manual epilation of hairs. Near the end of therapy, the remaining infected and fluorescent hairs can be plucked out, or the involved area can be shaved closely. This will eliminate the infected distal end of the growing hair.

Inflammatory Type

Primary Lesions. Pustular, scaly round patches with broken-off hairs, causing bald areas.

Secondary Lesions. Bacterial-like infection is common. When the secondary reaction is marked the area becomes swollen and tender. This inflammation is called a *kerion*. Minimal scarring sometimes remains.

Distribution. Any scalp area. Concurrent body ringworm infection is common.

Course. Duration much shorter than the noninflammatory type of infection. Spontaneous cures will result after 2 to 4 months in majority of cases, even if untreated.

Etiology. The inflammatory type of scalp ringworm is most commonly caused by *M. canis*, occasionally by *M. audouini*, rarely by *M. gypseum*, *T. mentagrophytes* and *T. verrucosum*. Except for *M. audouini* in the species are zoophilic, that is, passed from infected animals or soil.

Contagiousness. High incidence in children and farmers. Endemic except for cases due to *M. audouini*.

Laboratory Findings. Microscopic examination of the infected hairs in 20 percent potassium hydroxide solution shows an ectothrix arrangement of the spores. The hairs infected with *M. canis* and *M. audouini* fluoresce with a bright yellowish-green color under the Wood's light.

Differential Diagnosis (see chart on p. 172).

Prophylactic Treatment

1. Same as for noninflammatory cases but less stringent.

Active Treatment

1. Griseofulvin oral therapy (as above under noninflammatory type)

2. Local therapy. For some mild cases of the inflammatory type, or where drug expense is a factor, local therapy can be used with good results.

Sulfur, ppt.   5%
Sterosan or Vioform ointment,
q.s.   15.0
Sig: Apply locally b.i.d. The scalp and the hair should be shampooed nightly.

3. If kerion is severe, with or without griseofulvin therapy:

A. Boric acid or Burow's solution wet packs

Sig: 1 tablespoon of boric acid crystals, or 1 Domeboro tablet, to 1 quart of warm water. Apply soaked cloths for 15 minutes twice a day.

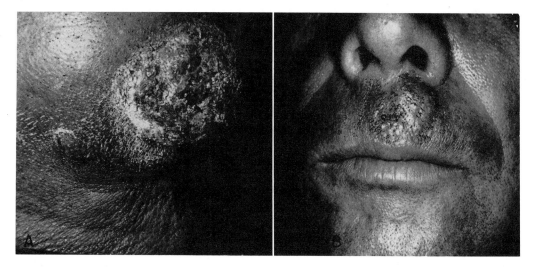

Fig. 15-6. Tinea of the beard area. (*A*) Of the chin. (*B*) Of the upper lip due to *T. mentagrophytes.*

B. Antibiotic therapy orally helps to eliminate secondary bacterial infection.

TINEA OF THE BEARD

Fungal infection is a rare cause of dermatitis in the beard area. Farmers occasionally contract it from infected cattle (Fig. 15-6). Any presumed bacterial infection of the beard that does not respond readily to proper treatment should be examined for fungi.

Primary Lesions. Follicular pustular lesions, or sharp bordered ringworm-type lesions, or deep boggy inflammatory masses.

Secondary Lesions. Bacterial infection is common. Scarring is unusual.

Etiology (see table, p. 160).

Differential Diagnosis

Bacterial folliculitis: acute onset, rapid spread; no definite border; responds rather rapidly to local therapy; no fungi found on examination of hairs or culture (p. 119).

Treatment

Farmer with a quarter-sized boggy inflammatory, pustular mass on chin of 3-weeks' duration.

1. Have veterinarian inspect cattle if farmer is not aware of source of infection.

2. Boric acid wet packs

Sig: 1 tablespoon of boric acid to 1 quart of hot water. Apply wet cloths to area for 15 minutes twice a day.

3. Sulfur, ppt.   5%
   Antifungal ointment, q.s.   15.0
   Sig: Apply locally b.i.d.

4. Griseofulvin oral therapy. The usual dose of griseofulvin for an adult is 250 mg. q.i.d. for 6 to 8 weeks or longer depending on clinical response, or negative Sabouraud's culture.

DERMATOPHYTID

During an acute episode of any fungal infection, an id eruption can develop over the body. This is a manifestation of an allergic reaction to the fungal infection. The commonest id reaction occurs on the hands during an acute tinea infection on the feet. To assume a diagnosis of an id reaction the following criteria should be followed: (1) the primary focus should be acutely infected with fungi, not chronically infected; (2) the id lesions must not contain fungi; and (3) the id eruption should disappear or wane following adequate treatment of the acute focus.

Primary Lesions. Vesicular eruption of the hands (primary on the feet); papulo-follicular eruption on body (primary commonly is scalp kerion); pityriasis-rosea-

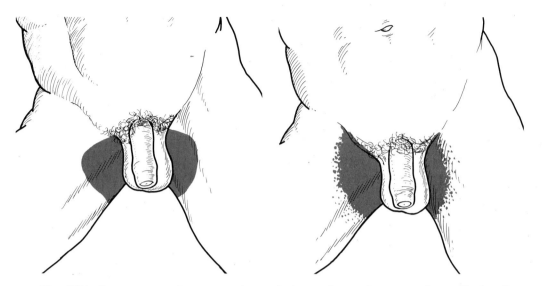

Fig. 15-7. Dermograms for comparison of tinea of crural area and moniliasis of crural area. (*Left*) Tinea of crural area. Note sharp border of lesions. *See also* Fig. 15-3 and Plate 42. (*Right*) Moniliasis of crural area. Note indefinite border with satellite pustulelike lesions at edge. Moniliasis can also involve the scrotum. *See also* Plate 44.

like id eruptions and others are seen less commonly.

Secondary Lesions. Excoriation and infection when itching is severe, which is unusual.

Treatment

1. Treat the primary focus of infection.
2. For a vesicular id reaction on the hands:

    A. Boric acid soaks

      Sig: 1 tablespoon of boric acid to 1 quart of cool water. Soak hands for 15 minutes twice a day.

3. For an id reaction on the body that is moderately pruritic.

    A. Linit starch or Aveeno oatmeal bath

      Sig: ½ of small box of Linit starch or 1 packet of Aveeno to 6 to 8 inches of cool water in a tub, once daily.

    B. Alcoholic white shake
      lotion (See Formulary
      p. 37)   120.0

      Sig: Apply locally b.i.d. Menthol 0.25% or phenol 0.5%, or camphor 2% could be added to this lotion.

4. For a severely itching generalized id eruption:

    A. Prednisone 5 mg. or related corticosteroid tablets   #20

      Sig: 1 tablet q.i.d. for 2 days then 1 t.i.d. for 4 days (or longer if necessary).

DEEP FUNGAL INFECTIONS

Those fungi that invade the skin deeply and go into living tissue are also capable of involving other organs. Only the skin manifestations of these deeply invading fungi will be the concern of this book.

The following diseases are included in this group of deep fungal infections. Other rarer deep mycotic diseases will be found in the Dictionary-Index and in Chapter 31, *Geographic Skin Diseases.*

Moniliasis
Sporotrichosis
Actinomycosis
North American blastomycosis

MONILIASIS
(Plates 43, 44 and 45)

Moniliasis is a fungal infection caused by *Candida albicans* which produces le-

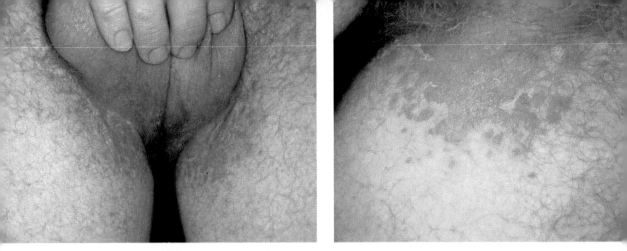

(*A & B*) Monilial intertrigo of crural area and closeup showing satellite lesions without the sharp border as seen in tinea cruris

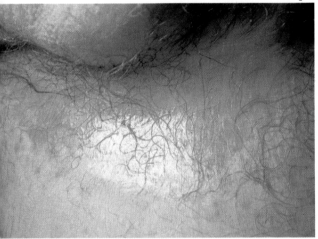

(*C*) Moist monilial intertrigo of crural area

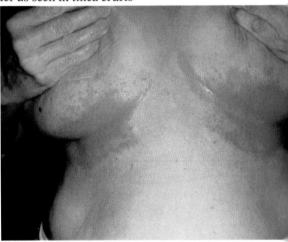

(*D*) Monilial intertrigo under breasts

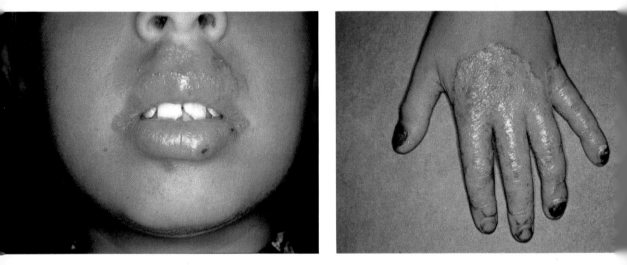

(*E & F*) Extensive moniliasis around the mouth and on dorsum of hand in child with Addison's disease

Plate 43. Monilial Infections. (*See also* Plate 51 for monilial paronychia and Plate 57 for infant monilial diseases.) (*G. S. Herbert Laboratories*)

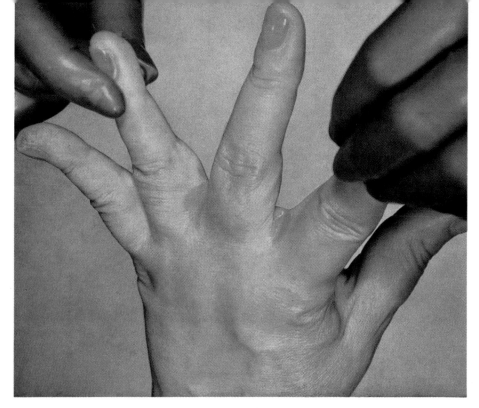

Plate 44. Monilial intertrigo of the webs of the fingers. (*Smith, Kline & French Laboratories*)

Plate 45. Monilial intertrigo under the breast. (Note the lack of a definite border to the eruption which distinguishes it from a tinea infection.) (*Smith, Kline & French Laboratories*)

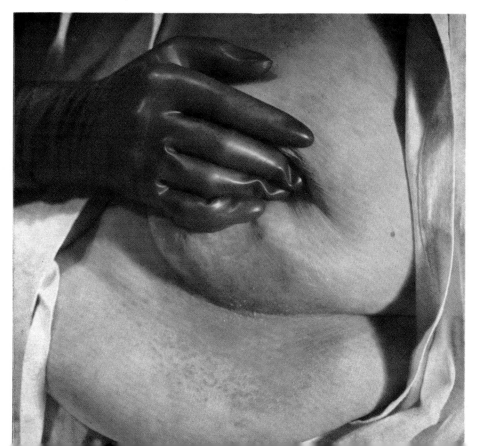

sions in the mouth, the vagina, the skin, the nails, the lungs, the gastrointestinal tract, or occasionally, a septicemia. The latter condition apparently has been seen in increasing frequency since the advent of the oral antibiotics. Since *C. albicans* exist commonly as a harmless skin inhabitant, the laboratory finding of this organism is not adequate proof of its pathogenicity and etiologic role. Monilia commonly seed pre-existing disease conditions. This book will be concerned with the *cutaneous* and the *mucocutaneous* monilial diseases. The following classification will be helpful.

1. Cutaneous moniliasis
    A. Localized diseases
        a. Monilial paronychia (Plate 51).
A common monilial infection which is characterized by development of painful, red swellings of the skin around the nail plate. In chronic infections the nail becomes secondarily thickened and hardened. Monilial paronychia is commonly seen in housewives and those individuals whose occupations predispose to frequent immersions of the hands in water. This nail involvement is to be differentiated from *superficial tinea of the nails* (the monilial infection does not cause the nail to lose its luster or to become crumbly, and debris does not accumulate beneath the nail), and from *bacterial paronychia* (this is more acute in onset and throbs with pain).

        b. Monilial intertrigo (Fig. 15-7 B and Plates 43 and 45). A moderately common condition characterized by well-defined, red, eroded patches, with scaly, pustular or pustulovesicular diffuse borders. The commonest sites are axillae, inframammary areas, umbilicus, genital area, and anal area, and webs of toes and fingers. Obesity and diabetes predispose to the development of this intertriginous type. It is to be differentiated from *superficial tinea infections*, which are not as red and eroded, and from *seborrheic dermatitis*.

    B. Generalized cutaneous moniliasis. (Plate 57) This rare infection involves the smooth skin, mucocutaneous orifices and intertriginous areas. It follows in the wake of general debility and is very resistant to treatment.

2. Mucous membrane moniliasis (Plate 43)
    A. Oral moniliasis (thrush and perlèche). Thrush is characterized by creamy white flakes on a red, inflamed mucous membrane. The tongue may be smooth and atrophic, or the papillae may be hypertrophic as in the condition labeled "hairy tongue." Perlèche is seen as cracks or fissures at the corners of the mouth, usually associated with monilial disease elsewhere and a dietary deficiency. A nonmonilial clinically similar condition is commonly seen in *elderly people with ill-fittting dentures* where the corners of the mouth override. Oral moniliasis is also to be differentiated from *allergic conditions*, such as those due to tooth paste or mouthwash.

    B. Monilial vulvovaginitis. The clinical picture is an oozing, red, sharply bordered skin infection surrounding an inflamed vagina that contains a buttermilklike discharge. This type of monilial infection is frequently seen in pregnant women and diabetics. It is to be differentiated from an *allergic condition*, or from *trichomonal vaginitis*.

    Laboratory findings for all of above monilial diseases: Skin or mucous membrane scrapings placed in 20 percent potassium hydroxide solution and examined with the high-power microscope lens will reveal small, oval, budding, thin-walled yeastlike cells with occasional mycelia. Culture on Sabouraud's media will produce creamy dull-white colonies in 4 to 5 days. Further cultural studies on cornmeal agar are necessary to identify the species as *Candida albicans*.

Treatment

Monilial paronychia of 2 fingers in a 37-year-old male bartender.

1. Advise patient concerning avoiding exposure of his hands to soap and water by wearing cotton gloves under rubber gloves, hiring a dishwasher, etc.
2. Sporostacin solution, or Onycho-Phytex liquid q.s.   15.0

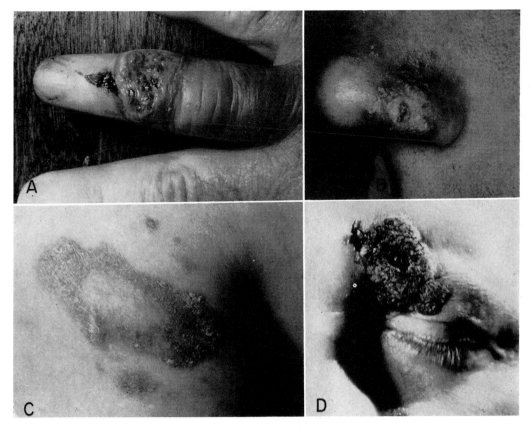

Fig. 15-8. Deep fungus infections. (*A*) Sporotrichotic chancre of the finger. (*B*) Sporotrichotic primary lesion of nose. (*C*) North American blastomycosis lesions on the posterior aspect of the shoulder. (*D*) North American blastomycosis lesion of eyebrow.

Sig: Apply to base of nail q.i.d. (Continue treatment for several weeks).

3. At night apply:

    Sulfur, ppt.   5%

    Benzoic and salicylic acid oint. (U.S.P.) q.s.   15.0

    Sig: Apply locally h.s. (or Sporostacin, Mycostatin, or Sterosan cream can be used as the base.)

Monilial intertrigo of inframammary and crural region in an elderly obese female.

1. Advise patient to wear pieces of cotton sheeting under breasts to keep the opposing tissues drier. Frequent bathing with thorough drying is helpful.

2. Fungizone lotion, or Nysta-Dome lotion, or

Sporostacin lotion or

Sulfur, ppt.   5%

Nonalcoholic white shake lotion q.s.   60.0

Sig: Apply locally t.i.d.

3. Powder can be used over lotion:

    Mycostatin Dusting Powder, q.s. 15.0

    Sig: Apply locally t.i.d.

Monilial vulvovaginitis in a 6-months pregnant woman.

1. Mycostatin vaginal tablets, 100,000 U.   #20

    Sig: Insert one tablet b.i.d. in vagina.

2. Fungizone lotion, or Nysta-Dome lotion, or

    Sporostacin lotion, or

    Sulfur, ppt.   5%

    Calamine lotion, q.s.   60.0

Sig: Apply locally b.i.d. to vulvar skin.

Important: Do not treat any monilial infection with oral or local antibacterial antibiotic, or with oral griseofulvin. This will intensify monilial infection. Know all of the ingredients of any salve or powder that you prescribe.

SPOROTRICHOSIS

Sporotrichosis is a granulomatous fungal infection of the skin and the subcutaneous tissues. Characteristically, a primary chancre precedes more extensive skin involvement (Fig. 15-8 A and B). Invasion of the internal viscera is rare. (Also see p. 328).

Primary Lesion. A sporotrichotic chancre develops at the site of skin inoculation, which is commonly the hand, less commonly the face or the feet. The chancre begins as a painless, movable, subcutaneous nodule that eventually softens and breaks down to form an ulcer.

Secondary Lesions. Within a few weeks subcutaneous nodules arise along the course of the draining lymphatics and form a chain of tumors that develop into ulcers. This is the classic clinical picture, of which there are variations.

Course. The development of the skin lesions is slow and rarely affects the general health.

Etiology. *Sporotrichum schenckii*, a fungus that grows on wood and in the soil. It invades open wounds and is an occupational hazard of farmers, laborers and miners.

Laboratory Findings. Cultures of the purulent material from unopened lesions readily grow on Sabouraud's media.

Differential Diagnosis. Consider any of the skin granulomas such as pyodermas, syphilis, tuberculosis, sarcoidosis and leprosy. An ioderma or bromoderma can cause a similar clinical picture.

Treatment

1. Saturated solution of potassium iodide   60.0 cc.
   Sig: On the first day, 10 drops t.i.d., p.c. added to milk or water. Second day, 15 drops t.i.d.; third day, 20 drops t.i.d. and increase until 30 to 40 drops t.i.d. are given. The initial doses may be smaller and the increase more gradual if one is concerned about tolerance. Watch for gastric irritation and ioderma. Continue this very specific treatment for 1 month after apparent cure.

ACTINOMYCOSIS

Actinomycosis is a deep fungal disease that characteristically causes the formation of a granulomatous draining sinus. The commonest location of the draining sinus is in the jaw region, but thoracic and abdominal sinuses do occur.

Primary Lesion. Red, firm, nontender tumor in jaw area that slowly extends locally to form a "lumpy jaw."

Secondary Lesions. Discharging sinuses that become infected with bacteria and, if untreated, may develop into osteomyelitis.

Course. General health is usually unaffected unless extension occurs into bone or deeper neck tissues. Recurrence is unusual if treatment is continued long enough.

Etiology. *Actinomyces israelii*, which is an anaerobic fungus that lives as a normal inhabitant of the mouth, particularly in individuals who have poor dental hygiene is causative. Injury to the jaw or a tooth extraction usually precedes the development of the infection. Infected cattle are not the source of human infection. The disease is twice as frequent in males as in females.

Laboratory Findings. Pinpoint-sized "sulfur" granules, which are colonies of the fungi, can be seen grossly and microscopically in the draining pus. A gram stain of the pus will show masses of interlacing gram-positive fibers with or without club-shaped processes at the tips of these fibers. The organism can be cultured anaerobically on special media.

Differential Diagnosis. Consider pyodermas, tuberculosis and neoplasm.

Treatment

1. Penicillin, 2,400,000 units intramuscularly daily until definite improvement is noted. Then oral penicillin in the same

dosage should be continued for 3 weeks after the infection apparently has been cured. In severe cases, 10 million or more units of penicillin given intravenously daily may be necessary.

2. Incision and drainage of the lumps and the sinuses.

3. Institute good oral hygiene.

4. In resistant cases, broad-spectrum antibiotics can be used alone or in combination with the penicillin.

NORTH AMERICAN BLASTOMYCOSIS

Two cutaneous forms of this disease are seen: primary cutaneous blastomycosis and secondary localized cutaneous blastomycosis.

Primary cutaneous blastomycosis occurs in laboratory workers and physicians following accidental inoculation. A primary chancre develops at the site of the inoculation, and the regional nodes enlarge. In a short time the primary lesion and nodes heal spontaneously, and the cure is complete.

The following discussion will be confined to the *secondary cutaneous form.* Systemic blastomycosis is rarer than the cutaneous forms.

Primary Lesion (secondary localized cutaneous form): Begins as a papule that ulcerates and slowly spreads peripherally with a warty, pustular, raised border. The face, the hands and the feet are involved most commonly (Fig. 15-8 C and D).

Secondary Lesion. Central healing of the ulcer occurs gradually with resultant thick scar.

Course. Takes months to develop large lesion. Therapy is moderately effective on a long-term basis. Relapses are common.

Etiology. The fungus *Blastomyces dermatitidis* is thought to invade the lungs primarily and the skin secondarily as a metastatic lesion. High native immunity prevents the development of more than one skin lesion. This immunity is low in the rare systemic form of blastomycosis where multiple lesions occur in the skin, the bones and other organs. This fungal disease affects adult males most frequently.

Laboratory Findings. Collect the material for a 20 percent potassium hydroxide solution mount from the pustules at the border of the lesion. Round budding organisms can be found in this manner or in a culture mount. A chest roentgenogram is indicated in every case.

Differential Diagnosis. Consider any of the granuloma-producing diseases such as tuberculosis, syphilis, iodide or bromide drug eruption, pyoderma and neoplasm.

Treatment

1. Surgical excision and plastic repair of early lesions is quite effective.

2. Amphotericin suppresses the chronic lesion more effectively than any other drug. It is administered by intravenous infusion daily in varying schedules which are described in larger texts or reviews.

BIBLIOGRAPHY

Hildick-Smith, G., Blank, H., and Sarkany, I.: Fungus Diseases and Their Treatment. Boston, Little, Brown & Co., 1965.

Wilson, J. W., and Plunkett, O. A.: The Fungous Diseases of Man. Berkeley, University of California, 1965.

16

Dermatologic Parasitology

This is a very extensive subject and includes the dermatoses due to 3 main groups of organisms: protozoa, helminths and arthropods.

The *protozoal dermatoses* are exemplified by the various forms of trypanosomiasis and leishmaniasis. (See p. 330)

Helminthic dermatoses include those due to roundworms (ground itch, creeping eruption, filariasis and other rare tropical diseases), and those due to flatworms (schistosomiasis, swimmer's itch and others). (Also see p. 320)

Arthropod dermatoses are divided into those caused by 2 classes of organisms: the arachnids (spiders, scorpions, ticks and mites) and the insects (lice, bugs, flies, moths, beetles, bees and fleas).

In this chapter we shall discuss scabies caused by a mite and pediculosis caused by lice. In Chapter 31, **Geographic Skin Diseases,** flea bites, chigger bites, creeping eruption, swimmer's itch and tropical dermatoses will be discussed.

SCABIES

This parasitic infestation is more prevalent in a populace ravaged by war, famine, or disease, when personal hygiene becomes relatively unimportant. In normal times scabies is rarely seen except in school children or in poorer people under crowded conditions. *Scabies should be ruled out in any generalized excoriated eruption.* (See Figs. 16-1 and 16-2.)

Primary Lesions. A minute burrow caused by the female of the mite *Sarcoptes scabiei.* The burrow measures approximately 2 mm. in length and can be hidden by the secondary eruption. Small vesicles may overlie the burrows.

Secondary Lesions. Excoriations of the burrows may be the only visible pathology. In severe, chronic cases bacterial infection may be extensive and take the form of impetigo, cellulitis and furunculosis.

Distribution. Most commonly, the excoriations are seen on the lower abdomen and the back with extension to the pubic and the axillary areas, the legs, the arms and the webs of the fingers. In this day of only mild cases of scabies the eruption is not commonly seen in the webs of the fingers.

Subjective Complaints. Itching is intense, particularly at night when the patient is warm in bed and the mite more

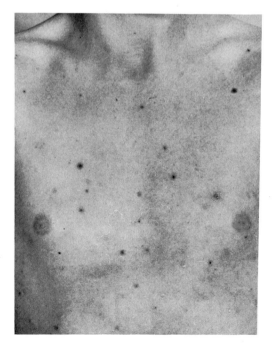

Fig. 16-1. Scabies lesions on a boy's chest. (*K.C.G.H.*)

active. However, many skin diseases itch worse at night, presumably due to a lower itch threshold when relaxation occurs.

Course. The mite can persist for months and years ("seven-year itch") in untreated, unclean individuals.

Contagiousness. Other members of the family may or may not have the disease, depending on the cleanliness of the household and the severity of the infestation.

Laboratory Findings. The female scabies mite and ova may be seen in curetted burrows examined under the low-power magnification of the microscope. Potassium hydroxide (20% solution) can be used to clear the tissue as with fungus smears. Skill is necessary to uncover the mite by curetting.

Differential Diagnosis

Pyoderma: examine the patient carefully to rule out concurrent parasitic infestation; positive history of high carbohydrate diet; only mild itching (p. 114).

Pediculosis Pubis: see lice and eggs on and around hairs; distribution different (p. 183).

Winter Itch: see no burrows; seasonal incidence; elderly patient usually; worse on legs and back (p. 71).

Dermatitis Herpetiformis: see vesicles, urticaria, excoriated papules, eosinophilia, no burrows (p. 192).

Neurotic Excoriations: nervous individual; patient admits picking at lesions; no burrows.

Parasitophobia: usually the patient brings in to the office pieces of skin and debris; showing the patient the debris under a microscope helps to convince him of the absence of parasites.

Treatment

1. Inspect or question concerning other members of family to rule out infestation in them.

2. Instruct patient to bathe thoroughly, scrubbing the involved areas with a brush.

3. Kwell lotion   60.0

Sig: Apply to the entire body from the neck down for 1 to 3 nights.

4. Do not bathe for 72 hours. Old clothes may be reworn.

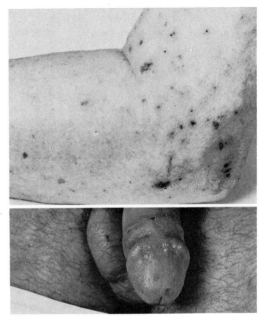

Fig. 16-2. Scabies. (*Top*) On arm. Note excoriations. (*K.U.M.C.*) (*Bottom*) On penis.

5. After 72 hours bathe carefully and change to clean clothes and bedding.

6. Washing, dry cleaning or ironing of clothes or bedding is sufficient to destroy the mite. Sterilization is unnecessary.

7. Itching may persist for a few days in spite of the destruction of the mite. For this apply:

A. Sulfur, ppt.   4%
   Camphor   1%
   Alcoholic white shake lotion,
     q.s.   120.0
   or
B. Eurax cream, q.s.   60.0

This cream has scabiecidal power and antipruritic action combined.

8. If itching persists for 1 to 2 weeks, re-examine patient carefully for burrows and retreat if necessary.

PEDICULOSIS

Lice infestation affects people of all ages but usually those in the lower-income strata because of lack of cleanliness and infrequent changes of clothing. Three clinical entities are produced, (1) infes-

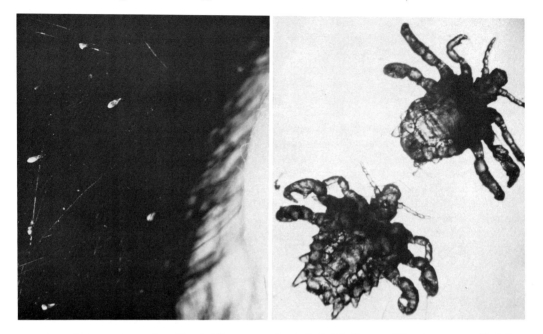

Fig. 16-3. Pediculosis. (*Left*) Nits on scalp hair behind ear. (*Dr. Lawrence Hyde*) (*Right*) Pubic louse or *Phthirus pubis* as seen with 7.5X lens of microscope. (*Dr. James Boley*)

tation of the hair by the head louse, *Pediculus humanus capitis*, (2) infestation of the body by *P. humanus corporis* and (3) infestation of the pubic area by the pubic louse, *Phthirus pubis* (Fig. 16-3). Since lice bite the skin and live on the blood, it is impossible for them to live without human contact. The readily visible oval eggs or nits are attached to hairs or to clothing fibers by the female. After the eggs hatch the newly born lice mature within 30 days. Then the female can live for another 30 days and deposit a few eggs daily.

Primary Lesions. The bite is not unusual but is seldom seen because of the secondary changes produced by the resulting intense itching. In the *scalp* and *pubic form* the nits are found on the hairs, but the lice are found only occasionally. In the *body form* the nits and the lice can be found after careful searching in the seams of the clothing.

Secondary Lesions. In the *scalp form* the skin is red and excoriated, with such severe secondary bacterial infection in some cases that the hairs become matted together in a crusty, foul-smelling "cap." Regional lymphadenopathy is common. A morbilliform rash on the body, an id reaction, is seen in long-standing cases.

In the *body form* linear excoriations and secondary infection, seen mainly on the shoulders, the belt-line and the buttocks, mask the primary bites.

In the *pubic form* the secondary excoriations are again dominant and produce some matting of the hairs. This louse can also infest body, axillary and eyelash hairs. An unusual eruption on the abdomen, the thighs and the arms, called *maculae cerulae* because of the bluish-gray, pea-sized macules, can occur in chronic cases of pubic pediculosis.

Differential Diagnosis of Pediculosis Capitis

Bacterial Infection of the Scalp: responds rapidly to correct antibacterial therapy (p. 116). *All cases of scalp pyoderma must be examined closely for a primary lice infestation.*

Seborrheic Dermatitis or *Dandruff:* the scales of dandruff are readily detached from the hair, while oval nits are not so easily removed (p. 87).

Hair Casts: resemble nits but can be pulled off more easily; no eggs seen on microscopic examination.

Differential Diagnosis of Pediculosis Corporis

Scabies: may see small burrows; distribution of lesions different; no lice in clothes (p. 182).

Senile or Winter Itch: history helpful; see dry skin, aggravated by bathing; will not find lice in clothes (pp. 72 and 71, respectively).

Differential Diagnosis of Pediculosis Pubis

Scabies: will not see nits; see burrows in pubic area and elsewhere (p. 182).

Pyoderma Secondary to Contact Dermatitis from condoms, contraceptive jellies, new underwear, douches: history important; acute onset; no nits (p. 114).

Seborrheic Dermatitis when in eyebrows and eyelashes: no nits found (p. 87).

Treatment

1. *Pediculosis capitis*
   A. Kwell lotion 60.0
   Sig: Shampoo and comb hair thoroughly, then when dry apply medicine. Shampoo again in 3 days and repeat application.
   B. For secondary scalp infection:
   a. Trim hair as much as is possible and agreeable with the patient.
   b. Shampoo hair twice a day with Dial Shampoo.
   c. Neosporin or other antibiotic ointment.
   Sig: Apply to scalp b.i.d.
   C. Change and clean bedding and headwear after 24 hours of treatment. Storage of headwear for 30 days will destroy the lice and the nits.
2. *Pediculosis corporis*
   A. Phenol 0.5%
   Calamine lotion, q.s. 120.0
   Sig: Apply locally b.i.d. for itching. (The lice and the nits are in the clothing.)
   B. Have the clothing laundered or dry cleaned. If this is impossible, dusting with 10% DDT or 10% lindane powder will kill the parasites. Care should be taken to prevent reinfestation. Storage of clothing for 30 days will kill both nits and lice.
3. *Pediculosis pubis:* Same as for scalp form.

17

Bullous Dermatoses

To medical students and practitioners alike, the bullous skin diseases are the most dramatic. One of these diseases, pemphigus, is undoubtedly greatly responsible for the aura that surrounds the exhibition and the discussion of an unfortunate patient with a bullous disease. Happy would be the instructor who could behold such student interest when a case of acne or hand dermatitis is being presented.

Three bullous diseases will be discussed in this chapter: *pemphigus, erythema multiforme bullosum* and *dermatitis herpetiformis*. However, other bullous skin diseases do occur, and in this introduction they will be differentiated from these three.

Bullous Impetigo. The name of *pemphigus neonatorum* has been attached to this pyodermic skin infection because of the resemblance of the large bullae in this disease to pemphigus. This term should be abandoned. Bullous impetigo is to be differentiated from the other bullous diseases by its occurrence in infants and children, rapid development of the individual bullae, presence of impetigo lesions in siblings, and rapid response to local antibiotic therapy (p. 114 and Pediatric Chapter).

Contact Dermatitis Due to Poison Ivy or Similar Plants. Bullae and vesicles are seen in linear configuration; history of pulling weeds or burning brush is usually obtained; past history of poison ivy or related dermatitis is common; duration of disease is only 7 to 14 days (p. 49).

Drug eruption, particularly from sulfonamides and iodides. Elicit drug history; eruption usually clears on discontinuing drugs; bullae appear rapidly (p. 60).

Epidermolysis Bullosa. (Plate 53) This rare chronic hereditary skin disease is manifested by the formation of bullae, usually on the hands and the feet, following mild trauma. The *simple form* of dominant inheritance can begin in infancy or adulthood with the formation of tense, slightly itching bullae at the sites of pressure, which heal quickly without scarring. Forced marches during war can initiate this disease in patients who have the heredity factor. Such cases are usually treated erroneously as athlete's foot. The disease is worse in the summer or may be present only at this time. The *dystrophic form* of recessive inheritance begins in infancy like the simple form, but as time elapses the bullae become hemorrhagic, heal slowly and leave scars which can amputate digits; death can result from secondary infection. Mucous membrane lesions are more common in the dystrophic form than in the simple form. Treatment is supportive. A lethal, non-scarring form is of recessive inheritance also, but is usually fatal within a few months. (See also p. 254 in Genodermatoses Chapter.)

Familial Benign Chronic Pemphigus (Hailey-Hailey Disease). This is a rare hereditary bullous eruption most common on the neck and in the axillae. It can be distinguished from pemphigus by its chronicity and benign nature, and by its histologic picture. Some consider this disease to be a bullous variety of keratosis follicularis (Darier's disease).

Porphyria. The congenital erythropoietic type and the chronic hepatic type (porphyria cutanea tarda) commonly have bullae on the sun-exposed areas of the body. See Dictionary-Index under *Porphyria* and Photosensitivity Chapter, p. 224.

Pemphigoid (Plate 60). A chronic bullous eruption most commonly occurring in elderly adults; usually not fatal. It is differentiated from true pemphigus by the histologic presence of subepidermal bullae without acantholysis and by the presence of immunofluorescent autoantibodies in the basement membrane; from erythema multiforme by its chronicity and the absence of iris lesions; and from dermatitis herpetiformis by the absence of response to sulfapyridine or Diasone therapy.

Benign Mucosal Pemphigoid (Fig. 17-1 and Plate 60). A disabling but nonfatal bullous eruption of the mucous membranes, most commonly involving the eyes. As the result of scarring, which is characteristic of this disease and separates it from true pemphigus, the eyesight is eventually lost. Over 50 percent of the cases have skin lesions. Histologically, the bullae are subepidermal and do not show acantholysis. There is no immunofluorescence by present techniques.

Incontinentia Pigmenti. The first stage of this rare disease of infants manifests itself with bullous lesions primarily on the hands and feet. See Dictionary-Index and Plate 57.

Toxic Epidermal Necrolysis. This rare disease is characterized by large bullae and a quite generalized Nikolsky sign where large sheets of epidermis become detached from the underlying skin. Prognosis is more serious in the adult form than in the childhood form. The cause can be unknown or can be due to drugs, severe bacterial infection or other toxic agents.

Impetigo Herpetiformis. One of the rarest of skin diseases, this is characterized by groups of pustules mainly seen in the axillae and the groin, high fever, prostration, severe malaise and generally a fatal outcome. It occurs most commonly in pregnant or postpartum women. It can be distinguished from pemphigus vegetans or dermatitis herpetiformis by the fact

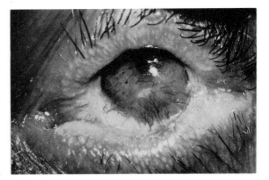

Fig. 17-1. Pemphigus, benign mucous membrane type, of eye. (*Drs. L. Calkins and A. Lemoine*)

that these diseases do not produce such general, acute, toxic manifestations.

In spite of high student and general practitioner interest in the bullous skin conditions, the diagnosis and the management of the 3 main diseases, particularly pemphigus and dermatitis herpetiformis, should be the problem of the dermatologist. Indeed, it is one of the greatest problems in the field of dermatology. It will be the purpose of the author in this chapter to present the salient features of these diseases, with therapy skimmed over lightly.

PEMPHIGUS VULGARIS
(Plates 1 F and 60)

Even though this disease is rare, most doctors see several cases of pemphigus early in their career. Pemphigus cases have to be hospitalized at one time or another during the course of the disease and, as a result, the hospital personnel and staff are exposed to this most miserable, odoriferous, debilitating skin disease. Prior to the advent of corticosteroid therapy the disease was eventually fatal (Fig. 17-2).

Primary Lesions. The early lesions of pemphigus are small vesicles or bullae on apparently normal skin. Redness of the base of the bullae is unusual. Without treatment the bullae enlarge and spread, and new ones balloon up on different areas of the skin or the mucous mem-

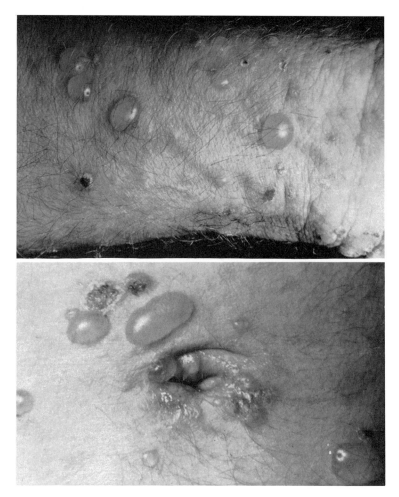

Fig. 17-2. Pemphigus vulgaris.

(*Top*) Pemphigus vulgaris bullae on wrist.

(*Bottom*) Pemphigus vulgaris bullae and crusted lesions around umbillicus. Same patient as above.

branes. Rupturing of the bullae leaves large eroded areas.

Secondary Lesions. Bacterial infection with crusting is marked and accounts in part for the characteristic mousy odor. Lesions that heal spontaneously or under therapy do not leave scars.

Course. When untreated, pemphigus can be rapidly fatal or assume a slow lingering course with debility, painful mouth and body erosions, systemic bacterial infection and toxemia. Spontaneous temporary remissions do occur without therapy.

Three variations of common pemphigus exist.

Pemphigus vegetans is characterized by the development of large granulomatous masses in the intertriginous areas of the axillae and the groin. Secondary bacterial infection, while present in all cases of pemphigus, is most marked in this form. Pemphigus vegetans is to be differentiated from a granulomatous ioderma or bromoderma (p. 60) and from impetigo herpetiformis (p. 187).

Pemphigus foliaceus appears as a scaly, moist, generalized exfoliative dermatitis. The characteristic mousy odor of pemphigus is dominant in this variant, which is also remarkable for its chronicity. The response to steroid therapy is less favorable in the foliaceus form than in the other types. (See also p. 334 for a Brazilian form.)

Pemphigus erythematosus clinically resembles a mixture of pemphigus, seborrheic dermatitis and lupus erythematosus. The distribution of the red, greasy, crusted and eroded lesions is on the butterfly area of the face, the sternal area, the scalp and occasionally in the mouth. The course is more chronic than for pemphigus vulgaris, and remissions are common.

Some dermatologists believe that pemphigus foliaceus and pemphigus erythematosus may be distinct diseases from pemphigus vulgaris and vegetans.

Etiology. Unknown, but autoimmunity is a factor.

Laboratory Findings. The histopathology of early cases is quite characteristic and serves to differentiate most cases of pemphigus from dermatitis herpetiformis and the other bullous diseases. Acantholysis, or separation of intercellular contact between the keratinocytes, is characteristic, and the bulla is intraepidermal. Antiepithelial autoantibodies against the intercellular substance have been found by direct and indirect immunofluorescent tests.

Differential Diagnosis. See Introduction to this chapter; also *dermatitis herpetiformis* and *erythema multiforme bullosum*.

Treatment

1. If possible, a dermatologist or an internist should be called in to share the responsibility of the care.

2. Hospitalization is necessary for the patient with large areas of bullae and erosions. Early cases of pemphigus can be managed in the office.

3. Triamcinolone, 4 mg., or related corticosteroids   #30

Sig: One tablet q.i.d. for 4 days; then reduce the dose slowly as warranted. (Very high doses may be needed to produce a remission in severe cases, along with ACTH intramuscularly or intravenously.)

4. Local therapy is prescribed to make the patient more comfortable and to decrease the odor by reducing secondary infection. This can be accomplished by the following, which must be varied for individual cases.

A. Potassium permanganate crystals
60.0

Sig: Place 2 teaspoons of the crystals in the bathtub with approximately 10 inches of lukewarm water. (To prevent crystals from burning the skin they should be dissolved completely in a glass of water before adding to the tub. The solution should be made fresh daily. The tub stains can be removed by applying acetic acid or "hypo" solution.)

B. Talc   120.0

Sig: Dispense in powder can.

Apply to bed sheeting and to erosions twice a day. (Called a "powder bed.")

C. Sulfur, ppt.   3%
Neo-Polycin or other antibiotic
ointment, q.s.   30.0

Sig: Apply to small infected areas b.i.d.

6. Supportive therapy should be used when necessary. This includes vitamins, iron, blood transfusions and oral antibiotics. Methotrexate therapy is also being used.

7. Nursing care of the highest caliber is a prerequisite for the severe case of pemphigus with generalized erosions and bullae. The nursing personnel should be told that this disease is not contagious or infectious.

DERMATITIS HERPETIFORMIS

Dermatitis herpetiformis is a rare, chronic, markedly pruritic, papular, vesicular and bullous skin disease of unknown etiology (Fig. 17-2, 17-3, 17-4). The patient describes the itching of a new blister as a burning itch which disappears when the blister top is scratched off. The severe scratching results in the formation of excoriations and papular hives which may be the only visible pathology of the disease. Individual lesions heal, leaving an area of hyperpigmentation which is very characteristic. The typical distribution of the blisters or excoriations is on the scalp, the sacral area, the scapular area, the forearms and the thighs. In severe cases, the resulting bullae may be indistinguishable from pemphigus. The duration of dermatitis herpetiformis varies from months to

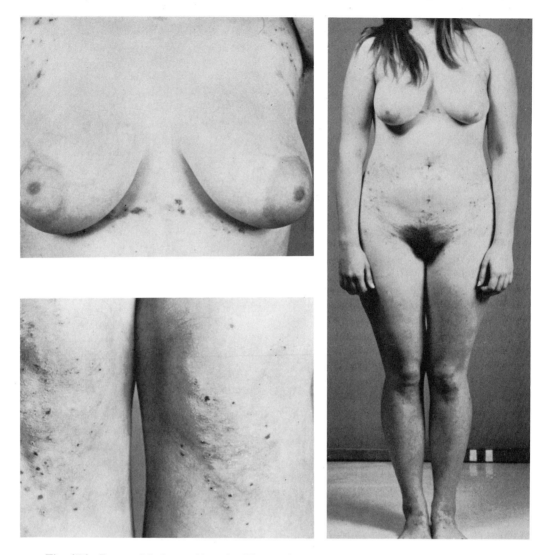

Fig. 17-3. Dermatitis herpetiformis. Front view showing excoriated vesicles on chest and knees. (*K.U.M.C.*)

as long as 40 years, with periods of remission scattered in between. Laboratory tests should include a biopsy which is quite characteristic, and a blood count which shows an eosinophilia.

Herpes gestationis (Plate 48) is dermatitis herpetiformis that occurs in relation to pregnancy. It usually develops during the 2nd or the 3rd trimester, and commonly disappears after birth, only to return with subsequent pregnancies. This variation of dermatitis herpetiformis may be related to an Rh incompatibility.

Differential Diagnosis of Dermatitis Herpetiformis

Pemphigus: see large, flaccid bullae; mouth involvement more commonly in pemphigus; debilitating course; biopsy quite characteristic, eosinophilia uncommon (p. 187).

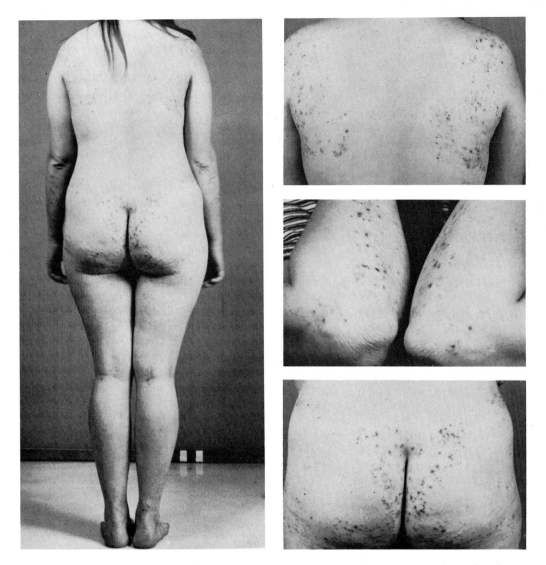

Fig. 17-4. Dermatitis herpetiformis. Back view (same patient as in Fig. 17-3) showing lesions distributed on scapular area, elbows and buttocks. (*K.U.M.C.*)

Erythema Multiforme Bullosum: bullae usually arise on a red irislike base; burning itch is absent; residual pigmentation is minor; course is shorter (p. 193).

Neurotic Excoriations: If this diagnosis is being considered, it is very important to rule out dermatitis herpetiformis, and usually this can be done by finding no scalp lesions, no blisters at any time, no eosinophilia.

Scabies: see no vesicles or bullae; see burrows, lesions in other members of family (p. 182).

Subcorneal pustular dermatosis: a chronic dermatosis characterized by an annular and serpiginous arrangement of pustules and vesico-pustules on the abdomen and the groin and in the axillae. Histopathologically, the pustule is found directly beneath the stratum corneum. Responds to sulfone therapy.

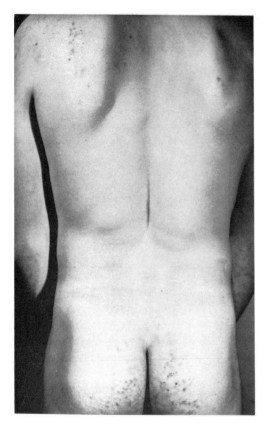

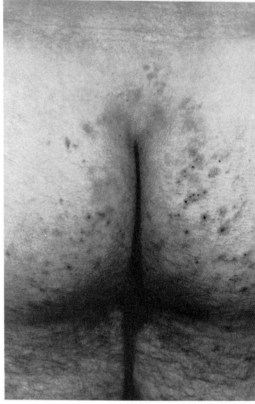

Fig. 17-5. Dermatitis herpetiformis. (*Top, left*) Showing typical distribution of excoriated papules on shoulders and buttocks. No vesicles or bullae present at this time. (*K.U.M.C.*) (*Top, right*) Showing close-up of buttocks lesions. (*K.U.M.C.*) (*Bottom*) Extensive excoriated papules on shoulder. (*K.C.G.H.*)

Treatment

A dermatologist should be consulted to establish the diagnosis and to outline therapy. This would consist of local and oral measures to control itching, and a course of one of the following quite effective drugs: sulfapyridine (0.5 Gm. q.i.d), Diasone (165 mg. q.i.d.) or Avlosulfon (dapsone 100 mg. q.i.d.). These initial doses should be decreased in relation to the patient's response. These drugs can be toxic, and the patient must be under the close surveillance of the physician. Corticosteroids are often used for a short period to give relief in acute flare-ups.

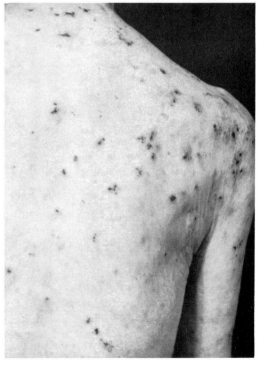

Fig. 17-6. Erythema multiforme bullosum. (*Top*) Bullae and iris lesions on hand.

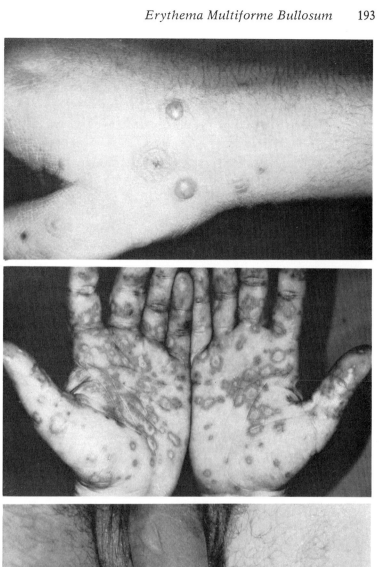

(*Middle*) Same patient with palmar lesions 5 days later.

(*Bottom*) Bullous lesions on penis.

ERYTHEMA MULTIFORME BULLOSUM

This entity has a clinical picture and course distinct from that of erythema multiforme (p. 80). Many drugs can cause an "erythema-multiforme-bullosum-like" picture, but then this manifestation should be labeled a "drug eruption." True erythema multiforme bullosum has no known cause (Fig. 17-2 C). Clinically, it differs from erythema multiforme by the development of large vesicles and bullae usually overlying red irislike macules. The lesions most commonly appear on the arms, the legs and the face but can occur elsewhere, including, on occasion, the mouth. Erythema multiforme bullosum can last from days to months. Slight malaise and fever may precede a new shower of bullae, but for the most part the patient's general health is unaffected. Itching may be mild or severe enough to interfere with sleep. When the characteristic iris lesions are absent, it is difficult to differentiate this bullous eruption from early pemphigus, dermatitis herpetiformis and bullous hives.

Treatment

These patients should be referred to a dermatologist or an internist to substantiate the diagnosis and initiate therapy. Corticosteroids orally and by injection are the single most effective drugs in use today. For widespread cases that must be hospitalized, the local care is similar to that for pemphigus.

BIBLIOGRAPHY

Katz, S. I., and Inderbitzin, T. H.: Autoantibodies in pemphigus and pemphigoid. Progress in Derm., *4*:17, 1969.

Lever, W. F.: Pemphigus and Pemphigoid. Springfield, Charles C Thomas, 1965.

Sams, W. M.: Bullous pemphigoid. Arch. Derm., *102*:485, 1970.

18

Exfoliative Dermatitis

As the term implies, exfoliative dermatitis is a generalized scaling eruption of the skin. The causes are many. This diagnosis never should be made without additional qualifying etiologic terms.

This is a rather rare skin condition, but many general physicians, residents and interns see these cases because they are frequently hospitalized. The purpose of hospitalization is 2-fold: (1) to perform a diagnostic work-up, since the cause in many cases is difficult to ascertain, and (2) to administer intensive therapy under close supervision.

Classification of the cases of exfoliative dermatitis is facilitated by dividing them into primary and secondary forms.

PRIMARY EXFOLIATIVE DERMATITIS

These cases develop in apparently healthy individuals from no ascertainable cause.

Skin Lesions. Clinically, it is impossible to differentiate this primary form from the one in which the etiology is known or suspected. Various degrees of scaling and redness are seen, ranging from fine generalized granular scales with mild erythema to scaling in large plaques with marked erythema and lichenification. Generalized adenopathy is usually present. The nails become thick and lusterless, and the hair falls out in varying degrees.

Subjective Complaint. Itching in most cases is intense.

Course. The prognosis for early cure of the disease is poor. The mortality rate is high in older patients due to generalized debility and secondary infection.

Etiology. Various authors have studied the relationship of lymphomas to cases of exfoliative dermatitis. Some believe the incidence to be low, but others state that from 35 percent to 50 percent of these exfoliative cases, particularly those in patients over the age of 40, are the result of lymphomas. However, years may pass before the lymphoma becomes obvious.

Laboratory Findings. There are no diagnostic changes, but the usual case has an elevated white blood cell count with eosinophilia. Biopsy of the skin is not diagnostic in the primary type. Biopsy of an enlarged lymph node, in either the primary or the secondary form, will reveal *lipomelanotic reticulosis.*

Treatment. A male, age 50, has had a generalized, pruritic, scaly, erythematous eruption for 3 months.

1. A general medical work-up is indicated, either in the office or in the hospital. A focus of infection in the teeth, the tonsils, the gallbladder or the genitourinary tract should be ruled out.

2. A high protein diet should be prescribed, because these patients have a high basal metabolic rate and catabolize protein.

3. Bathing instructions are variable. Some patients prefer a daily cool bath in a colloid solution for relief of itching (1 box of soluble starch or 1 cup of Aveeno to 10 inches of water), but for most cases generalized bathing dries the skin and intensifies the itching.

4. Provide extra blankets for the bed. These patients lose a lot of heat through their red skin and consequently feel chilly.

5. Locally, an ointment is most desired, but some prefer an oily liquid. Formulas for both follow:

   A. White petrolatum   240.0
   Sig: Apply locally b.i.d. (As time

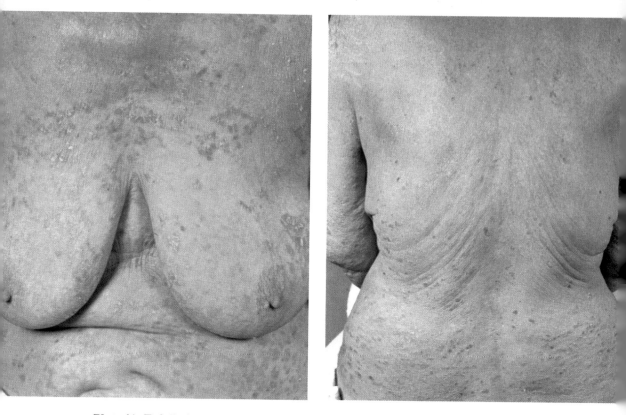

Plate 46. Exfoliative dermatitis due to psoriasis. The primary scaly lesions of psoriasis can be seen on the back and the chest. (*K.U.M.C.*) (*Texas Pharmacal*)

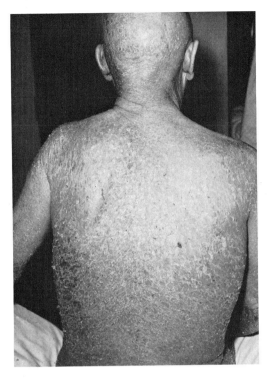

Fig. 18-1. Secondary exfoliative dermatitis. Generalized scaling in patient with leukemia.

progresses more antipruritic effect can be gained by adding menthol 0.25%, or camphor 2%, or phenol 0.5%, or coal tar solution 1% to 5%. Watch for sensitivity to these chemicals, with intensification of itching and erythema.)

    B. Zinc oxide   40%
        Olive oil q.s.   240.0

        Sig: Apply locally with hands or a paint brush b.i.d. (Antipruritic chemicals can also be added to this.)

    6. Oral antihistamine, for example:
        Temaril, 2.5 mg.   #20
        Sig: 1 tablet q.i.d. for itching.

SUBSEQUENT CARE

1. Systemic steroids. For resistant cases the corticosteroids have consistently provided more relief than any other single form of therapy. Any of the preparations can be used, for example:

        Triamcinolone (Kenacort or Aristocort), 4 mg.   #30

        Sig: 1 tablet q.i.d. for 5 days; then 1 tablet b.i.d. or as indicated.

2. Systemic antibiotics may or may not be indicated.

SECONDARY EXFOLIATIVE DERMATITIS
(Plate 46)

The majority of patients with secondary exfoliative dermatitis have had a previous skin disease which became generalized because of overtreatment or for unknown reasons. There always remains a few cases of exfoliative dermatitis in which the cause is unknown but suspected.

Skin Lesions. The clinical picture of this secondary form is indistinguishable from the primary form unless some of the original dermatitis is present. It is important to look for such diagnostic evidence at the edge of an advancing early exfoliative dermatitis or on mildly involved areas.

Course. The prognosis in the secondary form is better than for the primary form, particularly if the original cause is definitely known and more specific therapy can be administered.

Etiology and Treatment. A list follows of the commoner causes of secondary exfoliative dermatitis. The treatment of these cases consists of a combination of that listed above for the primary form of exfoliative dermatitis plus the cautious institution of stronger therapy directed toward the original causative skin condition. This therapy should be reviewed in the section devoted to the specific disease.

Contact dermatitis (p. 49)
Drug eruption (p. 60)
Psoriasis (p. 97)
Atopic eczema (p. 56)
Pyoderma with id reaction (p. 114)
Fungal disease with id reaction (p. 174)
Seborrheic dermatitis (p. 87)
Lymphoma (Fig. 18-1) (p. 281) A useful rule is that 50 percent of all patients over the age of 50, who have an exfoliative dermatitis, have a lymphoma.

BIBLIOGRAPHY

Anderson, P. C., and Loeffel, E. D.: Erythrodermatitis, a review of 40 cases. Missouri Med., *67*:252, 1970.

19

Pigmentary Dermatoses

There are two variants of pigmentation of the skin: hyperpigmentation and hypopigmentation. The predominant skin pigment to be discussed in this chapter is melanin, but other pigments can be present in the skin. A complete classification of pigmentary disorders appears at the end of this chapter.

The melanin-forming cells and their relationship to the tyrosine-tyrosinase enzyme system are discussed on p. 4.

The common clinical example of abnormal hyperpigmentation is chloasma, but secondary melanoderma can result from many causes. The commonest form of hypopigmentation is vitiligo, but secondary leukoderma does occur.

CHLOASMA

Clinical Lesions. An irregular hyperpigmentation of the skin that varies in shades of brown (Fig. 19-1).

Distribution. Usually on the sides of the face, the forehead and the sides of the neck.

Course. Slowly progressive, but remissions do occur. More obvious in the summer.

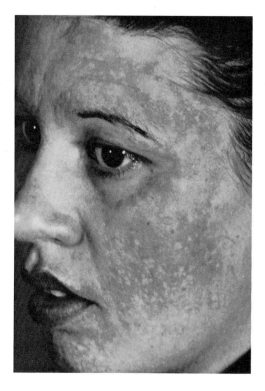

Fig. 19-1. **Chloasma.** This hyperpigmentation became prominent during pregnancy. (*K.C.G.H.*)

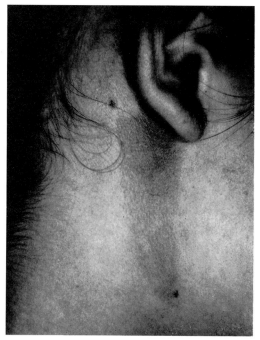

Fig. 19-2. **Secondary hyperpigmentation.** An example of berlock dermatitis on neck due to a photosensitivity reaction from a perfume.

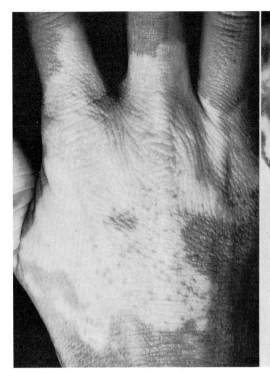

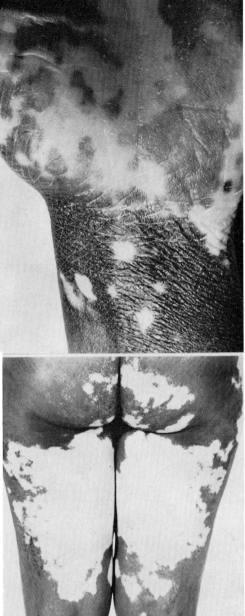

Fig. 19-3. Vitiligo. (*Top, left*) On dorsum of hand of a white patient. Central brown dots show result of 2½ months of 8-MOP therapy. (*Top, right*) On wrist and palm of Negro patient. (*Bottom*) On posterior aspect of thighs of a Negro patient.

Etiology. Unknown, but some cases appear during pregnancy (called "mask of pregnancy") or with chronic illness. There appears to be an increased incidence of chloasma in women taking contraceptive hormones. To be nosologically correct, such cases should be labeled *Drug Eruption, hyperpigmentation, due to hormones.* A lay term for chloasma is "liver spots," but there is no association with liver pathology. The melanocyte-stimulating hormone of the pituitary may be excessive and affect the tyrosine-tyrosinase enzyme system.

Differential Diagnosis. Rule out the causes of *secondary melanoderma* (see end of this chapter). (Fig. 19-2.)

Treatment

1. Do not promise great therapeutic results to the patient. Most cases associated with pregnancy fade or disappear completely following delivery.

   2. Benoquin ointment (Elder)   30.0

     Sig: Apply locally b.i.d. Stop if irritation develops.

The active chemical in this ointment, monobenzyl ether of hydroquinone, was discovered following an investigation of

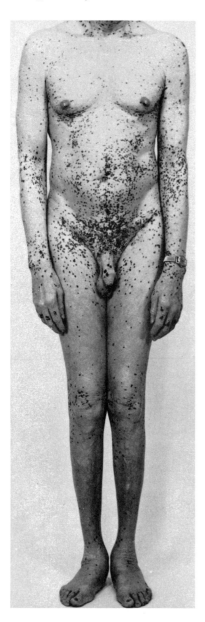

Fig. 19-4. Secondary hypopigmentation. A marked example of loss of pigment that occurred in a Negro male following healing of an exfoliative dermatitis. Corticosteroids were used in the therapy.

the cause of an occupational leukoderma which occurred in Negroes exposed to rubber-aging compounds in the rubber industry.

Allergic contact reactions to this drug occur in an appreciable number of cases. If this happens, the 5 percent Benoquin lotion or the even milder Eldoquin lotion can be substituted, or a salve containing 5 percent ammoniated mercury in white petrolatum. Since therapy is not very effective, if you have a patient who is not too concerned, the suggestion of using only cosmetic covering is adequate advice.

VITILIGO

Clinical Lesions. Irregular areas of depigmented skin occasionally seen with a hyperpigmented border (Fig. 19-3).

Distribution. Most commonly on the face and the dorsum of hands and feet, but can occur on all body areas.

Course. Slowly progressive, but remissions and changes are frequent. More obvious during the summer because of the tanning of adjacent normal skin.

Etiology. Unknown. Heredity is a factor in some cases.

Differential Diagnosis. Rule out causes of secondary hypopigmentation (see end of this chapter). (Fig. 19-4.)

Treatment

An attractive young woman with large depigmented patches on her face and dorsum of hands asks if something can be done for her "white spots." Her sister has a few lesions.

1. Cosmetics. The use of the following covering or staining preparations is recommended: pancake type cosmetics, such as Covermark by Lydia O'Leary; walnut juice stain; or potassium permanganate solution in appropriate dilution. Many patients with vitiligo become quite proficient in the application of these agents. If the patient desires a more specific treatment, the following can be suggested with certain reservations:

2. Psoralen derivatives. For many years Egyptians along the Nile River chewed certain plants to cause the disappearance of the white spots of vitiligo. Extraction of the chemicals from these plants revealed the psoralen derivatives to be the

active agents, and one of these, 8-methoxy-psoralen (8 MOP), was found to be the most effective. This chemical is now manufactured in this country under the name of Oxsoralen (Elder) in 10 mg. capsules and also a topical liquid form. The results of the necessary long-term therapy with this chemical have been so disappointing that I do not prescribe it any more. Its greatest usefulness has been and continues to be as a research tool.

A short 2-week course of these capsules (20 mg. per day) has been advocated for the purpose of acquiring a better and quicker suntan. The value of such a course has been questioned.

Trisoralen (Elder) is a synthetic psoralen in 5 mg. tablets. The recommended dosage is 2 tablets taken 2 hours before measured sun exposure for a long term course. Detailed instructions accompany the package. Some dermatologists feel this therapy to be quite effective.

CLASSIFICATION OF PIGMENTARY DISORDERS

A. Melanin hyperpigmentation or melanoderma
1. Chloasma
2. Incontinentia pigmenti
3. Secondary to skin diseases
   a. Chronic discoid lupus erythematosus (Fig. 20-1)
   b. Tinea versicolor
   c. Stasis dermatitis
   d. Many cases of dermatitis in Negroes and other dark-skinned individuals
   e. Scleroderma
4. Secondary to external agents
   a. X-radiation
   b. Ultraviolet
   c. Sunlight
   d. Tars
   e. Photosensitizing chemicals as in cosmetics causing development of the clinical entities labeled as Riehl's melanosis, poikiloderma of Civatte, berlock dermatitis (Fig. 19-2) and others.

5. Secondary to internal disorders
   a. Addison's disease
   b. Chronic liver disease
   c. Pregnancy
   d. Hyperthyroidism
   e. Internal carcinoma causing malignant form of acanthosis nigricans
   f. Hormonal influence on benign acanthosis nigricans
   g. Intestinal polyposis causing mucous membrane pigmentation (Peutz-Jehgers syndrome)
   h. Albright's syndrome
   i. Schilder's disease
   j. Fanconi's syndrome
6. Secondary to drugs such as ACTH, estrogens, progesterone, melanocyte-stimulating hormone

B. Nonmelanin pigmentations
1. Argyria due to silver salt deposits
2. Arsenical pigmentation due to ingestion of inorganic arsenic as in Fowler's solution and Asiatic pills
3. Pigmentation from heavy metals such as bismuth, gold, and mercury
4. Tattoos
5. Black dermographism, the common bluish-black or green stain seen under watches and rings in certain people from the deposit of the metallic particles reacting with chemicals already on the skin
6. Hemosiderin granules in hemochromatosis or bronze diabetes
7. Bile pigments from jaundice
8. Yellow pigments following atabrine and chlorpromazine ingestion
9. Carotene coloring in carotinosis
10. Homogentisic acid polymer deposit in ochronosis

C. Hypopigmentation
1. Albinism
2. Vitiligo
3. Leukoderma or acquired hypopigmentation
   a. Secondary to skin diseases such as tinea versicolor, chronic dis-

coid lupus erythematosus (Fig. 20-1), localized scleroderma, psoriasis, secondary syphilis, pinta, etc.

b. Secondary to chemicals such as mercury compounds and monobenzyl ether of hydroquinone

c. Secondary to internal diseases, such as hormonal diseases, and in Vogt-Koyanagi syndrome

d. Associated with pigmented nevi (leukoderma acquisitum centrifugum or Sutton's disease)

BIBLIOGRAPHY

Kenney, J. A.: Vitiligo treated with psoralens. Arch. Derm., *103*:475, 1971.

20

Collagen Diseases

The diseases commonly included in this group are lupus erythematosus, scleroderma and dermatomyositis. The skin manifestations are usually a dominant feature of these diseases, but in some cases, particularly acute L. E., skin lesions may be absent. Rheumatoid arthritis and periarteritis nodosa are often included in the collagen disease group but only occasionally are accompanied by skin lesions, usually of the erythema-multiforme-like group (p. 80).

The onset of the collagen diseases is insidious, and the prognosis as to life is serious. It is not unusual to attach the label of "collagen disease" to a patient who has only minimal subjective and objective findings (malaise, weakness, vague joint and muscle pains, biologic false-positive serology and high sedimentation rate) with the realization by the physician that months and years will have to elapse before a more exacting diagnosis of one of the above diseases can be made.

LUPUS ERYTHEMATOSUS
(Plate 47)

Systemic L. E. and chronic discoid L. E. are clinically dissimilar but basically related diseases. The two diseases differ in regard to characteristic skin lesions, subjective complaints, other organ involvement, L. E. cell test findings, response to treatment, and eventual prognosis.

	Chronic Discoid L. E.	Systemic L. E.
Primary lesions	Red, scaly, thickened, well-circumscribed patches with enlarged follicles and elevated border	Red, mildly scaly, diffuse, puffy lesions. Purpura also seen
Secondary lesions	Atrophy, scarring and pigmentary changes	No scarring. Mild hyperpigmentation
Distribution	Face, mainly in "butterfly" area, but also on scalp, ears, arms and chest. May not be symmetrical	Face in "butterfly" area, arms, fingers and legs. Usually symmetrical
Course	Very chronic with gradual progression; slow healing under therapy; no effect on life	Acute onset with fever, rash, malaise and joint pains. Most cases respond rather rapidly to steroid and supportive therapy, but the prognosis for life is poor
Season	Aggravated by intense sun exposure or radiation therapy	Same
Sex incidence	Almost twice as common in females	Same
Systemic pathology	None obvious	Nephritis, arthritis, epilepsy, pancarditis, hepatitis, etc.
Laboratory findings	Biopsy characteristic in classic case. L. E. cell test negative, as are other laboratory tests	Biopsy less useful. L. E. cell test positive. Leukopenia, anemia, albuminuria, increased sedimentation rate, positive antinuclear antibody test, and biologic false-positive serologic test for syphilis

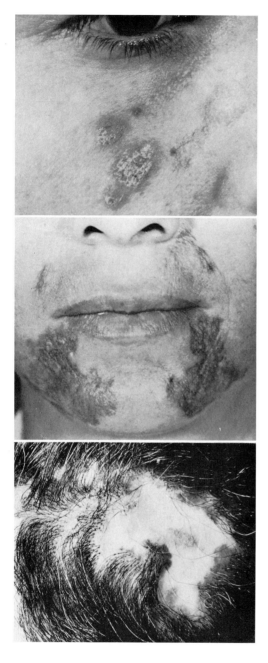

Fig. 20-1. Chronic discoid lupus erythematosus. (*Top*) Typical active red, scaly patches on cheek. (*Center*) Marked hyperpigmentation and scarring following healing. (*Bottom*) Permanent hair loss and atrophic hypopigmentation following healing in Negro's scalp.

However, rare cases of clinically classic chronic discoid L. E. show laboratory evidence of the pathology seen with the acute form of L. E. and can terminate as the disseminated disease. Certain early borderline cases are difficult to categorize, but eventually the majority of these subacute forms develop into the acute disseminated disease. The variations of the acute and the chronic forms of L. E. are shown in the chart on page 203.

CHRONIC DISCOID LUPUS ERYTHEMATOSUS
(Fig. 20-1 and Plate 60)

Differential Diagnosis

Systemic L. E. (see chart, p. 203)

Actinic Dermatitis: many cases are grossly and histologically similar to acute or chronic L. E. but get history of presence only in summer; see faster response to antimalarial drugs and locally applied sun-screening agents.

Seborrheic Dermatitis: lesions greasy, red, scaly, associated with scalp dandruff; see in eyebrows and scalp without hair loss; rapid response to antiseborrheic local therapy (p. 87).

Any Cutaneous Granulomas: such as sarcoidosis (p. 133), secondary and tertiary syphilis (p. 135) and lupus vulgaris (p. 131).

Cases with scarring alopecia are to be differentiated from *alopecia cicatrisata* (p. 226), *old tinea capitis of endothrix type* (p. 170), *lichen planus* (p. 107) and *folliculitis decalvans* (p. 226).

Treatment

Young female patient with two red, scaly, dime-sized lesions on right cheek of 3 months' duration.

1. Laboratory work-up should include a complete blood count, urinalysis, serology, L. E. cell test (Fig. 20-2), sedimentation rate and, uncommonly, a biopsy. The tests should be normal, but the biopsy rather characteristic of chronic discoid L. E. The assistance of a dermatologist to corroborate the diagnosis might be indicated.

Fig. 20-2. L. E. cells under low power (*top*) and high power (*bottom*) lens of microscope. (*Drs. Sloan Wilson and Wm. Larsen*)

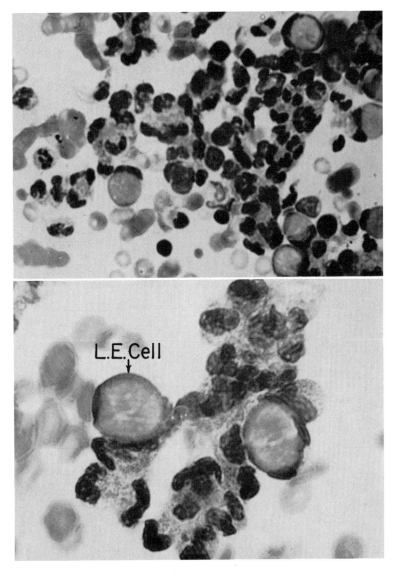

L.E. Cell

2. Lidex cream (0.05%)   15.0

Sig: Apply b.i.d. locally to lesions. More effective if covered with an occlusive bandage (Blenderm) or dressing (Saran wrap).

3. Uval   75.0
     or
     Skolex cream   30.0
     or
     A-fil cream   30.0

Sig: Apply to face as sun screen for protection. (Effect of cream lasts for 4 to 6 hours.)

Chloroquine and related anti-malarial type drugs are very effective for this disease. However, because of an irreversible retinitis that has developed in a few patients on long-term therapy, this therapy is not advised, except when used by a physician very knowledgeable of the effects of these drugs.

SYSTEMIC LUPUS ERYTHEMATOSUS (Fig. 20-3)

Differential Diagnosis

Chronic discoid L. E. (see preceding chart)

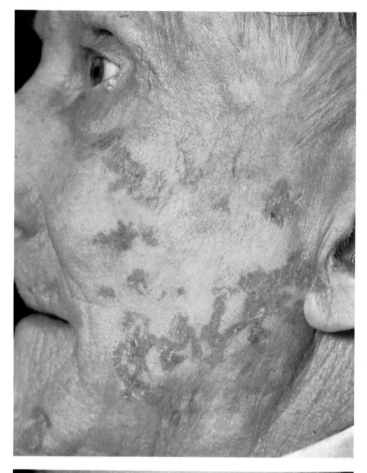

Plate 47. Lupus erythematosus (*Top*) Chronic discoid lupus erythematosus on the cheek of an elderly male. (*K.C.G.H.*)

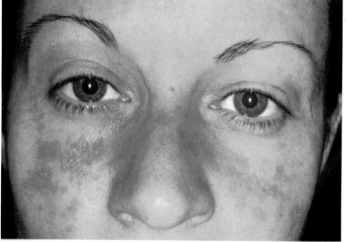

(*Bottom*) Acute disseminated lupus erythematosus showing classic "butterfly" eruption. (*Dr. S. Wilson & W. Larson*) (*Smith, Kline & French Laboratories*)

Actinic Dermatitis: skin lesions may be very similar in appearance, usually only in summer; find no altered laboratory studies; more rapid response to antimalarial drugs.

Seborrheic Dermatitis: associated with scalp dandruff; responds to local anti-seborrhea therapy (p. 87).

Contact Dermatitis: due to cosmetics, paint sprays, vegetation, hand creams, etc.; acute onset with no systemic symptoms; history helpful (p. 49).

Dermatomyositis: muscle soreness and weakness, negative L. E. cell test (p. 209).

Drug Eruption Due to Apresoline: can simulate acute L. E.; take history.

Treatment

Young female patient with diffuse red, puffy eruption on cheeks, nose, forehead and at base of fingernails of 1 week's duration. Complains of malaise, fever, joint pains, headache and ankle edema which has become progressively worse in the past 3 weeks.

The patient should be hospitalized and, following careful diagnostic work-up, should be treated with corticosteroids and any other supportive therapy as indicated for the organs involved. Sulfonamide therapy is contraindicated. Preferably, such patients should be in the hands of an internist, with assistance from the other specialties as needed.

SCLERODERMA

As with lupus erythematosus, there are two forms of scleroderma that are clinically unrelated except for some common histopathologic changes in the skin. *Localized scleroderma (morphea)* is a benign disease. *Diffuse scleroderma* is a serious disease.

LOCALIZED SCLERODERMA

Morphea is an uncommon skin disease of unknown etiology with no systemic involvement.

Primary Lesions. These are single or multiple, violaceous, firm, inelastic macules and plaques that enlarge slowly. The progressing border retains the violaceous hue, while the center becomes whitish and

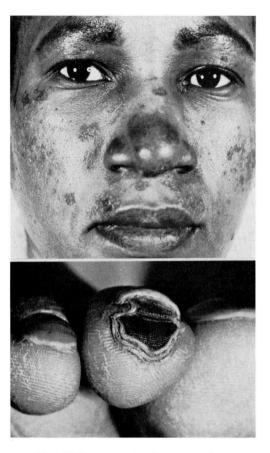

Fig. 20-3. **Systemic lupus erythematosus.** (*Top*) Scaly, dark red lesions in Negro woman with positive L. E. cell test. (*K.U.M.C.*) (*Bottom*) Gangrene of toe due to Raynaud's phenomenon in fatal case. (*Dr. Robert Jordan*)

slightly depressed beneath the skin surface. Bizarre lesions occur, such as long linear bands on extremities, saber-cut type lesions in scalp, or lesions involving one side of the face or the body, causing hemiatrophy.

Secondary Lesions. Mild or severe scarring after healing is inevitable. Scalp lesions result in permanent hair loss. Ulceration is rare.

Distribution. Trunk, extremities and head most frequently involved.

Course. Disability is confined to the area involved. Lesions tend to involute slowly and spontaneously. Relapses are rare.

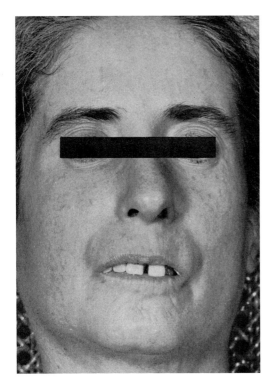

Fig. 20-4. Diffuse scleroderma. Note apparent immobility of the skin and lack of facial lines.

Differential Diagnosis. Guttate macular form from *lichen sclerosis et atrophicus* (histopathology rather characteristic); plaque type from *traumatic scars* (history important, no violaceous border); and *idiopathic atrophoderma* (rare, no induration).

Treatment. No therapy is necessary or effective. Time is the healer.

DIFFUSE SCLERODERMA

This uncommon systemic disease of unknown etiology is characterized by a long course of progressive disability due primarily to lack of mobility of the areas and the organs that are affected. The skin becomes hidebound, the esophagus and the gastrointestinal tract semirigid, the lungs and the heart fibrosed, the bones resorbed, and the overlying tissue calcified (Fig. 20-4).

Primary Lesions. There is usually a long prodromal stage of swelling of the skin with progressive limitation of movement. The early stage may or may not be associated with Raynaud's phenomenon, which is worse in the winter.

Secondary Lesions. As months and years pass the limitation of movement becomes marked, particularly of the hands, the feet and the face. The skin becomes atrophic, hidebound, develops sensory, vasomotor and pigmentary changes and, finally, ulcerations.

Distribution. The skin of the hands, the feet and the face is involved early, and in some rare cases the changes are confined only to the extremities ("acrosclerosis"). In the majority of patients, however, the entire skin becomes involved along with the internal organs.

Course. The prognosis is grave, and most cases die of the disease after years of disability. However, spontaneous or therapy-induced remissions can occur.

Sex Incidence. More common in females.

Laboratory Findings. Histologic examination of the skin shows generalized atrophy and hyalinization. The atrophic skeletal muscles lack the inflammatory component seen in dermatomyositis. The sedimentation rate is elevated early in the course of the disease. Other abnormal findings are related to the organs involved.

Differential Diagnosis

Dermatomyositis: find muscle tenderness, weakness, few skin changes; muscle biopsy rather characteristic (p. 209).

Early Rheumatoid Arthritis: swelling of joints and overlying skin; x-ray pictures helpful in determining diagnosis, as is time itself.

Treatment

No specific therapy is known. Protection of the skin from trauma, cold and infection is important. Physiotherapy may prevent contractures. Sympathectomy produces temporary benefits in some patients. Chelating agents are reported helpful for patients with extensive calcification. Bismuth orally or intramuscularly is an old form of treatment of doubtful value. Corticosteroids are not very beneficial.

DERMATOMYOSITIS

The rarest of the three collagen diseases is characterized by an acute or insidious onset of muscle pain, weakness, fever, arthralgia and in some cases a puffy erythematous eruption usually confined to the face and the eyelids. Progression of the disease results in muscle atrophy and contractures, skin telangiectasia and atrophy, and generalized organ involvement with death in 50 percent of cases. Dermatomyositis has a relationship to adenocarcinoma that is unexplained.

Laboratory Findings. These include increased sedimentation rate, rather characteristic muscle changes on biopsy study, albuminuria, anemia, positive antinuclear antibody test, negative L. E. cell test, and negative serologic test for syphilis.

Degeneration of the muscles is accompanied by creatinuria.

Differential Diagnosis: *Systemic lupus erythematosus, diffuse scleroderma, photosensitivity reactions, erysipelas, polyneuritis, myasthenia gravis* and others.

Treatment. Removal of an associated adenocarcinoma (present in 20% of cases of dermatomyositis) may result in a remission. Corticosteroid therapy, often in high doses as for systemic L. E., may cause a remission.

BIBLIOGRAPHY

Dubois, E. L.: Lupus Erythematosus. New York, McGraw-Hill, 1966.

Symposium: Cutaneous manifestations of systemic disease. N.Y. State J. Med., *63*: Nos. 21 and 22, 1963.

Tufanelli, D. L.: Lupus erythematosus. [Review] Arch. Derm., *106*:553, 1972.

21

The Skin and Internal Disease

It is not possible to separate the skin and its diseases from the internal organs and their diseases. The physician who fails to recognize this union will end up treating a disease and not a patient. Even the common contact dermatitis from the poison ivy plant affects various people differently, and the person as a whole must be taken into consideration when treating the disease. This is the art of medicine, the learning of which comes slowly.

This union of the skin organ and the internal organs becomes most apparent when studying certain diseases that have both skin and internal components. Some internal diseases have skin manifestations, and a few skin diseases have internal manifestations. This close interrelationship can be extremely interesting and complex, but since these conditions do not form a common part of everyday office practice they will be presented here in summary form. For further reading consult the Bibliography at the end of this chapter.

DERMATOSES DUE TO INTERNAL DISEASE

The skin manifestations of internal diseases may be *specific* or *nonspecific*. The *specific* skin changes contain the same pathologic process as the internal disease. An example is the lymphoblastomatous infiltrate in the skin of a patient with a lymphoblastoma.

More often, however, the skin changes are *nonspecific*. They do not contain the primary disease process. Therefore, these nonspecific skin changes are not diagnostic of the internal disease but when considered with other changes may be helpful in establishing the diagnosis.

The most important and common internal conditions and their related dermatoses are listed as follows:

Puberty State. In males at puberty the beard, the pubic and other body hair begins to grow in characteristic patterns which differ from the hair growth in females. Both sexes at this time notice increased activity of the apocrine glands with axillary perspiration and "B.O.," and increased development of the sebaceous glands with the formation of varying degrees of seborrhea and the comedones, the papules and the pustules of acne. Certain skin diseases disappear around the onset of puberty, such as the infantile form of atopic eczema, tinea of the scalp, and urticaria pigmentosa.

Pregnancy State. Certain physiologic skin changes occur, such as increased perspiration; hyperpigmentation of the abdominal midline, nipples, vulva, face (chloasma), and generally in some brunettes, with nevi and freckles also becoming more prominent; hypertrichosis which may be unnoticed until the excess hair begins to shed after delivery; and striae of breasts, abdomen and thighs. The skin diseases of pregnancy are dermatitis herpetiformis (herpes gestationis) (Plate 48), impetigo herpetiformis, vulvar pruritus, often due to monilial infection, palmar erythema, spider hemangiomas and pedunculated fibromas. The following dermatoses are usually better or disappear during pregnancy: psoriasis, acne (can be worse), alopecia areata and possibly diffuse scleroderma.

Menopause State. Common physiologic changes in the skin of women during menopause include hot flashes, increased perspiration, increased hair growth on the

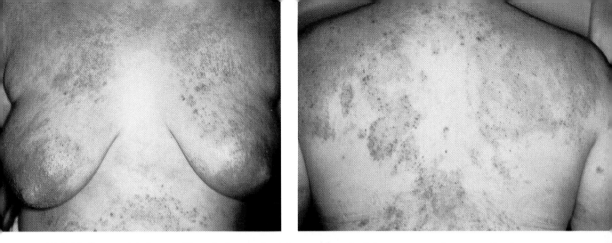

(*A & B*) Dermatitis herpetiformis (gestationis) associated with pregnancy in two patients

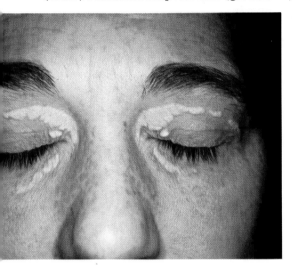

(*C*) Xanthelasma

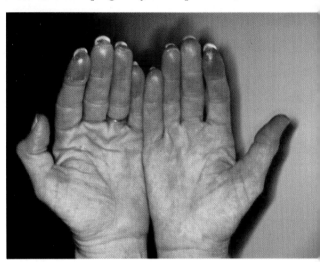

(*D*) Raynaud's disease with gangrene

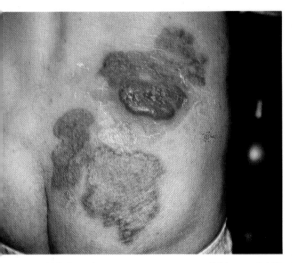

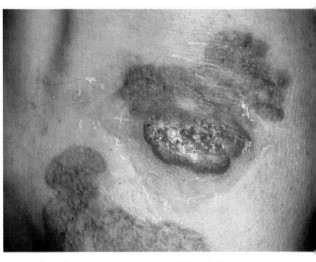

(*E*) Pyoderma gangrenosum of hip and (*F*) closeup showing active and scarred, healed areas (this case not associated with ulcerative colitis)

Plate 48. Dermatoses due to internal disease. (*Schering Corporation*)

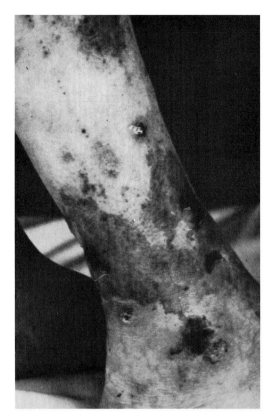

Fig. 21-1. Periarteritis nodosa with purpura and ischemic ulcers of the leg.

face, and varying degrees of scalp hair loss. Other skin conditions associated with the menopause are chloasma, pedunculated fibromas, localized neurodermatitis, vulvar pruritus, keratoderma climactericum (palmar psoriasis) and rosacea.

Geriatric State. (See Chapter 30, Geriatric Dermatoses, p. 303). The diffuse atrophy of the skin that occurs in the aged individual is partially responsible for the dryness which results in senile pruritus and winter itch. Other changes include excessive wrinkling and hyperpigmentation of the skin. Specific dermatoses noted with increased frequency are seborrheic and senile keratoses, epitheliomas, senile purpura, pedunculated fibromas and capillary senile hemangiomas (p. 273).

Rheumatic Fever. See nonspecific changes of increased sweating which results in prickly heat; also petechiae, urticaria, erythema nodosum, erythema multiforme, and rheumatic nodules.

Periarteritis Nodosa (Fig. 21-1). See periarteritic nodules which are specific, and nonspecific purpura, erythema and gangrene.

Thromboangiitis Obliterans (Buerger's Disease). See superficial migrating thrombophlebitis, pallor or cyanosis, gangrene and ulceration.

Ulcerative Colitis. A characteristic ulcerative disease of the skin called *pyoderma gangrenosum* (Plate 48) is associated quite frequently with ulcerative colitis, but the skin lesions can occur without this association. The ulcers are deep and foul smelling, spread rapidly and characteristically have undermined edges with necrotic holes.

Fröhlich's Syndrome. Due to hypopituitarism in the male. Find feminine type smooth skin and scant hair growth, particularly in pubic and axillary regions, well-developed scalp hair, obesity and small thin fingernails.

Acromegaly. Due to hyperpituitarism and excess growth-stimulating hormone. See skin changes due to overgrowth of the skeletal system; coarsened skin, deepened lines, increased sweating and oiliness, acne, increasing number of nevi, hyperpigmentation and hypertrichosis.

Cushing's Syndrome. Due to basophile ademona of the pituitary gland. See purplish atrophic striae, hyperpigmentation, hypertrichosis in females and preadolescent males, and increased incidence of pyodermas.

Hyperthyroidism. The skin is moist and warm, and has an evanescent erythema, hyperpigmentation (hypopigmentation rarely), seborrhea, acne, toxic alopecia and nail atrophy. Localized myxedema of the pretibial areas of the legs can develop and appears to be related to exophthalmos.

Hypothyroidism. The skin in generalized myxedema is cool, dry, scaly, thickened and hyperpigmented. Also see toxic alopecia with hair that is dull, dry and coarse, and increased incidence of pyodermas.

Addison's Disease. The most important

dermatosis is hyperpigmentation which is first seen on areas of friction, pressure and irritation. Sweating is increased, and the axillary and pubic hair is shed.

Diabetes Mellitus (Plate 49). Due to the increased amount of carbohydrate in the skin of patients with diabetes, skin infections occur with much higher frequency than in nondiabetic individuals. These infections include boils, carbuncles, ulcers, gangrene, moniliasis, tinea of the feet and the groin with or without secondary bacterial infection, and infectious eczematoid dermatitis. Other dermatoses seen are pruritus, xanthoma diabeticorum and necrobiosis lipoidica diabeticorum.

Lipidoses. This complex group of metabolic diseases causes varying skin lesions, depending somewhat on the basic metabolic fault. Thannhauser's classification will be used to summarize these skin manifestations (see References).

1. *Hypercholesteremic xanthomatoses* include the lesions of xanthelasma of eyelids (Fig. 21-2 and Plate 48), and papular, nodular, and plaquelike xanthomas on the extensor surfaces of the extremities. These latter lesions are seen in xanthoma tuberosum and also occur secondary to liver disease or hypothyroidism.

2. *Hyperlipemia* of the idiopathic type or secondary to diabetes mellitus, chronic pancreatitis or nephrosis is characterized by the sudden development of eruptive xanthomatoses consisting of single or multiple yellowish papules, nodules or plaques most commonly seen on the flexor surfaces of the extremities and on the trunk, the face and the scalp. Pruritus may be severe.

3. *Normocholesteremic xanthomatoses* include xanthoma dissemination, Schüller-Christian syndrome, Letterer-Siwe disease and eosinophilic granuloma. Xanthelasma and flexural xanthomas occur. Vesicular lesions can be seen in cases of Schüller-Christian syndrome, and a seborrheic-dermatitis-like picture in Letterer-Siwe disease (Fig. 29-5).

4. *Extracellular lipid accumulations* occur in lipoid proteinosis, extracellular cholesterosis and necrobiosis lipoidica diabeticorum. Skin lesions of the latter occur

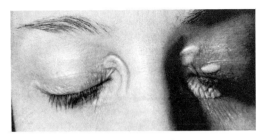

Fig. 21-2. Xanthelasma in woman with high blood cholesterol.

mostly in women on the anterior tibial area of the leg and are characterized by sharply circumscribed, yellowish plaques with a bluish border. Diabetes is present in the majority of cases.

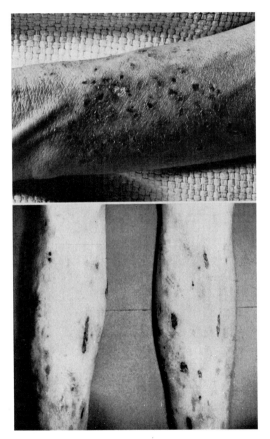

Fig. 21-3. Skin manifestations of nervous disorders. (*Top*) Neurotic excoriations on the forearm. (*K.U.M.C.*) (*Bottom*) Factitial dermatitis on the legs. (*Dr. David Morgan*)

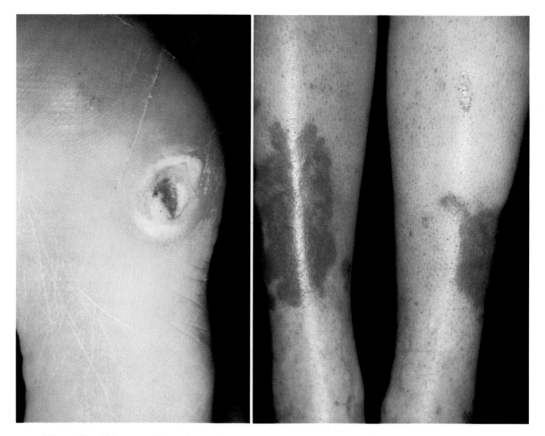

Plate 49. Skin manifestations of diabetes mellitus. (*Left*) Mal perforans of sole of foot of 3 years' duration. (*Right*) Necrobiosis lipoidica diabeticorum on anterior tibial area of legs. (*Dermik Laboratories, Inc. and Smith Kline and French Laboratories*)

5. *Disturbances of phospholipid metabolism* include Niemann-Pick disease and Gaucher's disease. Both develop a yellowish discoloration of the skin.

Vitamin Deficiencies. Dermatoses due to lack of vitamins are rare in the United States. However, a common question asked by many patients is, "Doctor, don't you think my trouble is due to lack of vitamins?" The answer in 99 percent of the cases is "No!"

VITAMIN A. Phrynoderma is the name for generalized dry hyperkeratoses of the skin due to chronic and significant lack of vitamin A. Clinically, the skin resembles the surface of a nutmeg grater. Eye changes are often present, including night blindness and dryness of the eyeball.

Large doses of vitamin A (25,000 to 50,000 units t.i.d.) are used in the treatment of patients with Darier's disease, pityriasis rubra pilaris, comedone acne and xerosis (dry skin). The value of this therapy has not been proved.

Hypervitaminosis A, due to excessively high and persistent intake of vitamin A in drug or food form, causes hair loss, dry skin, irritability, weight loss, and enlargement of the liver and the spleen.

VITAMIN B GROUP. Clinically, a patient with a true vitamin B deficiency is deficient in all of the vitamins of this group. Thus the classic diseases of this group, beriberi and pellagra, have overlapping clinical signs and symptoms.

VITAMIN B_1 (THIAMINE). This deficiency is clinically manifested by beriberi. The cutaneous lesions consist of edema and redness of the soles of the feet.

VITAMIN B_2 (RIBOFLAVIN). A deficiency

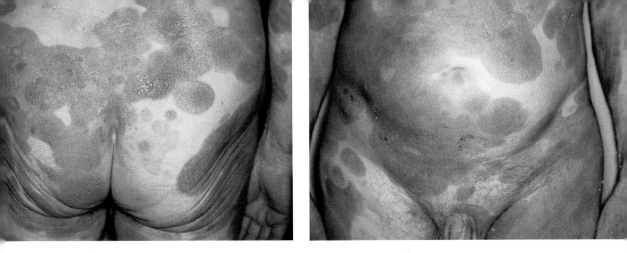

(A) Mycosis fungoides in plaque stage of buttocks and (B) abdomen of 79 year old male

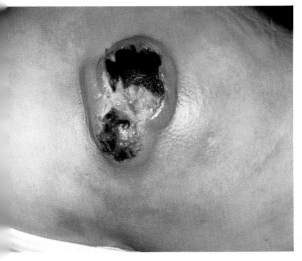

(C) Mycosis fungoides in tumor stage on thigh

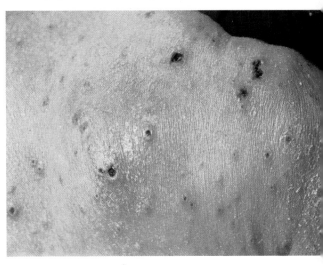

(D) Non-specific pyoderma with lymphocytic leukemia

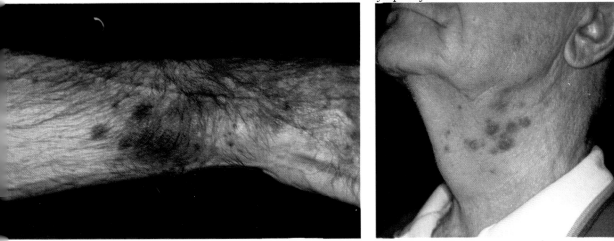

(E) Purpura of arm and (F) folliculitis of neck in same patient with myelogenous leukemia

Plate 50. Dermatoses associated with lymphomas. (*Syntex Laboratories, Inc.*)

of this vitamin has been linked with red fissures at the corners of the mouth and glossitis. This can occur in marked vitamin B_2 deficiency, but most cases with these clinical lesions are due to contact dermatitis or malocclusion of the lips from faulty dentures.

NICOTINIC ACID. This deficiency leads to pellagra, but other vitamins of the B group are contributory. The skin lesions are a prominent part of pellagra and include redness of the exposed areas of hands, face, neck and feet, which can go on to a fissured, scaling, infected dermatitis. Local trauma may spread the disease to other areas of the body. The disease is worse in the summer and heals with hyperpigmentation and mild scarring. Gastrointestinal and neurologic complications are serious.

The B group vitamins are administered with benefit to patients who have rosacea. Vitamin B_{12} in doses of 1,000 micrograms subcutaneously is somewhat effective for cases of severe seborrheic dermatitis.

VITAMIN C (ASCORBIC ACID). Scurvy is now a rare disease, and the skin lesions are not specific. They include a follicular papular eruption, petechia and purpura.

VITAMIN D. No skin lesions have been attributed to lack of this vitamin. Vitamin D and vitamin D_2 (calciferol) have been used in the treatment of lupus vulgaris.

VITAMIN E. It has been reported that vitamin E is effective in treating pseudoxanthoma elasticum and epidermolysis bullosa (Ayres and Mihan).

VITAMIN K. Hypoprothrombinemia with purpura from various causes responds to vitamin K therapy.

VITAMIN P (HESPERIDIN). With vitamin C (Hesper-C Bitabs), vitamin P is beneficial for chronic purpuric eruptions of the Schamberg's variety.

Internal Cancer. (Plate 50) Skin lesions may develop from internal malignancies either by metastatic spread or by the occurrence of nonspecific eruptions. The most interesting of the *nonspecific dermatoses* is the rare entity, *acanthosis nigricans.* The presence of the velvety, papillary, pigmented hypertrophies of this disease in the axillae, the groin and other moist areas of an adult will indicate an internal cancer, usually of the adbominal viscera, in over 50 percent of cases. A benign form of acanthosis nigricans exists in children and becomes most manifest at the age of puberty. This benign form is not associated with cancer.

A *dermatitis herpetiformis-like eruption* with vesicles and intense pruritus is seen occasionally in patients with an internal malignancy or lymphoma.

Purpuric lesions and pyodermas also occur as nonspecific changes in patients with malignancies (Plate 50).

Specific skin lesions showing the malignancy or lymphoma on biopsy occur in *mycosis fungoides, leukemia, lymphomas* and in *metastatic skin lesions* from internal malignancies.

Neuroses and Psychoses. A common belief among many members of the medical profession is that the majority of skin diseases are due to "nerves" or are a neurotic manifestation. This old idea is undoubtedly based on the familiar sight of the scratching skin patient; he just looks "nervous"; and it makes one nervous and itchy merely by looking at him. It is hard to know which came first for most patients, the itching or the nervousness. In my practice I tend to de-emphasize the nervous element but not ignore it. My answer to patients and doctors who question the role of nerves in a particular case is to say that they play a definite role in many skin eruptions, but rarely are "nerves" the precipitating cause of a dermatosis. If a patient has an emotional problem and also has an itching dermatitis, a flare-up of the problem will intensify his itch as it would aggravate another patient's duodenal ulcer or migraine headache.

Therapy of patients with skin disease where "nerves" are thought to play a dominant part can well be handled by the calm, receptive, attentive, interested general physician. Simple local therapy prescribed with the confidence of a competent physician will often establish in the patient the necessary faith that will cure his complaint. Occasionally, these patients will not respond to such therapy, and a rare case might benefit from special psychiatric care.

The following list will divide the psychocutaneous diseases into those thought to be (1) related to psychoses, (2) related to neuroses, and (3) those with questionable psychic relationship.

1. Dermatoses Related to Psychoses

Factitial dermatitis (Fig. 21-3 B). The patient denies that he is producing the skin disease. This is not to be confused with neurotic excoriations.

Skin lesions due to compulsive movements. An example is the chronic biting of an arm in a feeble-minded patient.

Delusions of parasitism, cancer, syphilis, etc. Various "proofs" are often presented by the patient to substantiate his existing belief.

Trichotillomania in adults. A rare cause of hair loss.

2. Dermatoses Related to Neuroses

Neurotic excoriations (Figs. 3-2 and 21-3 A). The patient admits picking or scratching the lesions. (See p. 193.)

Phobias. A fear that the patient will contract a disease, i.e., syphilophobia, acarophobia, cancerophobia, bacteriophobia, etc.

Trichotillomania of children. Not as serious as in adults. The physician's index of suspicion must be high to diagnose this disease (p. 225).

Neurodermatitis (Plate 16). The primary cause can be an insect bite, contact dermatitis due to a permanent wave, psoriasis, stasis dermatitis, or many other conditions that can initiate the scratching habit. The habit then outlives the disease, and the neurodermatitis cycle develops.

3. Dermatoses of Questionable Psychic Cause

Hyperhidrosis of palms and soles
Dyshidrosis
Alopecia areata
Lichen planus

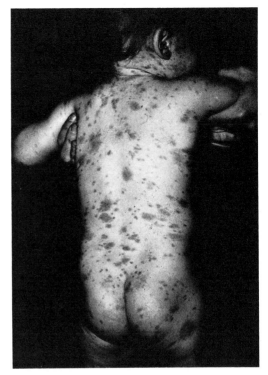

Fig. 21-4. Urticaria pigmentosa in a 9-month-old boy. (*See also* Plate 58.)

Chronic urticaria
Rosacea
Atopic eczema
Psoriasis
Aphthous stomatitis
Primary pruritus, local or generalized

INTERNAL MANIFESTATIONS OF SKIN DISEASE

The purpose of the author in this section is to list some of the internal phenomena that occur with certain diseases that primarily involve the skin. The collagen diseases belong in this group, particularly *lupus erythematosus* and *scleroderma*, but they have been discussed earlier in this book.

Rosacea. Eye lesions, such as keratitis, conjunctivitis and blepharitis, are seen rather commonly. Stomach achlorhydria or hypoacidity is of doubtful significance.

Atopic Eczema. This is one manifestation of a triad of atopic conditions, the

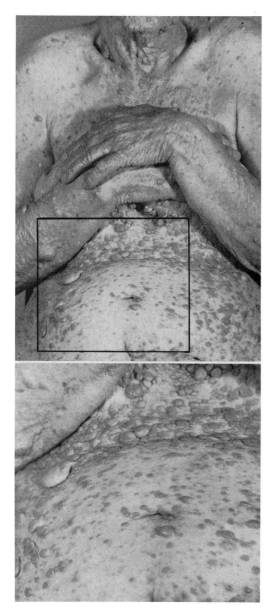

Fig. 21-5. Neurofibromatosis.

other two being bronchial asthma and hayfever. Eye cataracts are seen with severe forms of atopic eczema but only rarely. Blood eosinophilia is common.

Psoriasis. This chronic papulosquamous eruption is associated with arthritis in a small number of cases. The psoriasis usu-ally exists as one of the more severe forms of the disease, such as the exfoliative type, and frequently precedes the development of the arthritis. Most observers believe that the joint lesions are a form of rheumatoid arthritis.

Urticaria Pigmentosa or Mastocytosis (Fig. 21-4 and Plate 58). This rare maculopapular disease, mainly of children, is characterized by urtication of the lesions following scratching. The skin lesions are composed of mast cells, and mast cell infiltrates are found in bone, liver, lymph nodes and the thymus. The childhood form usually disappears spontaneously after a few years. The form in adults can last for years and eventuate in a lymphoma.

Pseudoxanthoma Elasticum. This rare but characteristic skin disease of yellowish papules or plaques, mainly of the body folds, is a degeneration of the elastic tissue. Systemically, angioid streaks of the retina are seen in 25 percent of cases and result in a slowly progressive loss of visual acuity. Other systemic manifestations, undoubtedly due to the degeneration of elastic tissue in the arteries, include mental changes, intermittent claudication, absence of peripheral pulses, and intestinal hemorrhage.

Incontinentia Pigmenti (Plate 57). This disease is another example of the widening of clinical horizons. The pathology noted in the first early cases was a whorled hyperpigmentation of skin found in infants. Histologically, melanin was seen in the corium. This suggested that the epidermis was incontinent. It was later learned that when cases were seen at birth or soon after, the earliest stages of the disease were vesicular and bullous lesions, and then, lichenoid and warty lesions. The whorled hyperpigmentation was the third stage.

There is a familial or hereditary tendency in a few cases. Systemically, developmental defects have been found in an appreciable number of cases; these include faulty dentition, bone deformities, epilepsy and mental deficiency.

Neurofibromatosis (Fig. 21-5 and Plate 58). Also known as von Recklinghausen's disease, this hereditary condition classically consists of pigmented patches (café au lait spots), pedunculated skin tumors and nerve tumors. All of these lesions may not be present in a single case. Since internal nerves can be the site of the neurofibromas, deafness, paralysis, sensory disturbances and epilepsy may be associated with them. Malignant degeneration of the tumors is not unusual.

BIBLIOGRAPHY

Braverman, I. M.: Skin Signs of Systemic Disease. Philadelphia, W. B. Saunders, 1970.

Johnson, S. A. M. (ed.): The Skin and Internal Disease. New York, McGraw-Hill, 1967.

Symposium: Cutaneous manifestations of systemic disease. N.Y. State J. Med. *63:* Nos. 21 and 22, 1963.

Thannhauser, S. J.: Lipidoses, ed. 2. New York, Oxford University Press, 1950.

Wiener, K.: Skin Manifestations of Internal Disorders. St. Louis, C. V. Mosby, 1947.

——: Systemic Associations and Treatment of Skin Diseases. St. Louis, C. V. Mosby, 1955. These two older texts are remarkable for their completeness.

22

Diseases Affecting the Hair

The hair on an individual's scalp and body is a personal mark. Care of the scalp hair receives more attention, from both men and women, than any other part of the human anatomy. Thus it is easy to understand the psychological problems caused by a disease of the hair. Unfortunately, however, two of the commonest diseases of the hair, hereditary hair loss on the scalp and excessive growth on the face, cannot be prevented, contrary to magazine and newspaper ads (See p. 6.)

There are many rare diseases of the hair that will be defined at the end of this chapter.

GRAY HAIR

The congenital presence of completely gray or white hair (albinism) or patches of gray hair is quite rare. More commonly, grayness of the scalp hair is a slowly progressive process. Hereditary factors determine whether such grayness will begin in early or late adulthood or not at all. There is no proof that worry hurries this graying process.

Patchy gray hair can develop following nerve injuries. The new hair that grows in during the healing of alopecia areata is usually white or gray.

Treatment. The desirability of eliminating gray hair is confined mainly to women. Vegetable and chemical dyes and rinses (and bleaches to reverse the process) are used in fantastic quantities throughout the world and are safe if the individual is not irritated by or allergic to the agent used. When an allergy or irritation develops it is to be treated as contact dermatitis, usually with mild shampoos, 2 percent boric acid solution wet dressings and an appropriate water-washable corticosteroid salve.

HYPERTRICHOSIS

Excessive growth of hair (hypertrichosis or hirsutism) can be a definite psychological problem when it occurs on the face or the legs of women (Fig. 22-1). It would be a mistake for a physician to underestimate the seriousness attached to a woman's request for information regarding the treatment of such a problem. This form of hypertichosis is called the *essential type,* but other less common forms exist.

Congenital hypertrichosis is very rare and is characterized by the "dog-faced boys" seen in circus sideshows. This is a form of congenital ectodermal defect that is hereditary. The lanugo hairs of infancy are not replaced with the coarser adult hairs, and this results in a continuing growth of the long silken lanugo hairs.

Localized hypertrichosis is ordinarily seen in association with pigmented or nonpigmented intradermal nevi. This may consist of only 2 or 3 hairs, or the hairy growth may cover a large part of the body. After a small hairy nevus is removed by electrosurgery and the site healed, it is often necessary to remove the remaining excess long hairs by an electrosurgical method.

Endocrinopathic hypertrichosis is rare but must be ruled out when recently acquired hirsutism is noted. The menstrual history in a female can give valuable information. If menstruation is completely normal, it can be assumed that the patient does not have a pituitary, adrenal or ovarian tumor causing the excessive hair growth. If menstruation is abnormal and other findings are noted, such as obesity, deepening of the voice, enlargement of the clitoris, etc., then further clinical and laboratory studies are indicated.

Treatment of essential hypertrichosis in a 35-year-old attractive female. Examination reveals long dark hairs of the upper lip, the chin and the jaw areas.

1. Obtain a menstrual history. If it is completely normal, as we shall assume that it is in this patient, she can be assured that she has no abnormal internal reason for this excessive growth. If the menstrual history is not normal, proceed with further studies as indicated.

2. Question the patient regarding similar excess hair growth (do not use the word "beard") in her family. Other female members will usually be found to have this condition. This unalterable hereditary influence should be stressed.

3. Attempt to talk the patient into the fact that the excess hair she has is normal for her, is more noticeable to herself than others, and that treatment is not very satisfactory. If this cannot be accomplished, and it usually cannot be, then proceed to a discussion of the forms of treatment. The following suggested types of therapy begin with the easiest, the least expensive and the least injurious.

4. Bleaching the hairs. This can be done by using any of the many available proprietary preparations; it is not permanent but is simple, effective and seldom irritating.

5. Plucking the hair. If the area of excess hair growth is not too large this is a temporary, not too simple, but effective method which can result in a folliculitis. Plucking the hair does not increase hair growth.

6. Depilatories dissolve the hair shaft

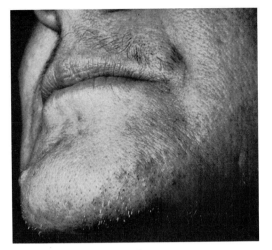

Fig. 22-1. Hypertrichosis of chin and upper lip in a 50-year-old woman.

and offer a temporary, simple, effective and somewhat irritating method.

7. Epilating waxes produce a mass plucking effect, and offer a temporary though somewhat painful, effective form of hair removal. Folliculitis can follow.

8. Electrosurgical removal of the hairs is the only permanent method. (X-rays can also cause permanent removal of hairs but adequate dosage seriously damages the skin. The use of x-rays to epilate hair permanently is a form of malpractice.) Electrosurgical treatments can be carried out by electrolysis or by electrocoagulation (see p. 45). This latter method is faster but can result in scarring if not done carefully. Either procedure should be done by a skilled technician, who can be found in any large city. This form of

---

FACTS REGARDING HAIR

1. **Shaving, cutting or plucking the hair does not affect the hair growth.**
2. **Frequent shampooing does not damage normal scalp hair.**
3. **Excessive brushing of the hair can be harmful.**
4. **Hair growth or loss in normal individuals is a physiologic process that cannot be altered by cosmetic applications.**
5. **Graying of the hair cannot occur overnight.**

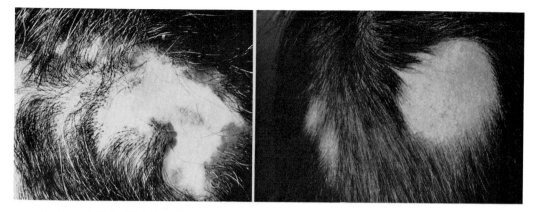

Chronic Discoid L.E. (Negro)   Tinea of the Scalp

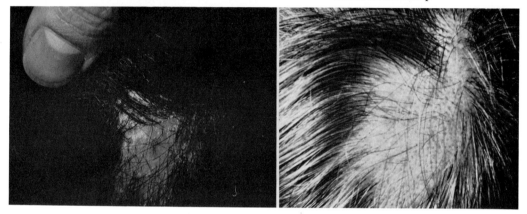

Alopecia Cicatrisata   Traumatic Alopecia

Fig. 22-2. Hair loss due to various causes. The case of traumatic alopecia was caused by the accidental catching of the scalp hair in a rotary massaging instrument used on the patient's back.

hair removal is effective, slighty painful, very time-consuming if large areas are to be treated, and quite expensive. Scarring should be minimal or nonexistent when the procedure is done by a skilled technician. All of these facts should be stated to the patient.

HAIR LOSS

Hair loss (alopecia) in the scalp is important mainly because it is so obvious (Fig. 22-2). Hair loss on other parts of the body is unusual, but when present it is commonly associated with scalp alopecia.

There are two types of scalp hair loss, *diffuse* and *patchy*. Patchy alopecias can

be of the nonscarring or of the scarring variety. In the scarring variety the hair cannot regrow because of a destroyed follicle. A complete classification follows, but only the more common alopecias will be discussed.

CLASSIFICATION

Diffuse Hair Loss

1. Male-pattern hair loss
2. Female-pattern hair loss
3. Temporary hair loss in females
4. Hair loss due to infection: pneumonia, exanthems and typhoid
5. Hair loss due to chemicals and

drugs: severe reactions to locally applied chemicals, oral ingestion of thallium, nitrogen mustard, methotrexate, heparin and excess vitamin A

6. Hair loss due to endocrinopathy: hypothyroid and hypopituitary states

7. Hair loss associated with other diseases: exfoliative dermatitis, systemic lupus erythematosus, dermatomyositis, lymphomas, etc.

8. Congenital ectodermal defects: hair loss only, or associated with congenital loss of nails, teeth and cutaneous glands

Patchy Nonscarring Hair Loss

1. Alopecia areata
2. Tinea of the scalp
3. Trichotillomania
4. Secondary syphilis
5. Traumatic marginal alopecia

Patchy Scarring Hair Loss

1. Tinea infection of the scalp of the rare severely infected form
2. Bacterial infection of the scalp
3. Alopecia cicatrisata
4. Hair loss associated with other diseases: chronic discoid lupus erythematosus, scleroderma, lichen planus, neoplasms, zoster, etc.
5. Hair loss due to physical and chemical agents: overdose of x-rays, third-degree burns, trauma, caustics

DIFFUSE HAIR LOSS

1. Male-Pattern Hair Loss. This very common condition results in the expenditure of hundreds of thousands of dollars every year for medicines that promise the presumably unfortunate male a head of thick, luxuriant hair. Contrary to the statements in the most convincing "hair-restoring" ads, there is no "cure" for this hereditary disease.

Clinically, the earliest hair loss extends back on both sides of the forehead in an M-shape to meet a slowly enlarging area of similar hair loss on the vertex of the scalp. The degree of hair loss varies with the individual, as does the age at which it begins.

ETIOLOGY: The dominant factors are heredity, age of the individual, and hormones. The heredity and the age, of course, cannot be altered. Hormonal therapy in safe dosage has no beneficial effect. Castrated males do not have this male-pattern hair loss, but castration is not recommended as a form of treatment.

DIFFERENTIAL DIAGNOSIS

Alopecia areata: patchy hair loss with exclamation-point hairs (see below)

Trichotillomania: patchy and bizzare areas of hair loss (see below)

TREATMENT: A 27-year-old male with receding hairline and a slight amount of scaling on his scalp.

1. Question the patient about his heredity. Usually there is a history that the father began to lose his scalp hair when he also was in his twenties. Explain about this unalterable factor of heredity.

2. Tell the patient that treatment is of no value, contrary to the hair-restoring ads.

3. Suggest the use of a dandruff-removing shampoo such as Selsun Suspension to keep the scalp as healthy as possible. *Dandruff, unless it becomes severely secondarily infected, does not cause hair loss.*

2. Female-Pattern Hair Loss. This mild diffuse hair loss occurs in a small percentage of women, most commonly after the age of 50. The loss begins on the vertex of the scalp and is never complete. It probably is related to a relative increase in the male hormone. There is no effective form of therapy.

3. Temporary Hair Loss in Females. A moderately common complaint from a young female patient is that for 6 months her hair has been "falling out in handfuls." Examination reveals a good head of hair but some diffuse thinning. The patient is otherwise healthy.

ETIOLOGY: This temporary hair loss can follow the use of an anesthetic, the birth of a baby or a nervous upset, or have no apparent cause. During pregnancy the hair growth is often increased, but this fact is not obvious to the patient. However, when the patient returns to the unpregnant state and the luxuriant hair

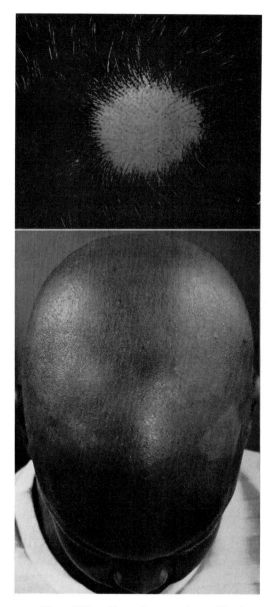

Fig. 22-3. Alopecia areata. (*Top*) Single area on vertix of scalp. Exclamation point hairs are barely visible. (*Bottom*) Total alopecia of 4-year-old Negro girl.

growth begins to shed she becomes alarmed. This cycle of events should be explained to the patient.

TREATMENT consists of pointing out the causative factor and reassuring the patient that she will not become bald.

Usually the hair loss will slowly cease, and the normal hair pattern, though somewhat less thick, will be re-established.

PATCHY NONSCARRING HAIR LOSS

1. Alopecia Areata. This common disease of unknown cause results in serious psychological problems when it occurs over large areas of the scalp (Fig. 22-3).

PRIMARY LESION. See loss of hair in a slowly enlarging area or areas. *No scaling or evidence of infection is present.* The hair breaks off at a point approximately 2 to 3 mm. above the scalp surface. The broken hairs are aptly called "exclamation-point hairs" because they appear to be thicker at the top and thin at the base like the top part of an exclamation point (!). These "exclamation-point hairs" are pathognomonic of alopecia areata and are found in all active cases, usually at the periphery of the bald patch. When healing begins the new hairs are commonly white but eventually they regain their normal color.

DISTRIBUTION. Any hairy area of the body can be affected. The commonest areas are the scalp, the eyebrows, the eyelashes and the beard.

PROGNOSIS. The great majority of cases of alopecia areata that have one or several small patches will regrow their hair in 6 to 12 months time with no treatment. Recurrences are quite common. Prepubertal cases have a poorer prognosis for permanent "cure." Total loss of the scalp hair and/or the body hair (alopecia totalis) carries with it a very poor prognosis for eventual return of the hair.

AGE GROUP. This disease occurs most commonly in young adults, and less commonly in children.

ETIOLOGY. The cause is unknown. Some cases appear to be due to a focus of infection (teeth, prostate, sinuses, gallbladder, genitourinary tract, etc.), and some may be due to emotional problems. The factor of heredity is evident in some cases.

DIFFERENTIAL DIAGNOSIS

Tinea of the Scalp: no exclamation-point hairs; mainly in children; see scaliness, usually some infection; Wood's light usually shows fluorescence; fungi found on KOH slide preparation of hair or culture media (p. 170).

Trichotillomania: no exclamation-point hairs, irregular areas of hair loss, "nervous" child (see below).

Secondary Syphilis: no exclamation-point hairs; see other secondary skin lesions; serologic test for syphilis is positive (p. 134).

Chronic Discoid Lupus Erythematosus: no exclamation-point hairs; in the active lesions see redness, enlarged hair follicle opening and scaliness, but in the healed stage see atrophic hyperpigmented or depigmented patches with absent hair follicles (p. 204).

Alopecia Cicatrisata (Fig. 22-2): no exclamation-point hairs; find small area of hair loss with no inflammation and no change over many years time; hair follicles are atrophic (p. 226).

Folliculitis Decalvans: no exclamation-point hairs; see folliculitis and eventual destruction of the hair follicle (p. 226).

TREATMENT. A young female patient presents herself in your office with two 3 x 2 cm. sized areas of hair loss of 2 weeks' duration. Her father died 1 week prior to onset of the disease. Examination reveals exclamation-point hairs at the periphery of both lesions. She is able to comb her hair so as to cover the bald areas.

1. Reassure the patient (1) that it would be exceedingly rare for her to lose all of her hair; and (2) that the lesions might enlarge some but that within 6 to 8 months' time all of her hair will be back. Tell her that the new hair may come in white at the beginning, but the natural color will soon return.

2. Treat her dandruff, if she has any, with Fostex Cream Shampoo or Selsun Suspension Shampoo. (Selsun Suspension rarely, if ever, causes hair loss.)

3. Kenalog Spray Can (large) Sig.: Spray sparingly on the area t.i.d. (This is moderately effective, gives them a "treatment," and is non-messy.)

4. Have her return if necessary for reassurance.

Subsequent visit with considerable extension of the bald areas. No specific therapy is known. Injections of vitamins or the oral administration of a tranquilizer might satisfy the patient and allow you to follow her more closely until the hair begins to regrow.

Treatment of recurrent severe cases or cases of alopecia totalis

1. The prognosis is poor for return of hair in these severe cases, and the patient should be told this. A statement of the truth can prevent useless migration of the patient from one physician to another.

2. A wig may be desired by the patient, and this purchase can be encouraged.

3. Corticosteroid therapy. This therapy causes regrowth of hair in some of the severe cases but should not be initiated without careful examination of the patient and a thorough discussion with the patient regarding the side-effects and the expense of months of therapy.

This therapy can be administered in 3 ways—orally, by intralesional injection and by intramuscular injection.

Orally, an adequate dose usually produces side-effects, since the therapy must be continued for a long term. On cessation of therapy, most cases relapse.

Intralesional injections for small areas in the scalp are effective. See p. 73 for technic. Atrophic areas causing a washboardlike effect are a common side-effect. I have not been impressed with this type of therapy.

Intramuscular injection of 10 mg. of triamcinolone parenteral suspension (Kenalog 40 I.M.) once a week for 6 to 8 weeks, then less frequently, has been quite beneficial for severe widespread cases.

2. Tinea of the Scalp. This is characterized by broken-off hairs, scaliness and occasionally infection, fluorescence under Wood's light, the finding of the organism in KOH preparations of the hair and growths on Sabouraud's media: usually it is seen in children. (See p. 170 and Plate 58 and Figs. 15-5 and 22-2.)

3. Trichotillomania. This rare form of hair loss must be thought of when exclamation-point hairs, scaliness and in-

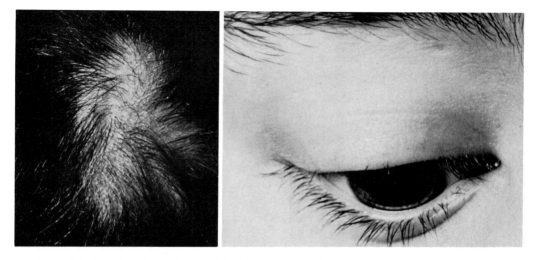

Fig. 22-4. Trichotillomania. (*Left*) Of the scalp of a 9-year-old boy. (*Right*) Of the eyelashes of a 10-year-old girl.

fection are not seen (Fig. 22-4 and Plate 58). Children are usually affected. It can occur in the scalp, the eyebrows and the eyelids. The emotional problems of the patient and the parents are responsible for this disease, and these problems may be simple or serious. The patient and the parents may or may not be aware of the "pulling tendency." These cases should be handled by a dermatologist and, in severe cases, by a psychiatrist.

4. Secondary Syphilis. Alopecia due to secondary syphilis is uncommon. The usual form of hair loss due to syphilis is the patchy moth-eaten form (Fig. 13-3 A), but very rarely a diffuse hair loss occurs. The absence of exclamation-point hairs differentiates it from alopecia areata, which it resembles closely.

PATCHY SCARRING HAIR LOSS

1. Tinea of the Scalp. The rarer forms of tinea that are accompanied by severe kerion formation may result in small spots of permanent hair loss as a result of destruction of the hair follicles. The organisms *Microsporum canis, M. gypseum, Trichophyton mentagrophytes* and *T. tonsurans* are the ones most frequently responsible for scarring (see p. 170).

2. Bacterial Infection of the Scalp. Any deep bacterial process can destroy the hair follicle and produce patches of permanent hair loss. These deep infections can be due to pyogenic bacteria, tuberculosis, leprosy and syphilis, but all of these are rare causes of hair loss.

Folliculitis decalvans is the name given to a rare form of hair loss, apparently due to bacterial infection, that progresses slowly for many years with recurrent crops of infection at the spreading border. Atrophic scarring remains in the center. This diagnosis should not be made until at least two attempts have failed to grow a fungus on culture media. Favus of the scalp due to *Trichophyton schoenleini* can mimic this disease.

3. Alopecia Cicatrisata. This very rare form of permanent hair loss is characterized by no history or evidence of scaling or infection (Fig. 22-2). The cause is unknown and treatment is ineffective.

OTHER DISORDERS AFFECTING THE HAIR

The following hair disorders, except for *ingrown hairs*, are quite rare and will be discussed briefly.

Ingrown Hair (Pili Incarnati). This common condition, seen particularly in

Negroes, is usually associated with pseudofolliculitis of the beard.

Fragility of the Hair Shaft (Fragilitas Crinium). Longitudinal splitting and fraying of the hair shaft which represents structural weakness of the hair. The commonest form is terminal splitting of the hair shaft seen in women who have allowed their hair to grow very long. This fragile hair can be associated with trichorrhexis nodosa, monilethrix and ringed hair.

Trichorrhexis Nodosa. A condition of the scalp, and also the beard and the pubic hair of adults, characterized by the clinical appearance of nodular swellings along the shaft which under the microscope are shown to be transverse fractures of the hair shaft suggesting the appearance of the bristles of two brooms interlocked.

Twisted Hairs (Pili Torti). Beaded Hair (Monilethrix). Ringed Hair (Pili Annulati). These 3 conditions may be different clinical manifestations of altered hair growth from hereditary and congenital causes. The terms are self-defining.

Trichostasis Spinulosa. A rather common condition in adults due to hyperkeratosis of the hair follicle opening and seen most commonly in patients with acne, keratosis pilaris and seborrheic dermatitis. The follicular plug contains 10 to 50 short lanugo hairs.

True **knotted hairs** rarely occur, but **pseudoknotted hair (trichonodosis)** occurs somewhat more frequently.

Progressive **kinking** of the scalp hair and **woolly hair** are additional rare genetic diseases.

BIBLIOGRAPHY

Behrman, H. T.: The Scalp in Health and Disease. St. Louis, C. V. Mosby, 1952.

Savill, Agnes, and Warren, Clara: The Hair and Scalp, ed. 5. Baltimore, Williams & Wilkins, 1962.

23

Diseases Affecting the Nails

The nails are affected by (1) primary nail diseases, (2) any dermatitis that involves the surrounding skin and (3) many internal diseases.

The structure of the nails is discussed on page 6.

A frequent misconception among patients is that nutrition plays an important part in the production of nail disorders. Lack of calcium and vitamins is mentioned most by patients. No little amount of verbal persuasion is necessary to correct this assumption. The questionable role of gelatin therapy for the improvement of fragile nails will be considered under that disorder.

PRIMARY NAIL DISEASES

Only the most common primary nail diseases will be included in this chapter. The terminology for the rare primary conditions is very complex and will be defined at the end of this chapter.

CONTACT REACTIONS
(Plate 51)

Changes in the nails, mainly the fingernails, from cosmetic applications are related to the constant attempts by manufacturers to discover a nail polish or covering that will adhere to and become a part of the nail for the life of the individual, or at least for the duration of a certain fad. Several years ago such a cosmetic panacea was discovered in the form of a base coat, but the nail rebelled with the development of thickening and loosening of the nail plate. More recently, the use of artificial nails and a press-on type covering resulted in splitting of the distal ends of the nail.

These nail-bed reactions are not related to, and should be differentiated from, the allergic sensitivity manifested by some women to chemicals in the nail polish. The fingernails, interestingly enough, do not react to this allergy, but the sensitivity shows up on the eyelids and the neck as a contact dermatitis (see p. 49).

NAIL-BITING

This common nervous habit of some children and fewer adults is very difficult to stop. Often the less attention that is paid to this tic the better, with the resulting cessation of the biting. The local application of distasteful chemicals to the nails seldom helps.

INFECTIONS

Primary nail infections can occur from several causes.

Bacterial and *monilial infections* (Plate 51) can cause a paronychial reaction; the monilial infections are chronic and very resistant to therapy (p. 178).

Green nails (Plate 51) is a unique and distinctive infection from which *C. albicans* and *Ps. aeruginosa* can be cultured. Complete débridement is necessary for a cure.

INGROWN NAILS

The mechanism of this disorder is the growth of the lateral edge of the nail plate, usually of the big toe, into the adjacent skin groove. Tight-fitting shoes and improper nail-trimming initiate the process. The result is a foreign-body type reaction with pain, redness, swelling and infection.

Prophylactic management is simple: the toenail never should be trimmed in a semilunar manner but should be trimmed straight across so the corner lies above the skin groove.

Active treatment of an acute process consists of hot soaks and local application

Fig. 23-1. Primary nail diseases. (*Top*) Tinea of the nails due to *T. rubrum.*

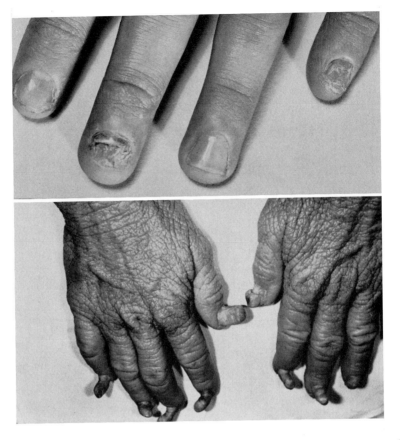

(*Bottom*) Onychogryphosis (claw nails) of unknown cause. (*Dr. Chester Lessenden*)

of an antiseptic tincture. After the pain has lessened, the placement of a pledget of cotton gently under the nail may be sufficient to raise the pointed corner up above the skin surface. More resistant cases are treated by removing the overlying skin by excision and suture, or by removing the lateral section of the nail back to the nail base with or without destruction of the base by electrosurgery.

HANG NAILS

Some patients are prone to develop small cutaneous tags from the lateral and posterior skin folds. Accidental or intentional pulling on these skin flaps tears into the deeper skin with resultant bleeding and a painful raw area that is susceptible to bacterial infection. This can be prevented by removal of the hang nail with scissors.

Treatment of the infection, which may develop into a *bacterial paronychia,* is with hot soaks, local application of antiseptic tinctures or ointments, avoidance of covering dressings, and, in severe cases, use of systemic antibiotics.

LEUKONYCHIA

The common "white spots" of the nail plate have been responsible for many interesting homespun etiologic labels. Medically speaking, we cannot do much better regarding the cause. (I've always thought they followed the telling of white lies.) The histogenesis is also not known, but current theories propose that the white spots are due to tiny air bubbles in the nail or due to the presence of incompletely keratinized cells, probably the result of minor injury. No treatment is indicated.

Hereditary leukonychia is very rare and involves all the finger- and toe-nails (Plate 51).

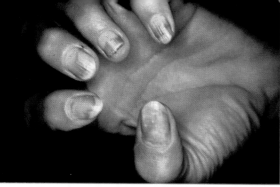

(A) Onycholysis contact reaction
to nail hardener

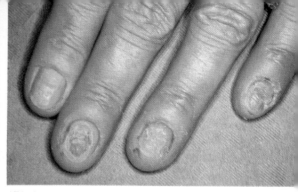

(B) Onychotillomania or picking
of nail plate

Plate 51. Nail disorders. (*Westwood Pharmaceuticals*)

(C) Traumatic, habit-tic injury to plate

(D) Tinea due to *T. rubrum*

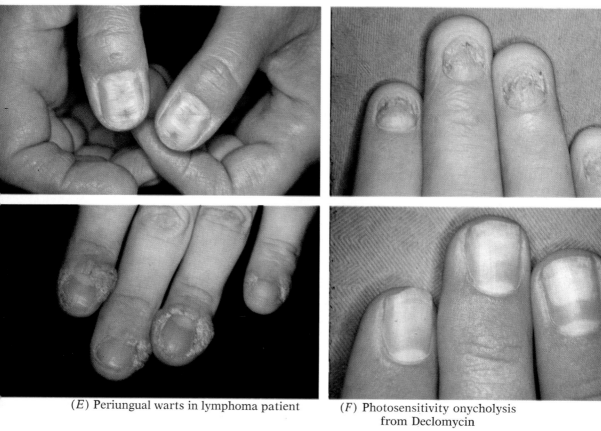

(E) Periungual warts in lymphoma patient

(F) Photosensitivity onycholysis
from Declomycin

(G) Monilial paronychia

(H) Green nails from monilial and
pseudomonas infection

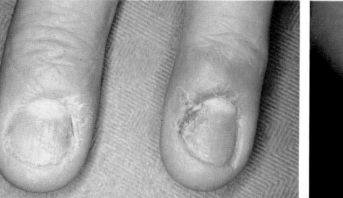

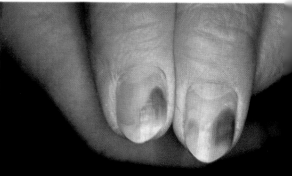

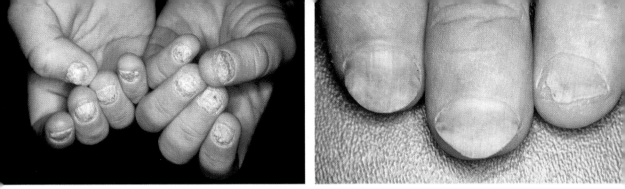

(I & J) Psoriasis of nails showing crumbling, pitting, and distal detachment of plates

Plate 51. Nail disorders *(Continued)*

(K & L) Lichen planus showing pterygium and plate atrophy on closeup of fingernails

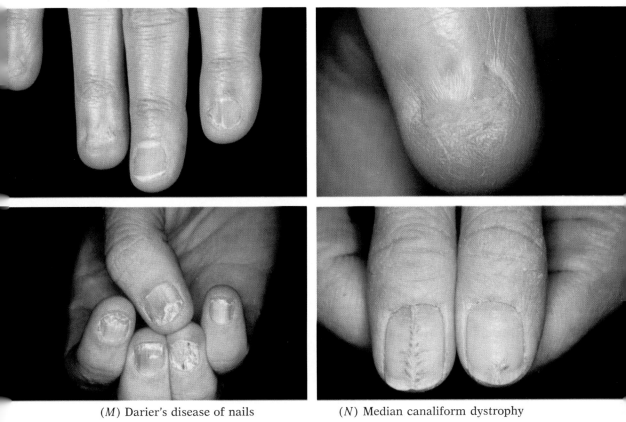

(M) Darier's disease of nails

(N) Median canaliform dystrophy

(O) Beau's lines due to hyperpigmentation in Negro following x-radiation

(P) Hereditary leukonychia totalis and partial onycholysis

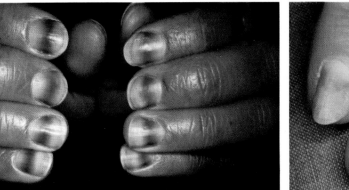

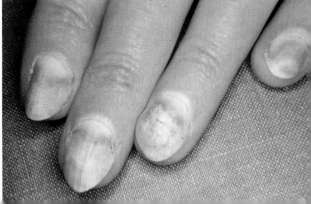

FRAGILE NAILS

The distal splitting of fingernails is a common complaint of women. In most instances the cause cannot be determined, but some cases are due to the "permanent" type of nail polishes or the solvents used in removing the polish.

The only therapy that appears to be even worthy of a trial is the daily oral ingestion of one envelope of Knox Gelatin mixed with fruit juices or water. This treatment should be kept up for at least 3 months to receive benefit, since it takes that long for the nail to grow out to the fragile end.

NAIL DISEASE SECONDARY TO OTHER DERMATOSES

The nail, as one of the skin appendages, is susceptible to diseases of the skin adjacent to the nail or dermatoses on distant areas. It is important to remember that a dermatitis of the skin can be made to heal rather rapidly, but that any concurrent nail involvement will take approximately 3 months to grow out with the nail. The "scar" remains on the nail much longer than on the skin.

TINEA OF THE NAILS
(Plate 51)

Disturbance of nail growth due to fungi is the most commonly observed nail problem (Fig. 23-1). A major percentage of the male population have one or more thickened toenails which almost invariably are caused by fungi. Females have onychomycosis of the toenails less frequently, and both sexes have fingernail involvement only rarely. Tinea of the nails is discussed in detail on page 165.

WARTS
(Plate 51)

Verrucae can occur anywhere on the body, but one of the most difficult warts to treat is the type that grows around the nail and under the nail plate. If the wart is large and extends rather far under the nail, a deformed nail may result from the removal. The patient should be told about this possibility in advance. The management of these problem warts is discussed on page 152.

ECZEMATOUS ERUPTIONS OF THE FINGERS

These eczematous skin eruptions include *contact dermatitis, atopic eczema* and *nummular eczema.* The nail becomes involved when these dermatoses affect the adjacent skin. When the skin dermatitis heals the nail will heal also, but, as stated previously, the mark of the dermatitis on the nail will take 3 months to disappear completely.

An unusual reaction of the nail is the development of a *highly polished nail surface* in some patients with severely itching *atopic eczema.* This is due to the habit of some atopics of constantly rubbing the skin with the flat nail surface instead of scratching with the distal end of the nail.

PSORIASIS
(Plate 51)

An astute clinician can occasionally diagnose psoriasis by merely examining the nails. Often the only sign of psoriasis will be the nail changes for which the patient seeks medical advice. Psoriasis can cause any and all of the dystrophic changes of the nails. The commonest changes are small pinpoint pits, with or without distal detachment of the nail. A proximal red halo frequently is present around the distal detachment. In severe psoriatic nail involvement there is complete disintegration of the plate surface with massive subungual proliferation. Even these severe changes are usually asymptomatic.

Treatment of psoriasis of the nails is very unsatisfactory. If psoriasis is present on other areas and responds to therapy, the nails may also clear up. Cordran tape applied over the nails is moderately effective.

OTHER DERMATOSES
(Plate 51)

Nonspecific nail changes can occur along with *lichen planus, alopecia areata, Darier's disease, epidermolysis bullosa, ichthyosis, pityriasis rubra pilaris* and other dermatoses.

NAIL DISEASE SECONDARY TO INTERNAL DISEASE

Changes in the nails can reflect internal disease. The great majority of these changes are nonspecific.

BEAU'S LINES
(Plate 51)

Beau's lines, or transverse furrows of the nails, may develop with any of a large group of cutaneous and systemic disturbances (Fig. 23-2). The latter include many of the acute infectious febrile diseases, such as malaria, syphilis and pulmonary tuberculosis, and coronary disease, pregnancy, collagen diseases and emotional shock.

Beau's lines are due to a temporary growth disturbance in the nail plate. A simile is the alteration in the annual growth rings of trees when affected by drought, fire, or pestilence. The width of Beau's lines varies directly with the duration of the internal disease. As stated before, the "scar" of this nail alteration will take approximately 3 months to grow out. Many are the awesome, astute, detective-like, laity-impressing deductions made by the clever physician when these lines are noted. A proper and impressive statement on finding Beau's lines approximately halfway down all of the fingernails is, "I see that you had a rather severe illness about 6 weeks ago."

HIPPOCRATIC NAILS

Clubbed nails and fingers are classically associated with chronic lung and heart disorders (Fig. 23-3). These changes apparently are due to the prolonged anoxemia present. Equally common is a congenital and hereditary form of hippocratic nails seen in healthy individuals.

OTHER CONDITIONS OF THE NAILS

The following rarer conditions of the nails will be defined briefly.

Anonychia. Total congenital absence of the nail.

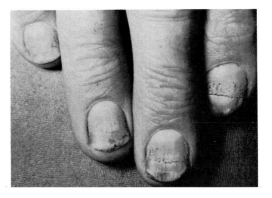

Fig. 23-2. Beau's lines following exfoliative dermatitis due to arsenic in Fowler's solution.

Median Canaliform Dystrophy. Appears in a fir tree configuration in the middle of the nail plate. The cause is unknown and the defect can spontaneously disappear.

Onychatrophia. Simple atrophy of the nails which may be congenital, hereditary, traumatic, or due to any severe local or systemic disease.

Habit-Tic Nail Deformity (Plate 51). This is seen on one or both thumbnail plates, where by habit, which may be denied by the patient, usually the middle fingernail is used to traumatize the cuticle area of the thumbnail. The result is a fir tree-like ridging of the nail plate.

Softened Nails (Hapalonychia). A rare atrophic condition usually concurrent with the aging process.

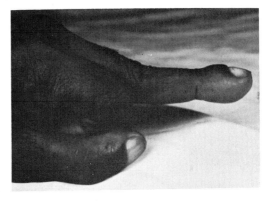

Fig. 23-3. Hippocratic or clubbed nails and fingers in Negro male with cardiovascular syphilis.

Spoon Nails (Koilonychia). Usually a congenital defect but seen with certain systemic diseases and occasionally with *Plummer-Vinson syndrome.*

Thickening of the Nail Plates (Onychauxis). Usually the result of continued trauma, as from ill-fitting shoes.

Claw Nails (Onychogryphosis). A marked thickening of the nails, particularly the toenails, where the nail plate becomes elongated and twisted. Trauma is the most important cause (Fig. 23-1).

Distal Separation of the Nails (Onycholysis). A spontaneous separation of the nail plate from the underlying bed which begins at the distal end and slowly progresses proximally. Occurs with systemic diseases and from irritating local causes.

A *photosensitivity onycholysis* can occur following systemic Declomycin or other tetracycline therapy (Plate 51).

Miscellaneous Nail Disorders. Nail picking (onychotillomania) (Plate 51), racket nails, longitudinal single nail groove, enlargement and adherence of the cuticle (pterygium), reeded nails with longitudinal splitting (onychorrhexis), horizontal splitting of the nails (onychoschizia), shedding of the nail (onychomadesis).

BIBLIOGRAPHY

Pardo-Castello, V., and Pardo, O. A.: Diseases of the Nails. ed. 3. Springfield, Charles C Thomas, 1960.

Samman, P. D.: The Nails in Disease. ed. 2. Springfield, Charles C Thomas, 1972.

24

Diseases of the Mucous Membranes

The mucous membranes of the body adjoin the skin at the oral cavity, nose, conjunctiva, penis, vulva and anus. Histologically, these membranes differ from the skin in that the horny layer and the hair follicles are absent. Disorders of the mucous membranes are usually associated with existing skin diseases or internal diseases.

Only two of the most common diseases of the mucous membranes will be discussed here. At the end of the chapter will be found a listing of the uncommon affections of these areas.

GEOGRAPHIC TONGUE

This is an extremely common condition of the tongue that usually occurs without symptoms (Fig. 24-1). Rarely the lesions are sensitive to sour or salty foods. When these lesions are noticed for the first time by the individual, they may initiate fears of cancer.

Clinical Appearance. Irregularly shaped (maplike or geographic) pale red patches on the tongue. Close examination reveals that the filiform papillae are flatter or denuded in these areas. The patches slowly migrate over the tongue surface and heal without scarring.

Course. Come and go but may be constantly present in some individuals.

Etiology. Unknown, but the lesions seem to be more extensive during a systemic illness.

Subjective Complaints. Usually none, but some patients complain of burning and tenderness, especially on eating sour or salty foods.

Differential Diagnosis

Syphilis, secondary mucous membrane lesions (very similar clinically, but acute in onset, usually more inflammatory; see other cutaneous signs of syphilis; dark-

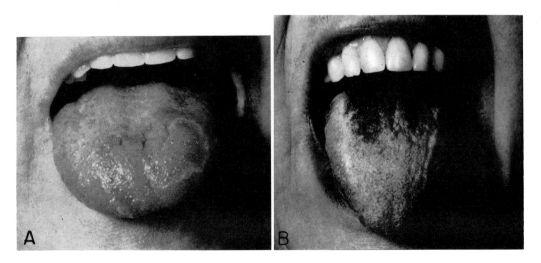

Fig. 24-1. Mucous membrane diseases. (*A*) Geographic tongue. (*B*) Black hairy tongue.

235

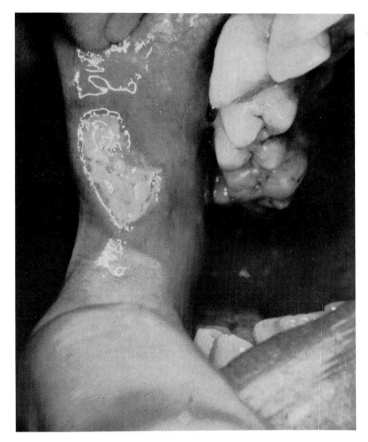

Fig. 24-2. Periadenitis mucosa necrotica recurrens.

field examination and serology would be positive, p. 134).

Treatment

1. Reassure patient that these are not cancerous lesions.
2. There is no effective or necessary therapy. However, if patient complains of burning and tenderness, prescribe:

Kenalog in Orabase   15.0
Sig: locally t.i.d.

APHTHOUS STOMATITIS

Canker sores are extremely common, painful, superficial ulcerations of the mucous membranes of the mouth.

Course. One or more lesions develop at the same time and heal without scarring in 5 to 10 days. Can recur at irregular intervals.

Etiology. Unknown. But certain foods, especially chocolate, nuts and fruits, can precipitate the lesions or may even be causative. Some cases in women recur in relation to menstruation. A viral etiology has not been proved. A pleomorphic, transitional L-form of an alpha-hemolytic streptococcus (*S. sanguis*) has also been implicated as etiologic.

Differential Diagnosis

Syphilis, secondary lesions (clinically similar; less painful; see other signs of syphilis; darkfield examination and serology would be positive, p. 134).

Treatment. Most persons who get these lesions have learned that very little can be done for them and that the ulcers will heal in a few days.

Kenalog in Orabase (prescription needed) applied locally before meals will relieve some of the pain.

Tetracycline Therapy. An oral suspension in a dosage of 250 mg. per teaspoonful (or the powdery contents of a 250 mg. capsule in a teaspoon of water) kept in the mouth for 2 minutes and then swallowed, and done 4 times a day, is quite healing.

HERPES SIMPLEX

This viral infection can occur as a group of umbilicated vesicles on the mucous membranes of the lips, the conjunctiva, the penis and the labia. Frequently recurring episodes of this disease can be quite disabling. Refer to page 145.

FORDYCE CONDITION

This is a physiological variant of oral sebaceous glands where more than the normal number exist. When they are suddenly noticed, the individual becomes concerned as to the diagnosis.

OTHER MUCOSAL LESIONS AND CONDITIONS

CAUSES

Mucosal lesions can also be due to:

Physical Causes. Sucking of lips, pressure sores, burns, actinic or sunlight cheilitis (Fig. 25-1), tobacco, other chemicals, and allergens.

Infectious diseases from viruses, bacteria, spirochetes, fungi and animal parasites. Gangrenous bacterial infections are called *noma*. *Ludwig's angina* is an acute cellulitis of the floor of the mouth due to bacteria, abscesses and sinuses; may be due to dental infection. *Trench mouth*, or *Plaut-Vincent's disease*, is an acute ulcerative infection of the mucous membranes caused by a combination of a spirochete and a fusiform bacillus.

Systemic Diseases. These include lesions seen with *hematologic diseases* (leukemia, agranulocytosis from drugs or other causes, thrombocytopenia, pernicious anemia, cyclic or periodic neutropenia, etc.), *collagen diseases* (lupus erythematosus and scleroderma), *pigmentary diseases* (Addison's disease, Peutz-Jeghers syndrome, etc.) and *autoimmune diseases* which cross over in several categories but include pemphigus and pemphigoid, and possibly benign mucosal pemphigoid.

Drugs. *Dilantin sodium* causes a hyperplastic gingivitis; *bismuth* orally and intramuscularly causes a bluish-black line at the edge of the dental gum (Plate 14); certain drugs cause hemorrhage and secondary infection of the mucous membranes.

Metabolic Diseases. Mucosal lesions are seen in primary systemic amyloidosis, lipoidosis, reticuloendothelioses, diabetes, etc.

Tumors, Local or Systemic. These include leukoplakia, squamous cell epithelioma, epulis and cysts.

RARER CONDITIONS OF ORAL MUCOUS MEMBRANES

Halitosis, or fetor oris, is a disagreeable odor of the breath.

Periadenitis Mucosa Necrotica Recurrens. (Fig. 24-2.) Also known as Sutton's disease, this is a painful, recurrent, ulcerating disease of the mucous membranes of the oral cavity.

Foot and Mouth Disease. A virus disease of animals and occasionally man, characterized by a painful, self-limited vesicular stomatitis.

Koplik's Spots. Bright red pinpoint-sized lesions on the mucous membranes of the cheek; seen in patients before the appearance of the rash of measles.

Burning Tongue (Glossodynia). A rather common complaint, particularly of middle-aged women; usually accompanied by no visible pathology. The etiology is unknown, and therapy is of little value; but the many diseases and local factors that cause painful tongue must be ruled out from a diagnostic viewpoint.

Black Tongue (Hairy Tongue, Lingua Nigra). (Fig. 24-1.) Overgrowth of the papillae of the tongue apparently caused by an imbalance of bacterial flora due to the use of antibiotics and other agents.

Moeller's Glossitis. A painful, persistent, red eruption on the sides and the tip of the tongue that persists for weeks or months, subsides, and then recurs. The etiology is unknown.

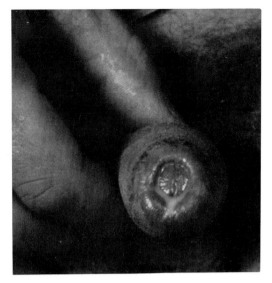

Fig. 24-3. Fusospirochetal balanitis.

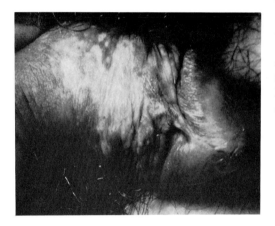

Fig. 24-4. Balanitis xerotica obliterans.
(*Dr. David Morgan*)

Furrowed Tongue (Grooved Tongue, Scrotal Tongue). A tongue that is usually larger than normal, containing deep longitudinal and lateral grooves of congenital origin or due to syphilis.

Glossitis Rhomboidea Mediana. A rare disorder characterized by a smooth reddish lesion, usually in the center of the tongue. This term is poor because there is no inflammation, and the reddish plaque may not always be in the center.

Sjögren's Syndrome. A very rare entity characterized by dryness of all of the mucous membranes and of the skin in middle-aged women. This may be related to *Plummer-Vinson syndrome.*

Cheilitis Glandularis Apostematosa. A chronic disorder of the lips manifested by swelling and secondary inflammation due to hypertrophy of the mucous glands and their ducts.

RARER CONDITIONS OF GENITAL
MUCOUS MEMBRANES

Fusospirochetal Balanitis (Fig. 24-3). An uncommon infection of the penis characterized by superficial erosions. It must be differentiated from syphilis by a darkfield examination and blood serology.

Balanitis Xerotica Obliterans (Fig. 24-4). See Atrophies of the Skin in the Dictionary Index. It is to be differentiated from leukoplakia. The female counterpart is *lichen sclerosis et atrophicus.*

Lichen Sclerosis et Atrophicus. A rare atrophy of the skin (usually around neck) and of the genital mucous membranes. In children (Plate 58) it is the commonest chronic genital dermatitis. (See Atrophies of the Skin in the Dictionary-Index.)

Ulcus Vulvae Acutum. A rare self-limited disease mainly of virgins characterized by shallow ulcerated lesions of the vulva. Thought to be caused by *Bacillus crassus* or a virus.

BIBLIOGRAPHY

Modeé, J. S., et al: Oral Manifestations in Some Systemic Diseases. Medicina Cutanea, *4*:109-127, 1969. A very complete review in English.

25

Dermatoses Due to Physical Agents

Physical agents, such as heat, cold, pressure and radiant energy (x-rays, ultraviolet rays, gamma rays), can produce both irritative reactions and allergic reactions on the skin. The two common physical irritations of the skin are *sunburn*, due to ultraviolet radiation, and *radiodermatitis* due to ionizing radiation. Allergic reactions can also develop from these two physical agents and from the other agents listed above.

The following chapter on photosensitivity dermatoses also covers some of the sun reactions mentioned here.

SUNBURN

A sunburn can be mild and desired, or severe and feared. The most severe reactions come from prolonged exposure at swimming areas or when the unfortunate individual falls asleep under an ultraviolet lamp. The degree of reaction depends on several factors, including length and intensity of exposure, the individual's complexion and previous conditioning of the skin.

Certain drugs can increase the sensitivity of the skin to sunlight. The reaction can vary in intensity from a simple erythema, to a measleslike rash or to a severe bullous eruption. Consult page 68 for a list of these *photosensitizing drugs.*

Primary Lesions. Varying degrees of redness develop within 2 to 12 hours after exposure to the ultraviolet radiation and reach maximum intensity within 24 hours. Vesiculation occurs in severe cases along with systemic weakness, chills, malaise and local pain.

Secondary Lesions or Reactions. Scaling or peeling, though not desired by the sun devotee, is the aftermath of any overexposure. Vesiculation can be complicated by secondary infection. An increase in pigmentation is usually the desired end-result, but this tanning is not accomplished by overzealous exposure.

Lupus erythematosus of either the sys-

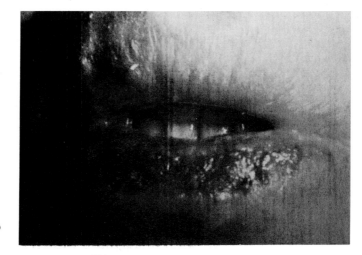

Fig. 25-1. Cheilitis due to sunlight sensitivity.

239

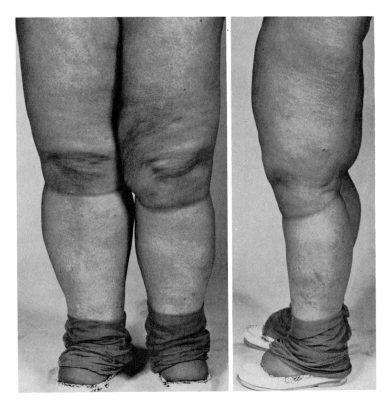

Fig. 25-2. Elephantiasis type of lymphedema following x-ray therapy of uterine malignancy.

temic or the chronic discoid type may be triggered by sun exposure in a susceptible person (p. 204). *Sunlight allergy (polymorphic light eruption* or *actinic dermatitis)* in susceptible individuals is manifested clinically by (1) plaquelike erythematous lesions, (2) contact-dermatitis-like lesions, (3) papular pruritic lesions and (4) erythema-multiforme-like lesions. These cases may be difficult to distinguish from lupus erythematosus, especially the discoid type. Short-term oral chloroquine therapy combined with protection from sunlight is quite effective.

Late Reactions to Sunlight. *Actinic* or *senile keratoses* appear mainly after the age of 50 but are seen in highly susceptible individuals in their 30's. Chronic sun and wind exposure on the part of a light-complexioned farmer, sailor or gardener will lead to the development of these superficial, red, scaling keratoses on exposed surfaces of the face, the lips (actinic cheilitis, Fig. 25-1), the ears, the neck and

the dorsum of the hands. *Prickle cell epitheliomas* arise in an appreciable percentage of these actinic keratoses (see pp. 264 and 269).

Prophylactic Treatment. The ultraviolet rays from the sun or from other sources can be either completely blocked or partially blocked from the skin surface.

1. Complete blocking of the sun rays is desired for prevention of actinic keratoses, a flare-up of lupus erythematosus, or a sun allergy reaction. Application of Uval, Solbar, A-fil Cream, Skolex Cream, or R.V.P. Ointment will accomplish this for 4 to 6 hours after a single application.

2. Partial blocking can be accomplished by the use of any of the many available proprietary "suntan" oils, lotions and creams. It is best to avoid the use of oily or greasy preparations, since a pustular or acnelike eruption can ensue in susceptible individuals. Sensible and gradual sun exposure of the skin is the best pre-

ventative for sunburn, but most people learn this the hard way.

Active Treatment. A young woman presents herself with a painful, erythematous, vesicular skin reaction on her face, back and thighs of 24 hours' duration following a holiday trip to the beach (first- and second-degree burns).

1. Boric acid crystals   60.0

Sig: 1 tablespoon to 1 quart of cool water. Apply cloths wet with the cool solution to the affected areas for as long a time as necessary to keep comfortable.

2. Menthol   0.25%

Nonalcoholic white shake lotion (see Formulary p. 37) q.s.   120.0

Sig: Apply locally t.i.d. to affected areas.

3. Blisters can be drained but should not be debrided.

SUBSEQUENT CARE. A day or two later, to soften the scales and to prevent secondary infection, prescribe:

1. Menthol   0.25%

Neosporin or other antibiotic ointment   15.0

White petrolatum   15.0

Sig: Apply locally t.i.d.

2. Warn the patient to exercise caution in resuming sun exposure to the now very sensitive skin.

RADIODERMATITIS

The hazards of ionizing radiation have reached the front page of the newspapers and the feature articles of most magazines. This is the Atomic Age. Some of the publicity is good, but it has made the pendulum swing to the side of general criticism of all forms of ionizing therapy as used in medicine. X-rays and other forms of such therapy are established as unique therapeutic modalities, but, as with all potent medicinal agents, they must be administered intelligently. When they are not so administered the result is varying degrees of damage to the skin and the underlying organs. We shall be concerned here with the skin changes, radiodermatitis.

Clinical Lesions. *Acute radiodermatitis* is divided into 3 degrees of severity similar to the reactions from thermal burns. The first degree is manifested by the slow development of erythema, hyperpigmentation and usually hair loss. A single dose of x-rays necessary to produce these changes is called an "erythema dose." All of the changes in the first degree are reversible.

The second degree is characterized by vesicle formation, erosions, hair loss, secondary infection and delayed healing. Atrophy and telangiectasis are the end-results.

The third degree of radiodermatitis includes ulceration, infection and greatly delayed healing. Epitheliomatous changes are very common in the chronic ulcer or scar.

Chronic radiodermatitis can follow acute radiation injury or develop slowly following repeated small radiation exposures (Figs. 25-2 and 25-3). *The dosage of ionizing radiation on the skin is cumulative; the effect of previous radiation therapy is never erased by the passage of time.*

Etiology. Many factors influence the development of radiodermatitis. These include the physical factors of kilovoltage, milliamperage, distance, filters and the half-value layer; the individual factors of health, age, complexion, type of lesion and size and depth of the area to be treated; and the treatment factors of dosage, number of treatments and interval between treatments.

Prophylactic Treatment. If all of the above etiologic factors are remembered, acute and chronic radiodermatitis will not develop following radiation therapy for benign conditions. However, certain degenerative changes are unavoidable when therapy must be directed toward the removal of a malignant condition. Ionizing therapy should be administered only by competently trained dermatologists or radiologists. It is most important for all concerned to remember that when a so-called complete course of radiation therapy has been given to a particular body area, no further radiation should be administered to this area at *any* future time.

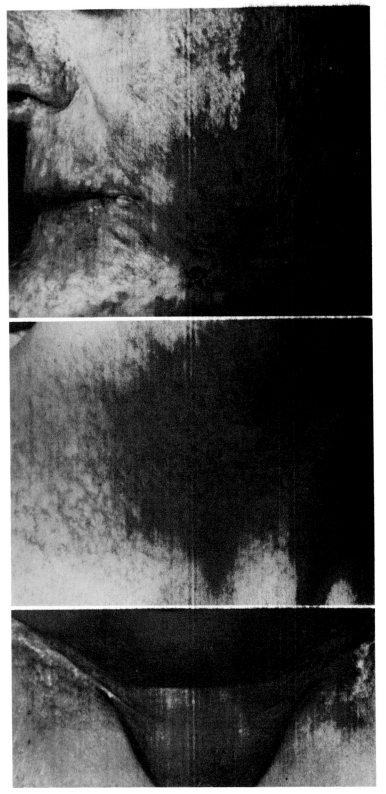

Fig. 25-3. Chronic radiodermatitis. (*Top*) Atrophy and scarring of face following permanent epilation of hypertrichosis by x-ray therapy given 30 years previously.

(*Center*) Telangiectasia on neck due to excessive x-ray dosage for acne with improper shielding.

(*Bottom*) On groin areas. This is the expected and normal atrophic reaction from x-ray therapy directed toward a uterine malignancy in a Negro woman. (*K.U.M.C.*)

Active Treatment. The acute cases of radiodermatitis can be treated symptomatically with bland local measures. Therapy of chronic radiodermatitis should be carried out by a dermatologist, a surgeon or a plastic surgeon. The damaged skin is markedly sensitive to other forms of irritation, such as wind, sunlight, injury, harsh cosmetics and local therapy.

BIBLIOGRAPHY

Cipollaro, A. C., and Crossland, P. M.: X-Rays and Radium in the Treatment of Diseases of the Skin, ed. 5. Philadelphia, Lea & Febiger, 1967.

26

Photosensitivity Dermatoses

James Kalivas, M.D.*

The most valuable clue to the diagnosis of a photodermatosis, or "light eruption," is the usually sharp demarcation between normal covered and abnormal exposed skin. At times, airborne contact dermatitis (as from ragweed pollen) may mimic the distribution of this disease, but the light eruption will tend to spare key areas like the submental region and the eyelid folds. Photo-testing may, however, be necessary to differentiate the two diseases. Often the patient does not realize that sunlight (ultraviolet) is evoking or aggravating the eruption. Once a presumptive diagnosis of light eruption is reached, the next step is to determine whether it is secondary to exogenous factors, or is primary (endogenous).

EXOGENOUS PHOTOSENSITIVITY

INTERNAL AGENTS

Most systemic photosensitizers tend to produce dose-proportionate, non-immunological, "phototoxic" reactions. (Plates 4 and 52.) This means that nearly all, except perhaps the blackest blacks, who take the drug can be potentially photosensitized. The most frequent offenders are demeclocycline (Declomycin), doxycycline (Vibramycin), chlorpromazine (Thorazine), hydrochlorothiazide (Hydro-Diuril, Esidrix), sulfonylureas (Orinase), and nalidixic acid (Neggram). In the drug eruption section on p. 68 is a more complete list of photosensitizers.

Clinically the eruption most often resembles an exaggerated sunburn, but may take the form of itching only in the exposed areas (from hydrochlorothiazide) or may be present as large bullae (from nalidixic acid). Nail detachment or onycholysis also occurs (Plate 51 and p. 234).

Treatment

1. The patient should avoid prolonged exposure to direct sunlight. This precaution may have to be observed for many months following a severe photodermatitis.

2. Chemical sunscreens are not terribly effective.

3. Topical steroids may afford some relief.

EXTERNAL AGENTS

Most topical photosensitizers tend to produce photoallergic reactions. These occur only in sensitized persons and characteristically are far out of proportion in severity to the amount of exposure received (Plate 52). The most important contact photosensitizers today are the halogenated salicylanilides found in such soaps as Zest, Lifebuoy, Phase III and Safeguard.

The most important topical phototoxic agents are the psoralens, which are found in such plant products as lime cologne, Shalimar perfume, parsnip, gas plant, figs, dill, and celery. Eruptions from these agents are typically followed by intense, bizzare hyperpigmentation. *Berlock dermatitis* is an example of this reaction (Fig. 19-2).

Clinically the eruption is usually eczematous in appearance, with prominent lichenification and scratch marks. Even after discontinuation of the offending soap or

---

* Associate Professor and Head of the Section of Dermatology, University of Kansas School of Medicine.

other agent, the eruption may linger for months and virtually disable the patient ("persistent light reactor").

Treatment

1. The patient should avoid sunlight and even strong fluorescent lighting insofar as possible. Sunscreens as a rule are only moderately effective. The better ones seem to be the benzophenones (Solbar, Uval, Pan-Ultra) and the para-aminobenzoic acid preparations (Presun, Pabanal, Pabafilm, etc.).

2. Topical steroids may afford some relief.

ENDOGENOUS PHOTOSENSITIVITY

Once the possibility of an exogenous photosensitizer has been ruled out by taking a careful history, the physician may then consider the so-called primary light-sensitive disorders. The two most common in this country are (1) the cutaneous porphyrias and (2) the collagen-vascular group. (Photosensitivity caused by melanin insufficiency as in vitiligo and albinism is discussed in Chapter 19 dealing with "Pigmentary Dermatoses.")

1. Porphyrias (*See* Dictionary Index)

Porphyria cutanea tarda (Plate 52 and p. 186): The most common porphyria with cutaneous manifestations is symptomatic porphyria, or porphyria cutanea tarda (PCT). Patients with this disorder are usually over forty, often drink heavily and often do not complain of undue sensitivity to sunlight. One may find associated diabetes mellitus in 25% of cases of PCT, and hepatic siderosis in 80% of cases. Over 90% of untreated patients with PCT have abnormal BSP retention.

Cutaneous lesions include hyperpigmentation in exposed areas, hypertrichosis (this may be the presenting complaint in women), blisters and erosions from abnormal fragility of the exposed skin, milia, periocular erythema, and scleroderma (may occur in unexposed areas). One does not find acute abdominal crises or primary neurological defects in PCT. These are

however seen in the much rarer *familial variegate porphyria*.

The **diagnosis** rests with demonstrating a greatly elevated urinary uroporphyrin excretion (>500 $\mu g/24$ hours). A tentative diagnosis may be made by finding the characteristic red fluorescence of a fresh-voided acidified urine sample under Wood's illumination.

Treatment

1. Phlebotomy. The treatment of choice is multiple, but not overzealous phlebotomies over a period of months. Generally, a lasting remission, both clinically and biochemically, may be achieved by withdrawal of 500 cc. of blood every 2 weeks for 3 to 4 times, then every 3 to 6 weeks for a total of 10 to 15 pints of blood.

2. Abstinence from alcohol should be urged. Also, although patients with PCT are not vulnerable to acute attacks from barbiturates, griseofulvin, sulfonamides, or oral contraceptives, etc. as are patients with variegate porphyria or acute intermittent porphyria (no skin changes in the latter), certain foreign substances, such as iron, diphenylhydantoin (Dilantin), and diethylstilbestrol, do seem to aggravate the disease and, with alcohol, should be avoided wherever possible.

Protoporphyria. The second most common cutaneous porphyria, protoporphyria, is inherited and usually begins in childhood. Children with this disorder complain bitterly of burning and stinging of the exposed areas after only minutes in the sun. For several days after exposure they may display marked erythema and edema of the face and hands. Sometimes urticaria and vesicles are seen. Photosensitivity may persist well into adult life, but between attacks there are usually few objective lesions. It is most often misdiagnosed as "solar urticaria" or "airborne contact dermatitis."

The **diagnosis** rests with demonstrating an elevated erythrocyte protoporphyrin concentration (>50 $\mu g/100$ ml of packed red cells). Fluorescence microscopy may

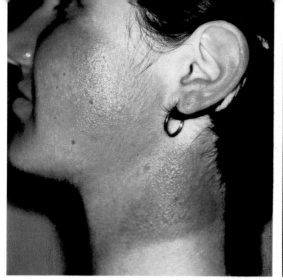
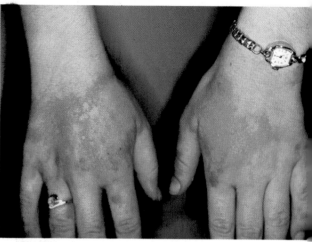

| (A) Photosensitivity dermatitis following Declomycin therapy | (B) Photosensitivity with residual hyperpigmentation from soap |

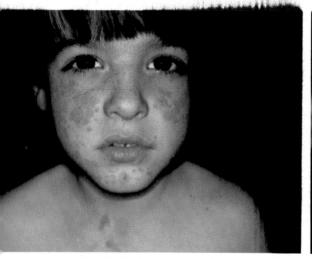

(C & D) Hydroa aestivale off and on for 4 years in 7-year-old boy; closeup of cheek

Plate 52. Photosensitivity dermatoses. (*Texas Pharmacal Co.*)

| (E) Papular polymorphic light eruption off and on for 15 years | (F) Porphyria cutanea tarda with blisters and hyperpigmentation |

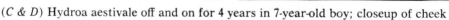
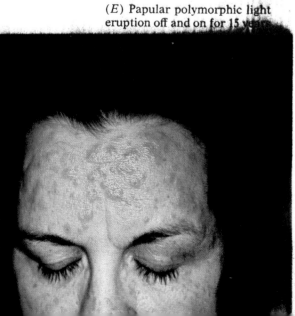
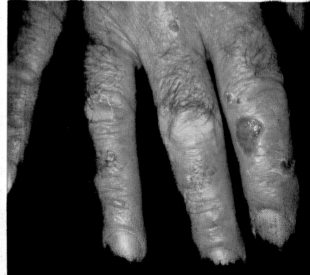

be used to screen blood smears for the disease.

Treatment. There is no reliable treatment available at present, although recent experience with large oral doses of carotene does offer some promise.

2. Collagen-Vascular disorders (See Chapter 20)

Polymorphous light eruption (PMLE) (Plate 52) will be included here, although opinion is divided as to whether it is truly related to lupus erythematosus. PMLE is characteristically seasonal (spring and summer), and it most commonly affects adolescents and young adults.

The skin lesions, as the name implies, are highly variable and may range from wheals (*idiopathic solar urticaria* is probably a variant of PMLE), to vesicles, to papules, to large plaques. Subjective symptoms are not as prominent as in protoporphyria. *Hydroa aestivale* may be a related variant of PMLE. (Plate 52)

Treatment

1. Topical sunscreens offer modest relief.

2. Oral antimalarials are usually highly effective in PMLE, but should not be used unless one is thoroughly familiar with the severe side effect of permanent retinal damage.

Lupus erythematosus (LE) (Plate 47): Both systemic and discoid LE may be exacerbated by sunlight, but only in about one-third of all cases. If the diagnosis is not apparent clinically, skin biopsy (more valuable in discoid LE) and/or laboratory tests (more valuable in systemic LE) may help clarify it.

Treatment. Sunscreens, topical steroids, and systemic antimararials have been used with some success. (See p. 204)

Dermatomyositis. Photosensitivity is usually less prominent in dermatomyositis than in lupus. Laboratory studies are usually necessary to verify the diagnosis.

Treatment. Sunscreens may be tried, but control of the underlying illness is usually of greater benefit. (See p. 209)

MISCELLANEOUS PHOTODERMATOSES

These include *solar urticaria* (see under polymorphous light eruption), *Hartnup disease, pellagra, xeroderma pigmentosum, Bloom's syndrome,* and *actinic reticuloid.* Poikiloderma approaching that seen in radiodermatitis may also be produced by ultraviolet, both on an acquired basis (*poikiloderma of Civatte*) (Fig. 30-2) and, rarely, on an inherited basis (*poikiloderma congenitale*). *Rosacea* (p. 95) often is aggravated by excessive sun exposure.

Except for rosacea and pellagra, effective treatment for all these conditions is nil to meager.

Actinic Keratoses (Plate 54 and p. 263). Also known as solar, or senile, keratoses, these dry, reddish, "sandpapery" excrescences are typically found on the face, ears, and hands of an elderly outdoorsman with a rufous telangiectatic complexion. Because they gradually undergo malignant transformation to *squamous cell carcinoma* in 20% of cases or more, they merit careful, thorough removal.

Treatment. 5-fluorouracil solution (Efudex 2% or 5%, Fluoroplex 1%) is probably the treatment of choice (see p. 265). It should be applied to all the sun-damaged areas (both abnormal and apparently "normal") b.i.d. for 2 to 4 weeks, or to the limits of tolerance, whichever occurs first. Patients should be warned in advance that a brisk inflammatory response will occur, and that this is desirable ("means the medicine is working"). Any remaining, thick keratoses which resist the fluorouracil treatment may be finished off with conventional techniques such as curettage and desiccation, caustic acid, liquid nitrogen, etc. (See p. 45).

Sunburn. Sunburn is usually the result, not of disease but of indiscretion. Some Caucasians, however, are remarkably deficient in melanin, which is the principal physiological sunscreen in man, and they burn with the briefest sun exposure. (Also see p. 239.)

Treatment

1. Prevention: Sunscreens are often of great value here. A variety are available commercially, but the *p*-aminobenzoic acid preparations are probably the most effective (e.g., Pabanol, Pabafilm, PreSun).

2. For the *acute sunburn*, soothing applications of cool tap water, milk, Burow's solution, or steroid lotions are helpful. Systemic analgesics and systemic steroids are sometimes necessary. Ultraviolet damage to the cornea requires expert ophthalmological management.

BIBLIOGRAPHY

Cripps, D. J.: Diseases aggravated by sunlight. Postgrad. Med., *41*: 557-567, 1967.

Daniels, F., Jr.: Diseases caused or aggravated by sunlight. Med. Clin. N. Am., *49*: 565-580, 1965.

Kalivas, J.: A guide to the problem of photosensitivity. JAMA, *209*: 1706-1709, 1969.

Willis, I.: Sunlight and the skin. JAMA, *217*: 1088-1093, 1971.

27

Genodermatoses

The genetic factor has a profound influence on normal man and diseased man. In normal man the skin has a certain color, thickness, hairyness and even odor that is inherited through the genes. The man with a skin disease reacts in a certain pattern because of a genetic inheritance. Such common skin problems as *acne, dandruff, atopic eczema* and *nevi* owe their presence to genetic patterns. The man with inherited allergies who gets *poison ivy dermatitis* or *pityriasis rosea* will have a more aggravated itchy response than the individual with these diseases who did not inherit an "allergic" itchy skin.

A concise summary of genetic disease occurs in a paper by Landau (see *Bibliography*). The following introductory material is quoted from this paper.

"The term "genetic disease" includes disorders transmitted by a known pattern of inheritance, syndromes associated with an abnormal chromosome pattern, and familial diseases for which no definite pattern of transmission has been determined."

Some genetic disorders, such as certain types of *ichthyosis* and *epidermolysis bullosa,* are also "congenital" since they are present at birth. Other genetic disorders, such as *pseudoxanthoma elasticum* and *hereditary angioneurotic edema,* are generally first detected after infancy and are genetic in origin but are not congenital.

Some significant advances have occurred in recent years in certain genodermatoses. For instance, careful clinical and histopathological studies have clarified 4 major types of ichthyosis. Two different types of autosomal recessive *oculocutaneous albinism* have been identified. A defect in the repair replication of DNA has been found in ultraviolet irradiated skin fibroblasts from patients with *xeroderma pigmentosum.* A gross deficiency has recently been detected of alpha-galactosidase in leukocytes of patients with *Fabry's disease.*

Two readily accessible parts of the skin provide information of genetic importance. The usefulness of dermatoglyphic interpretation has been well documented. The value of hair studies has only recently been appreciated. The hair is influenced in more than 30 different genetic diseases. Furthermore, the hair-root cells have been used in chromosome analysis, chromatin studies, and enzyme determinations.

PATTERNS OF INHERITANCE

The 3 most frequently encountered patterns of inheritance are autosomal dominant, autosomal recessive, and x-linked recessive.

A dominant condition is one in which those who have the mutant gene on only one member of the chromosome pair (heterozygotes) are clinically affected. Those who carry the gene on both members of the chromosome pair may, however, be very severely affected.

A recessive condition is one in which those who are clinically affected have the mutant gene on both members of the chromosome pair (homozygotes). The heterozygote shows no significant clinical abnormality, but may be detectable if the basic biochemical defect is known.

An x-linked condition is determined by a mutant gene on the x-chromosome. Most x-linked conditions are classified as recessive. The condition is always expressed in the male (hemizygotes). Females are generally heterozygous for the mutant gene, but may present some minor clinical manifestations. The heterozygous female is actually a mosaic, since one x-chromosome is randomly inactivated in each cell.

The risk figures are readily ascertained for the three common patterns of inheritance. With dominant conditions, the risk is one in two to the children of affected members of the family but little risk to later sibs of the first sporadic case in a family. With recessive conditions, the risk is one in four to later sibs of affected children, but little risk to anyone else in the family, even to children of index patients. With x-linked recessive conditions, the risk is one in two to sons of known heterozygous carrier women. If the mother is not a heterozygous carrier, all sons of a male with x-linked recessive condition will be unaffected, but all daughters will be carriers.

X-linked dominant conditions are extremely rare. Three examples with dermatological findings are *incontinentia pigmenti, focal dermal hypoplasia,* and *oral-facial-digital syndrome type 1.* The mutant gene in these conditions is considered to produce clinical manifestations in the heterozygous female and to be lethal in the hemizygous male.

A generalization that appears useful is that dominant conditions are less severe than recessive ones. A dominant mutation that precludes reproduction will disappear, but a recessive mutation can gain wide dissemination in heterozygous carriers even if it prevents reproduction in the homozygous state. Some examples of the lesser severity of the dominant forms of a condition are *ichthyosis vulgaris* compared with *non-bullous ichthyosiform erythroderma,* and *epidermolysis bullosa simplex* compared with *epidermolysis bullosa letalis.* Another generalization that has some merit is that dominant conditions tend to involve structural protein abnormalities, whereas recessive conditions tend to be errors of metabolism involving enzymes.

GENETIC COUNSELING

Genetic counseling should be an integral part of every medical practice, although some physicians may desire additional training in genetics. Current practice in genetic counseling consists of explaining the recurrence risks to the parents or the patient, placing these risks in proper perspective for them, but leaving to them the decision of whether or not to have further children."

There are many hereditary skin diseases. Ichthyosis is the most common one that is not discussed elsewhere in this book.

DOMINANT ICHTHYOSIS VULGARIS

Of the many types of ichthyosis, the dominant ichthyosis vulgaris form is the most common and will be considered here (Plate 53). A genetic classification of some of the other forms of ichthyosis will appear at the end of this section.

Primary lesions. Small white scales, often in association with keratosis pilaris-type lesions, are seen.

Secondary lesions. Rare. The scaling may be deep enough in some areas, particularly on the palms and soles, to result in small fissures.

Distribution. The arms and legs are the most severely affected, but the extent of involvement varies with individual cases. Some cases can have a considerable amount of scaling over the entire body.

Course. This common form of ichthyosis is worse in the winter. In most cases there is essentially no scaling in the summertime. There is a tendency for improvement after puberty or early adult life.

Differential Diagnosis

Xerosis or **acquired ichthyosis.** The most common cause of this dry skin problem is aging of the individual (see p. 72). If generalized dry skin develops in *young* adults it is an indication for a detailed investigation to rule out an internal malignancy such as Hodgkin's disease or lymphosarcoma or carcinomatosis. A vitamin A deficiency may also be a precipitating factor of dry skin. Hypothyroidism can also be a cause. Clinically, xerosis and ichthyosis vulgaris appear similar.

Treatment

1. It is important in the management of these cases of ichthyosis to explain that there is no cure for the problem (a fact

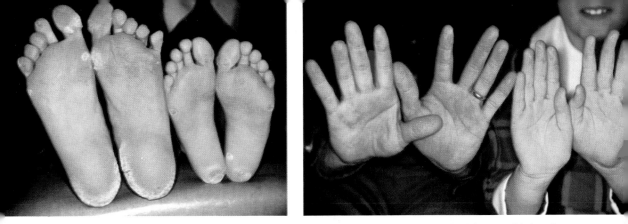

(A & B) Keratosis palmaris et plantaris of feet and hands of father and of 8-year-old daughter

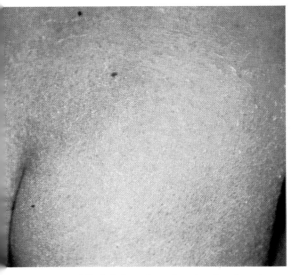

(C) Ichthyosis vulgaris, dominant type, of buttocks

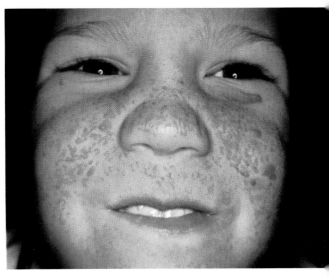

(D) Adenoma sebaceum in 4-year-old boy with epilepsy (tuberous sclerosis)

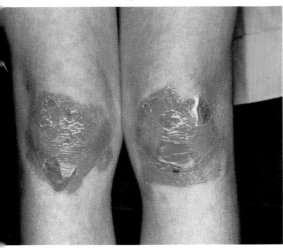

(E) Epidermolysis bullosa dystrophica, dominant type, of knees in girl age 5

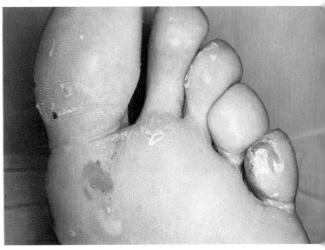

(F) Epidermolysis bullosa simplex, dominant type, in male age 23

Plate 53. Genodermatoses. *(Westwood Pharmaceuticals)*

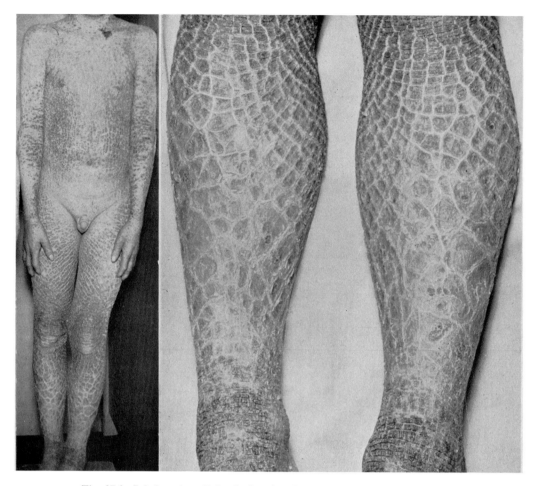

Fig. 27-1. Ichthyosis, x-linked, showing full body and close-up of legs.
(*Dr. David Morgan, K.C.G.H.*)

that the patient undoubtedly already suspects), but that there are ways to decrease the dryness of the skin in the wintertime.

Advise the patient to bathe only once a week. Suggest an emollient soap such as Dove, Aveeno bar, Basis soap, or Oilatum soap. Suggest the following emollients to be applied liberally on the skin:

Nivea Skin Oil or Cream
Keri Lotion or Cream
Lubriderm Lotion or Cream
Ultraderm Moisturizer
Neutraderm Lotion

or others.

White vaseline locally is appreciated by many who have the more severe form of this ichthyosis.

Salt-water baths have never been impressive to me, but some feel that daily bathing in a hypertonic salt-water solution is helpful.

2. Vitamin A orally appears to be beneficial for some cases. The dose should be 100 to 200 thousand units a day but for no longer than 3 months at a time.

3. Vitamin A acid (Retinoic acid) locally is helpful mainly for lamellar ichthyosis, but it also appears to be moderately helpful in some cases of dominant ichthyosis vulgaris. The proprietary preparation is Retin A. Warn that this causes a rather marked scaling and even redness of the skin. Intermittent therapy is usually well tolerated.

CLASSIFICATION OF ICHTHYOSIS

Ichthyosis vulgaris—autosomal dominant inheritance. See p. 250.

X-linked ichthyosis vulgaris—sex-linked recessive inheritance. This rare type is characterized by large brown scales that begin in very early infancy and persist throughout life. It occurs in males only. (Fig. 27-1.)

Lamellar ichthyosis—autosomal recessive inheritance. Rare. Diffuse erythema and scaling are present at birth and improve somewhat in later childhood. Retin A solution locally appears to be effective, but the toxicity has not been completely evaluated.

Non-bullous ichthyosiform erythroderma—autosomal recessive inheritance. Rare. This includes the Harlequin fetus (Plate 57) and several other uncommon forms of congenital ichthyosis. Rarely do these persons survive to adulthood. Systemic corticosteroids however may be life-saving for some with this type of ichthyosis.

Keratosis palmaris et plantaris (Fig. 27-2 and Plate 53)—Hereditary symmetrical thickening of the palms and the soles. It is noticed at an early age, and is seen alone or associated with ichthyosis or with congenital ectodermal defect.

Mal de Meleda—A hereditary ectodermal defect resembling keratosis palmaris et plantaris due to inbreeding of persons on the Mediterranean Isle of Mljet.

Keratosis Pilaris—This is a very common horny or nutmeg-grater type eruption on the posterior aspect of the upper arm and thighs. It is worse in the winter. Teenagers seem most aware of this rough skin and usually it becomes milder in adulthood. It appears to be an autosomal dominant condition. Therapy is really not effective but emollients help.

Keratosis punctata—A form of keratosis palmaris et plantaris characterized by the presence of numerous small crateriform pits on the palms and the soles. Common.

Ichthyosis hystrix—is a rare form of congenital "nevus" characterized by extensive horny, papillary, hyperpigmented elevations of the skin. This disease is not hereditary.

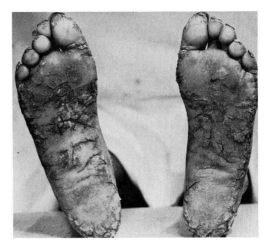

Fig. 27-2. Keratosis plantaris of patient with pityriasis rubra pilaris.

Bullous ichthyosiform erythroderma—is to be differentiated from ichthyosis. It is a rare ectodermal defect in which the skin is generally thickened, red, shiny, and shows a tendency to lichenification over the larger joints. Flaccid bullae occur in most cases early in the course of the disease, but may disappear later. The disease can be present at birth or develop later. This condition can be differentiated from ichthyosis in that it involves the flexural surfaces of the body, whereas ichthyosis usually does not. It is probably hereditary.

CLASSIFICATION OF GENODERMATOSES

The following list contains all but the rarest genodermatoses. Again it is important to emphasize that almost *every* skin disease is influenced by the genetic make-up of the individual.

The more comprehensive dermatologic texts should be consulted for further information on the following hereditary skin diseases. Also consult the Dictionary-Index of this book for the pages where these conditions are discussed further.

A. *Pigmentary Group*

Albinism is congenital and characterized by partial or universal loss of pigment of skin, hair and choroid. Life expectancy is shortened.

Piebaldism. The striking feature is a central white forelock overlying a depigmented area of the scalp. This white forelock is seen in 80 to 90 percent of the cases. Other areas of depigmentation may be present.

Vitiligo (See p. 200)

Freckles (ephelides). Small, brownish macules that develop around puberty and are accentuated by sunlight. They are to be differentiated from lentigines which develop earlier around the age of 2, are more widespread on the body and do not disappear in the winter.

Incontinentia pigmenti (See p. 218 and Plate 57). This is probably an x-linked dominant condition.

B. *Neurocutaneous Group*

Neurofibromatosis or *von Recklinghausen's disease.* (Fig. 21-5 and p. 219) This is transmitted as an autosomal dominant trait.

Tuberous sclerosis (Fig. 29-3 and p. 292). This is transmitted as an irregular dominant characteristic. Skin lesions include ash-leaf depigmentation, adenoma sebaceum of face (Plate 53), peri-ungual fibromas, and shagreen thickenings.

Encephalotrigeminal angiomatosis or *Sturge-Weber syndrome.* A syndrome of a port-wine mark, cavernous hemangioma of the side of the face and brain anomalies.

C. *Vascular Group*

Hereditary hemorrhagic telangiectasis or *Rendu-Osler-Weber syndrome.* An autosomal dominant condition with numerous telangiectases and spider hemangioma on the mucous membranes and the skin that frequently bleed or hemorrhage.

Angiokeratomas. Of the 3 forms of this group of diseases with skin angiomas (see p. 277) only the Fabry form or angiokeratoma corporis diffusum appears to be hereditary. It is a systemic phospholipid storage disease probably with recessive sex-linked inheritance.

Wiskott-Aldrich syndrome is very rare, but it combines typical atopic eczema lesions with thrombocytopenic purpura, bleeding and recurrent infections.

Congenital lymphedema or *Milroy's disease.* This uncommon solid persistent edema of the legs is prone to erysipelas-like inflammation.

D. *Diseases of the Corium*

Ehlers-Danlos Syndrome. Known also as cutis hyperelastica, this a rare congenital anomaly of the skin composed of marked fragility of the skin resulting in the formation of pseudotumors, hyperelasticity of the skin and abnormal hyperflexibility of the joints. It is probably of autosomal incompletely dominant inheritance with variable penetrance.

Cutis laxa is different from Ehlers-Danlos syndrome. In cutis laxa the skin hangs in permanent folds. Very rare.

Pseudoxanthoma elasticum, p. 218. Usually an autosomal recessive trait.

E. *Diseases with Prominent Epidermal Reactions*

Pityriasis rubra pilaris. One of the nutmeg-graterlike diseases. It appears mainly in young adults and is characterized by hard, reddish-yellow hyperkeratotic papules situated at the mouths of the hair follicles and the sweat ducts. Vitamin A therapy is helpful. Most cases are hereditary but some are acquired.

Familial benign chronic pemphigus or *Hailey-Hailey Disease*, p. 186.

Epidermolysis bullosa (p. 186 and Plate 53). There are 2 non-scarring forms:

1. *E. B. simplex*—dominant inheritance, a mild disease.

2. *E. B. letalis*—recessive inheritance. Death occurs usually in a few months.

Scarring forms:

1. *E. B. dystrophica* with dominant inheritance is mild.

2. *E. B. dystrophica* with recessive inheritance is very severe with extensive atrophy, scars and milia. All nails are dystrophic.

An acquired *non-hereditary form of epidermolysis bullosa* also exists.

Xeroderma pigmentosum. A rare condition that manifests itself early in life as a type of skin that is unusually sensitive to the effects of sunlight. Especially on the sun-exposed areas of the body, this results in early formation of freckles, telangiectasia, atrophy and actinic keratoses, which progress into basal and prickle cell epitheliomas or even melanomas and sarcomas. A defect in the repair replication of DNA has been found in these cases. A recessive condition with incomplete sex-linkage.

Acanthosis nigricans. A skin disease characterized by melanin hyperpigmentation and velvety hypertrophy occurring in the axillae mainly but also on the neck, the genitalia, the groin and other body folds. The *benign type*, appearing to be related to a hormonal imbalance, begins in childhood and becomes worse at the age of puberty. There is also evidence for an irregular dominant inheritance. The *malignant type* occurs in patients who usually have adenocarcinoma of the gastro-intestinal tract. *Pseudoacanthosis nigricans* is a clinically similar condition appearing in obese individuals and is entirely unrelated to the above two conditions.

Darier's disease (keratosis follicularis) (Fig. 27-3 & Plate 51 nails). A rare autosomal dominant skin disease usually beginning in early childhood. The disease is worse in the summer when the odor and the secondary bacterial infection become more pronounced. It is characterized by the presence of a diffuse papular eruption that usually coalesces to form a scaly, greasy dermatitis on the back, chest, face, neck and axillae. The eruption may be mild or severe and may or may not itch. It does not affect the patient's general health, but it may interfere with earning a living. Treatment with 150,000 units of vitamin A per day for 3- to 6-month periods is sometimes beneficial.

Ichthyosis, see p. 250.

Congenital ectodermal defect (Plate 58). A hereditary group of diseases that present many ectodermal defects such as keratoses of hands, feet and body, eye cataracts, decrease or absence of sweat and sebaceous glands, change in the nails and hair and, finally, dry skin that may be smooth or keratotic. Some cases are sex-linked recessive, others autosomal dominant and still others are autosomal recessive.

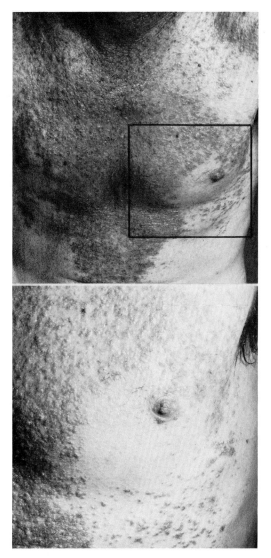

Fig. 27-3. Darier's disease. (*K.U.M.C.*)

Atopic eczema, p. 56. An allergic predisposition is inherited and may manifest itself as eczema, hay fever, asthma, migraine or just as an aggravated itch tendency.

Psoriasis, p. 97. There is a definite familiar tendency, but the hereditary influence is difficult to measure since many persons with mild psoriasis are not aware that they have the disease.

Lupus erythematosus, p. 204. Cases are increasingly being reported as familial.

F. *Metabolic Group*

Porphyria, p. 245.

A. *Erythropoietic porphyrias:*

1. *Erythropoietic protoporphyria* (p. 245) is a rare autosomal disease. Some cases may be clinically recognizable as *hydroa aestivale* (Plate 52).

2. Congenital porphyria is a very rare autosomal recessive disease that begins early in life with severe and even mutilating skin lesions.

B. *Hepatic porphyria*

1. Intermittent acute type is hereditary as autosomal dominant with prominent neurological symptoms. The only skin change is hyperpigmentation.

2. *Porphyria cutanea tarda* (p. 245 & Plate 52) has acquired and inherited elements, and is the commonest cutaneous form.

3. *Porphyria variegata* is rare in the United States, is an autosomal dominant disease and has light sensitivity and neurological problems.

Primary systemic amyloidosis is familial and very rare. (See Dictionary-Index)

Lipoid proteinosis is a very rare autosomal recessive disease characterized by deposition, even early in childhood, of a lipid-protein substance in the skin and in the tongue, vocal cord (hoarseness common) and other mucous membranes.

Primary hypercholesteremic xanthomatosis (p. 214) is characterized by fatty deposits in the eyelids (xanthelasma), knees and elbows, or any skin areas. Transmission is due to a single dominant gene of various expressivity.

Gout of the primary type is an autosomal dominant condition characterized by deposits of urate crystals in the ears and joints of the extremities.

G. *Tumors*

Seborrheic keratoses (p. 259 & Plate 59) are transmitted as a simple autosomal dominant trait.

Keloids (p. 272) appear to be familial as a simple autosomal dominant trait.

Nevi (p. 278) are probably genetically transmitted.

Trichoepithelioma (p. 283) is transmitted as an irregular autosomal dominant trait with partial limitation to the female sex.

Many nail, hair and mucous membrane disorders are hereditary. Common hair conditions include *male-pattern hair loss, gray hair* and *alopecia areata*.

BIBLIOGRAPHY

Baden, H. P., and Goldsmith, L. A.: Current advances in the treatment of ichthyosis. Prog. Derm., *6:*7, 1972.

Butterworth, T., and Strean, L. P.: Clinical Genodermatology. Baltimore, Williams & Wilkins, 1962. Unfortunately this excellent text is out of print.

Curth, H. O.: Genetics—A short glossary with illustrations. Cutis, *3:*470, 1967.

Landau, J. W.: The impact of genetic disease on the adolescent. Cutis, 7:151, 1971.

Schimke, R. N.: Heredity for clinicians. J. Kansas Med. Soc., *69:*1, 1968.

Wells, R. S., and Kerr, C. B.: Genetic classification of ichthyosis. Arch. Derm., *92:*1, 1965.

28

Tumors of the Skin

CLASSIFICATION

A patient comes into your office for care of a tumor on his skin. What kind is it? What is the best treatment? This complex problem of diagnosing and managing skin tumors is not learned easily. As an aid to the establishment of the correct diagnosis, all skin tumors (excluding warts which are due to a virus) will be classified (1) as to their *histologic origin*, (2) according to the patient's *age group*, and (3) on the basis of *clinical appearance*.

A complete histologic classification will be found at the end of this chapter, whereas only the more common tumors will be classified and discussed here. This histologic classification is divided into epidermal tumors, mesodermal tumors, nevus cell tumors, lymphomas and myeloses. In making a clinical diagnosis of any skin tumor, one should apply a histopathologic label. Whether the label is correct or not depends on the clinical acumen of the physician and whether the tumor, or a part of it, has been examined microscopically. *A histologic examination should be performed on any malignant skin tumor or on any tumor where a malignancy cannot be ruled out clinically.*

HISTOLOGIC CLASSIFICATION*

Epidermal Tumors

I. **Tumors of the Surface Epidermis**
  1. Nevoid tumors. Defined as benign neoplasms which probably arise from arrested embryonal cells.

* This partial classification and the complete one at the end of this chapter are modified from the one listed by Walter F. Lever: Histopathology of the Skin. ed. 4. Philadelphia, J. B. Lippincott, 1967.

  A. Seborrheic keratosis
    (b) Sebaceous cyst
  B. Pedunculated fibroma
  C. Cysts
    (a) Epidermal cyst
    (c) Milium
    (d) Dermoid cyst
    (e) Mucous cyst
  2. Precancerous tumors
  A. Senile or actinic keratosis and cutaneous horn
  B. Arsenical keratosis
  C. Leukoplakia
  3. Carcinoma: Squamous cell carcinoma
II. **Tumors of the Epidermal Appendages**
  Basal cell epithelioma

Mesodermal Tumors

I. **Tumors of Fibrous Tissue**
  1. Histiocytoma and dermatofibroma
  2. Keloid
II. **Tumors of Vascular Tissue:** Hemangiomas

Nevus Cell Tumors

I. **Nevi**
  1. Junction (active) nevus
  2. Intradermal (resting) nevus
II. **Malignant Melanoma**

Lymphoma and Myelosis

I. **Monomorphous Group**
II. **Polymorphous Group:** Mycosis fungoides

CLASSIFICATION BY AGE GROUPS

An age-group classification is helpful from a differential diagnostic viewpoint.

257

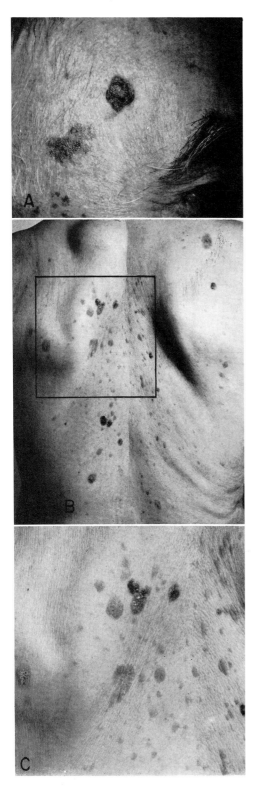

Viral warts will be considered in this classification because of the frequent necessity of differentiating them from other skin tumors. The most common tumors are listed first.

I. **Tumors of Children**
1. Warts (viral), very common
2. Nevi, junction type common
3. Hemangiomas
4. Granuloma pyogenicum
5. Molluscum contagiosum (viral)
6. Mongolian spot
7. Xanthogranuloma

II. **Tumors of Adults**
1. Warts (viral), plantar type common
2. Nevi
3. Cysts
4. Pedunculated fibromas
5. Histiocytomas
6. Keloids
7. Lipomas
8. Granuloma pyogenicum

III. **Additional Tumors of Older Adults**
1. Seborrheic keratoses
2. Senile or actinic keratoses
3. Papillary hemangiomas
4. Leukoplakia
5. Basal cell epitheliomas
6. Squamous cell carcinoma

CLASSIFICATION BASED ON
CLINICAL APPEARANCE

The clinical appearance of any tumor is a most important diagnostic factor. Some tumors have a characteristic color and growth that is readily distinguishable from any other tumor, but a large number, unfortunately, have clinical characteristics common to several similar tumors. A further hindrance to making a correct diagnosis is that the same histopathologic lesion may vary in clinical appearance. The following generalizing classification should be helpful, but, if in doubt, the lesion should be examined histologically.

Fig. 28-1. Seborrheic keratoses. (*A*) On forehead. (*B*) On back. Note lipoma over the left scapula. (*C*) Closeup of back lesions.

I. **Flat, skin-colored tumors**
   1. Flat warts (viral)
   2. Histiocytomas
   3. Leukoplakia
II. **Flat, pigmented tumors**
   1. Nevi, usually junction type
   2. Lentigo
   3. Histiocytoma
   4. Mongolian spot
III. **Raised, skin-colored tumors**
   1. Warts (viral)
   2. Nevi, usually intradermal type
   3. Cysts
   4. Lipomas
   5. Keloids
   6. Basal cell epitheliomas
   7. Squamous cell carcinoma
   8. Molluscum contagiosum (viral)
   9. Xanthogranuloma (yellowish)
IV. **Raised, brownish tumors**
   1. Warts (viral)
   2. Nevi
   3. Senile keratoses
   4. Seborrheic keratoses
   5. Pedunculated fibromas
   6. Basal cell epitheliomas
   7. Squamous cell carcinoma
   8. Malignant melanoma
   9. Granuloma pyogenicum
   10. Keratoacanthomas
V. **Raised, reddish tumors**
   1. Hemangiomas
   2. Granuloma pyogenicum
   3. Glomus tumors
VI. **Raised, blackish tumors**
   1. Seborrheic keratoses
   2. Nevi
   3. Granuloma pyogenicum
   4. Malignant melanomas
   5. Blue nevi

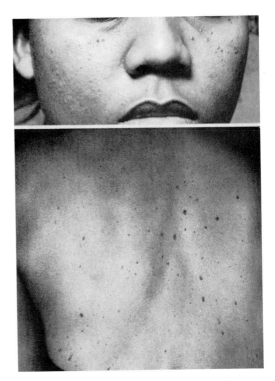

Fig. 28-2. Dermatosis papulosa nigra. On the face and the back of a Negro woman. (*K.U.M.C.*)

SEBORRHEIC KERATOSIS
(Plate 59)

It is a rare elderly patient who does not have any seborrheic keratoses. These are the unattractive "moles" or "warts" that perturb the elderly patient, occasionally become irritated but are otherwise benign (Fig. 28-1).

Dermatosis papulosa nigra is a form of seborrheic keratosis of Negroes that occurs on the face, mainly in women (Fig. 28-2). These small, multiple tumors should not be removed, because of the possibility of causing keloids.

Description. The size of seborrheic keratoses varies up to 3 cm. for the largest, but the average diameter is 1 cm. The color may be flesh-colored, tan, brown or coal black. They are usually elevated and have a greasy, warty sensation to touch.

Distribution. On face, neck, scalp, back and upper chest, and less frequently on arms, legs and lower part of trunk.

Course. They become darker in color and enlarge slowly. Trauma from clothing occasionally results in infection, and this prompts the patient to come to your office. Any inflammatory dermatitis around these lesions causes them to enlarge temporarily and become more evident, so much so that many patients suddenly note them for the first time. Malignant degeneration of seborrheic keratoses is doubted.

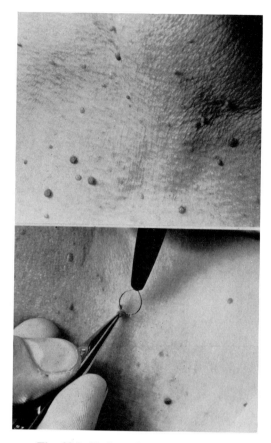

Fig. 28-3. Pedunculated fibromas. (*A, top*) On the neck of a woman. (*B, bottom*) A method of removal by grasping the skin tag with thumb forceps and applying a coagulating current to the base.

Etiology. Heredity is the biggest factor, along with old age. They are seen more commonly in patients with an oily, acne-seborrhea type of skin.

Differential Diagnosis

Actinic or Senile Keratoses (see p. 264 for chart).

Pigmented Nevi: longer duration, smoother surface, softer to touch; may not be able to differentiate clinically (p. 278).

Flat Warts: in younger patients, acute onset with rapid development of new lesions (p. 154).

Malignant Melanoma: very rare, usually with rapid growth, indurated; examine histologically.

Treatment. A 58-year-old female patient requests the removal of a warty, tannish, slightly elevated 2 by 2 cm. lesion on the right side of her forehead.

1. Examine the lesion carefully. The diagnosis usually can be made clinically, but if there is any question a scissors biopsy (p. 11) can be performed. It would be ideal if all of these seborrheic keratoses could be examined histologically, but this is not economically feasible or necessary.

2. A very adequate form of therapy is curettement, with or without local anesthesia, followed by a light application of trichloracetic acid as outlined under senile keratosis (p. 265). The resulting fine atrophic scar will hardly be noticeable in several months. Electrosurgery can be used, but this usually requires anesthesia. Surgical excision is an unnecessary and more expensive form of removal.

PEDUNCULATED FIBROMAS

Multiple skin tags are very common on the neck and the axillae of middle-aged, usually obese, men and women (Fig. 28-3). The indications for removal are twofold: cosmetic as desired and requested by the patient, and to prevent the irritation and the secondary infection of the pedicle that frequently develops from trauma of a collar, a scarf, etc.

Description. Pedunculated pinhead-sized to pea-sized soft tumors of normal skin color or darker. The base may be inflamed from injury.

Distribution. Neck, axillae, groin or less frequently on any area.

Course. Grow very slowly. May increase in size during pregnancy. Some become infected and drop off.

Differential Diagnosis

Filiform Wart: see digitate projections, more horny; also seen on chin area (p. 153).

Pedunculated Seborrheic Keratosis: see larger lesion, darker color, warty or velvety appearance (p. 259).

Neurofibromatosis: see lesions elsewhere, larger; can be pushed back into skin; also see café-au-lait spots; hereditary (p. 219).

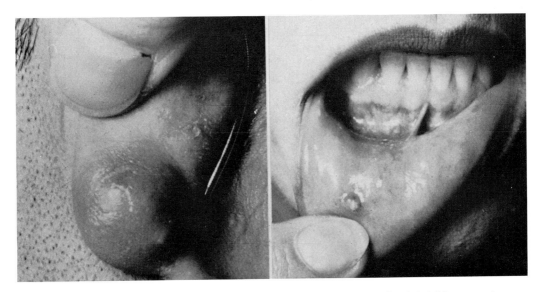

Fig. 28-4. Cysts. (*A, left*) Infected epidermal cyst of ear lobe. (*B, right*) Mucous retention cyst of lower lip.

Treatment. A 42-year-old woman has 20 small pedunculated fibromas of her neck and axillae which she desires removed. This should be done by electro-surgery. Without anesthesia gently grab the small tumor in a thumb forceps and stretch the pedicle (Fig. 28-3B). Touch this pedicle with the electrosurgery needle and turn on the current for a split second. The tumor separates from the skin, and no bleeding occurs. The site will heal in 4 to 7 days.

CYSTS

1. Epidermal cyst
2. Sebaceous cyst
3. Milium

The common skin cyst or wen that is clinically labeled a "sebaceous" cyst will turn out to be an epidermal cyst in 99.5 percent of cases when studied histologically. A true *sebaceous cyst*, from arrested embryonal cells or from a plugged sebaceous gland, is relatively uncommon. An *epidermal cyst* has a wall composed of true epidermis and probably originates from an invagination of the epidermis into the dermis and subsequent detachment from the epidermis (Fig. 28-4A). The

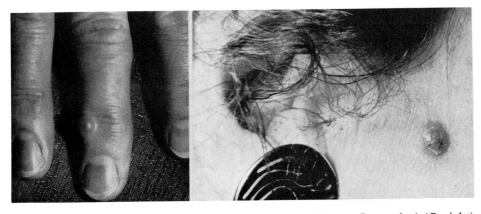

Fig. 28-5. Cysts. (*A, left*) Synovial cyst of finger. (*Dr. Chester Lessenden*) (*B, right*) Foreign body inclusion cyst on the cheek.

most common location for epidermal cysts is the scalp, where many such tumors of varying size can be found.

Milia are very common, white pinhead-sized, firm lesions that are seen on the face. They are formed by proliferation of epithelial buds following trauma to the skin (dermabrasion for acne scars), following certain dermatoses (pemphigus, epidermolysis bullosa and acute contact dermatitis) or from no apparent cause.

Differential Diagnosis of Epidermal and Sebaceous Cysts

Lipoma: rather difficult to differentiate clinically; more firm, lobulated; no cheesy material extrudes on incision; removal is by complete excision; clinically similar to *hibernoma.*

Dermoid Cyst: clinically similar; can also be found internally; usually a solitary skin tumor; histologically, contains hairs, eccrine glands, sebaceous glands, etc.

Mucous Cysts (Fig. 28-4B): translucent pea-sized or smaller lesions on the lips, treated by cutting off top of the lesion and carefully lightly cauterizing the base with a silver nitrate stick.

Synovial Cysts of the Skin (Fig. 28-5A): globoid, translucent, pea-sized swellings around the joints of fingers and toes.

Treatment of Epidermal and Sebaceous Cysts. Several methods can be used with success. The choice depends on the ability of the operator, and the site and the number of cysts. Cysts can regrow following even the best surgical care, because of incomplete removal of the sac.

1. A single 3-cm.-diameter cyst on the back should be removed by surgical excision and suturing. This can be done in two ways: either by incising the skin and skillfully removing the intact cyst sac, or by cutting straight into the sac with a small incision, shelling out the evacuated lining by applying strong pressure to the sides of the incision and suturing the skin. The latter procedure is simpler, requires a smaller incision and is quite successful.

2. A patient with several cysts in the scalp or a small cyst on an exposed area of the body can be treated in another simple way. A 2- to 3-mm. incision can be made directly over and into the cyst. Then the contents can be evacuated by firm pressure and the use of a small curette. In many instances the entire sac can be grasped firmly with a small hemostat and pulled out of the opening. If the entire sac is not removed at this time, a repeated attempt in one week, aided by the development of a mild infection, will usually be successful. No suturing or only a single suture is necessary. The resulting scar will be imperceptible in a short time.

3. If, during incision by any technic, a solid tumor is found instead of a cyst, the lesion should be excised completely and the material studied histologically. This diagnostic error is very common because of the clinical similarity of cysts, lipomas and other related tumors.

Treatment of Milia

1. Simple incision of the small tumors with a scalpel or a Hagedorn needle and expression of the contents by a comedone extractor are sufficient.

2. Another procedure is to remove the top of the milia lightly with electrodesiccation.

PRECANCEROUS TUMORS

1. Senile or actinic keratosis and cutaneous horn
2. Arsenical keratosis
3. Leukoplakia

SENILE (ACTINIC) KERATOSIS
(Plate 54)

This common skin lesion of light-complexioned, older persons occurs on the skin surfaces exposed to sunlight. A small percentage of these lesions slowly develop into squamous cell carcinomas. Another term, *actinic keratosis*, can be used when these tumors are seen in individuals in the 30-to-50 age group.

Description. Usually multiple, flat or slightly elevated, brownish or tan colored, scaly, adherent lesions measuring up to 1.5 cm. in diameter. Individual lesions may become confluent. A *cutaneous horn* is a very proliferative, hyperkeratotic form of senile keratosis that resembles a horn (Fig. 28-6A).

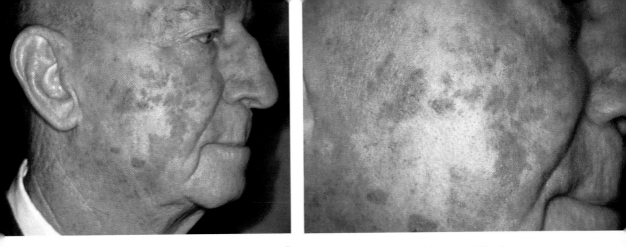

(A) Multiple actinic keratoses on face of 80-year-old fair complexioned farmer, (B) closeup

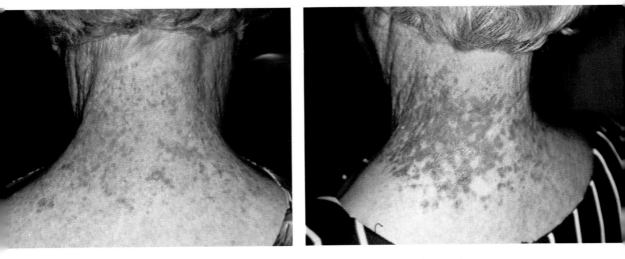

(C) Actinic keratoses of back of neck showing lesions before and (D) normal accentuation after 5 FU therapy b.i.d. for 2 wks.

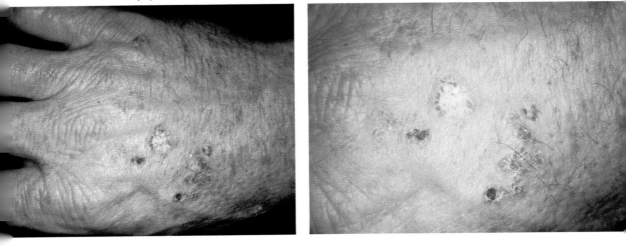

(E) Lesions on dorsum of hands, (F) closeup, in 44-year-old blue-eyed, outdoor worker

Plate 54. Actinic or senile keratoses. (*Dermik Laboratories Inc.*) (*Owen Laboratories Inc.*)

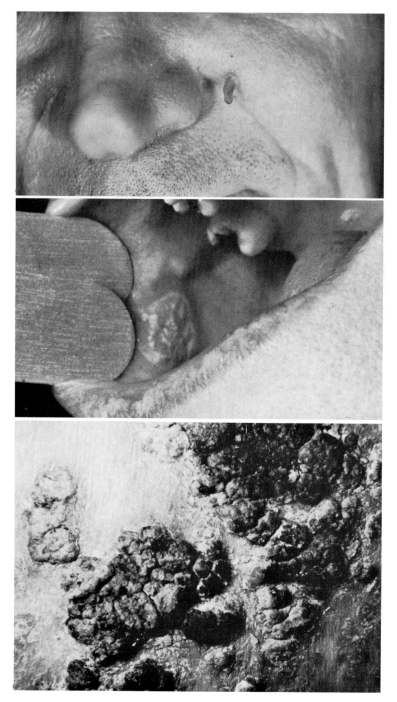

Fig. 28-6. Precanceroses. (*A, top*) Cutaneous horn on the cheek. There was no epithelioma at the base of this lesion.

(*B, center*) Biopsy-proved leukoplakia on the mucous membrane of the cheek. This was erroneously diagnosed clinically as lichen planus.

(*C, bottom*) Bowen's disease of thigh of 65-year-old male.

	Senile Keratosis	Seborrheic Keratosis
Appearance	Flat, brownish or tan scale firmly attached to skin	Greasy, elevated, brown or black; scale is warty and can be easily scratched away
Location	Sun-exposed areas	Face, back and chest
Complexion	Blue eyes, light hair, dry skin	Brown eyes, dark hair, oily skin
Subjective Complaints	Some burning and stinging	None
Precancerous	Yes	No

Distribution. Areas of skin exposed to sunlight, such as face, ears, neck and dorsum of hands.

Course. Lesion begins as a faint-red, slightly scaly patch that enlarges slowly peripherally and deeply over many years. A sudden spurt of growth would indicate a change to a squamous cell carcinoma.

Subjective Complaints. Patients often complain that these lesions burn and sting.

Etiology. Heredity and sun exposure are the two main causative factors. The blue-eyed, thin-skinned, light-haired farmer or sailor with a family history of such lesions is the best subject for multiple senile keratoses. Excessive sun exposure is important but not necessary.

Sex Incidence. Most commonly seen in men.

Differential Diagnosis

Seborrheic Keratosis (see chart)

Squamous Cell Carcinoma: any thickened lesion that has grown rapidly should be biopsied (p. 269).

Arsenical Keratosis: mainly on palms and soles.

Treatment. A 60-year-old farmer has 3 small senile keratoses on his face.

Examine the lesions carefully. *If there is any evidence of induration or marked inflammation, the lesion should be biopsied.* (See scissors technic, p. 11.)

There are two methods of removal of these keratoses.

For a single lesion, or only 3 or 4 lesions, I prefer a one-visit surgical treatment.

1. Surgical Method

Curettement followed by destruction of the base by acid or electrosurgery is very satisfactory. The technics are as follows. Local anesthesia is usually not necessary unless electrosurgery is used. Firmly scrape the lesion with the dermal curette, which will remove the mushy, scaly keratosis and bring you down to the more fibrous normal skin. Experience will provide the necessary "feel" of the abnormal versus the normal tissue. Some of the bleeding can be controlled by pressure or use of either one of the two following procedures: (1) with a cotton applicator apply a saturated solution of trichloracetic acid cautiously to the bleeding site; or (2) the bleeding base may be electrocoagulated. I prefer the acid technic because local anesthesia is not necessary for most patients, and healing is faster. Small lesions will heal in 7 to 14 days. No bandage is required; in fact, bandaging promotes infection.

Liquid nitrogen applied very lightly to the lesion is also a quite effective and rapid method of removal.

2. Fluorouracil Method

For the patient with multiple superficial senile or actinic keratoses, this therapy is very effective and will eliminate for some months or years the early damaged epidermal cells. Thus this fluorouracil therapy is really a cancer prevention routine.

Several preparations and strengths of solutions and creams are available but the following are most commonly indicated:

Fluroplex 1% cream	30.0
or	
Efudex 2% solution	10.0

Sig: Apply to area to be treated twice a day with fingers. It is wise to treat only a small area on the face at a time. Give instructions carefully and warn that it is natural for the skin to get quite red and irritated and sore after 4-5 days. Most commonly the course of therapy is for 2 weeks. Some patients must stop sooner and some need more time (or a stronger preparation) to get the desired effect.

After completion of the course of therapy the skin usually heals rapidly. A corticosteroid cream may be prescribed to hasten healing.

This therapy may have to be repeated in several months or years. If some keratoses are too thick to be removed by this fluorouracil method, then the surgical method as described first is indicated for these lesions.

3. Request the patient to return every 6 months for a check-up and treatment of new lesions as they develop.

4. For younger patients with these keratoses a sun-screen cream (Uval or Skolex Cream or A-fil Cream) should be prescribed for prevention of future lesions.

Treatment of a Cutaneous Horn. The same surgical technic as for senile keratosis. *To rule out cancer, every cutaneous horn should be sent with intact base for histopathologic examination.* The incidence of squamous cell carcinomatous change in the base of a cutaneous horn is appreciable.

Arsenical Keratosis

Prolonged ingestion of inorganic arsenic (Fowler's Solution, Asiatic Pills) can result in the formation many years later of small punctate keratotic lesions mainly seen on the palms and the soles. Progression to a squamous cell carcinoma can occur but is unusual.

Treatment. Small arsenical keratoses can be removed by electrosurgery; larger lesions can be excised and skin grafted if necessary. Vitamin A orally may be helpful.

Leukoplakia

Leukoplakia is a senile keratosis of the mucous membrane (Fig. 28-6B).

Description. A flat, whitish plaque localized to the mucous membranes of lips, mouth, vulva and vagina. Single or multiple lesions may be present.

Course. Progression to squamous cell carcinoma occurs in 20 to 30 percent of chronic cases.

Etiology. Smoking, sunlight and chronic irritation are the important factors in the development of leukoplakia. *Recurrent actinic cheilitis* may precede leukoplakia of the lips. The vulvar form may develop from *presenile* or *senile atrophy* of this area.

Differential Diagnosis

Lichen Planus: see a lacy network of whitish lesions mainly on the sides of the buccal cavity; when on lips, it may clinically resemble leukoplakia; see lichen planus elsewhere on body (p. 107).

Pressure Calluses From Teeth or Dentures: see evidence of irritation; differentiation may be possible only by biopsy.

On the vulva, *lichen sclerosis et atrophicus* or *kraurosis vulvae:* see no induration as in leukoplakia of this area; can extend onto skin of inguinal folds and perianal region; pruritus may or may not be present.

Treatment. Small patch of leukoplakia on lower lip of man who smokes considerably.

1. Examine lesion carefully. Biopsy any questionable area that shows inflammation and induration. If a squamous cell carcinoma is present, the patient should receive surgical or radiation therapy by a physician expert in this form of treatment.

2. Advise against smoking. The seriousness of continued smoking or other use of tobacco must be pointed out to the patient. Many early cases of leukoplakia disappear when smoking is stopped.

3. Eliminate any chronic irritation from teeth or dentures.

4. Protect the lips from sunlight with a sun-screen cream such as Skolex, A-fil Cream, A-fil Sunstick or Pan-Ultra Stick.

5. Electrosurgery preceded by local anesthesia is excellent for small persistent areas of leukoplakia. The coagulating current is effective. Healing is usually rapid.

EPITHELIOMAS AND CARCINOMAS

1. Basal cell epithelioma
2. Squamous cell carcinoma

Basal Cell Epithelioma
(Plates 1 C, 3 A, 55, and 59)

This is the commonest malignancy of the skin. Very fortunately, a basal cell epithelioma is not a metastasizing tumor, and the cure rate can be 100 percent if these lesions are treated early and adequately. Death from a basal cell epithelioma results from neglected cases, either by the patient or by the therapist.

Description. There are 4 clinical types of basal cell epithelioma: (1) nodulo-ulcerative, (2) pigmented, (3) fibrosing and (4) superficial.

The *nodulo-ulcerative basal cell epithelioma* is the commonest type. It begins as a small waxy nodule that enlarges slowly over the years. A central depression forms that eventually progresses into an ulcer surrounded by the pearly or waxy border. The surface of the nodular component has a few telangiectatic vessels which are highly characteristic.

The *pigmented type* is similar to the nodulo-ulcerative form, with the addition of brown or black pigmentation.

The *fibrosing type* is extremely slow growing, is usually seen on the face and consists of a whitish scarred plaque with an ill-defined border which rarely becomes ulcerated.

The *superficial form* may be single or multiple, is usually seen on the back and the chest and is characterized by slowly enlarging red scaly areas that on careful examination reveal a nodular border with telangiectatic vessels. A healed atrophic center may be present. Ulceration is superficial when it develops.

Distribution. Over 90 percent of the basal cell epitheliomas occur on the head and the neck, with the trunk next in frequency. These tumors are rarely found on the palms and the soles.

Course. Very slow growing, but sudden rapid growth periods do occur. Destructive forms of this tumor can invade cartilage, bone, blood vessels or large areas of skin surface, and result in death. The very rare cases of metastasizing basal cell epitheliomas probably represent wrong diagnoses.

Etiology. Basal cell epitheliomas develop most frequently on the areas of the skin exposed to sunlight and in blond or red-haired individuals. Trauma and overexposure to radium and x-radiation can cause basal cell epitheliomas. Long-term ingestion of inorganic arsenic can lead to formation of superficial basal cell epitheliomas. Most authors believe that a basal cell epithelioma is a carcinoma of the basal cells of the epidermis. Lever and others believe it not to be a carcinoma but a nevoid tumor derived from incompletely differentiated embryonal cells.

Age Group. Can occur from childhood to old age but is seen most frequently in male patients above the age of 50.

Differential Diagnosis. *Whenever the clinical appearance of a skin tumor suggests a basal cell epithelioma, the lesion should be studied histologically.*

Squamous Cell Carcinoma: see more rapid growth, firm scaly papule or nodule, more inflammation, no pearly telangiectatic border; biopsy may be necessary to differentiate.

Other lesions that can mimic a basal cell epithelioma are *keratoacanthomas, sebaceous adenomas, large comedones, warts, nevi, small cysts and scarring from injury or radiation.*

Superficial basal cell epitheliomas can resemble lesions of *psoriasis, seborrheic dermatitis, lupus vulgaris* and *Bowen's disease* (Fig. 28-6C).

Treatment. A 48-year-old female has an 8 x 8 mm. basal cell epithelioma on her forehead.

1. Inform the patient that she has a tumor of the skin that needs to be removed. (If the patient asks if the tumor is a cancer, I say that it is, and add that it is not like the cancer that develops inside the body.) Tell the patient that this tumor cannot spread into the body, but if it is not treated it can spread on the skin. State that removal of the lesion is almost 100 percent effective, but that periodic examinations will be necessary to check for any regrowth. If this tumor recurs it will regrow only at its previous site. Tell the pa-

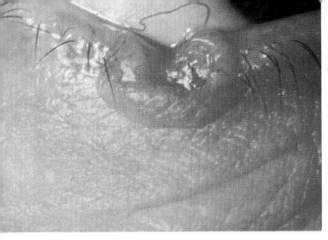

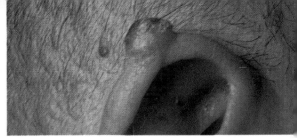

Of the lower eyelid. Note telangiectasia on the rolled edge of the ulcer. (Drs. Calkins and Lemoine)

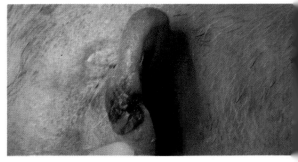

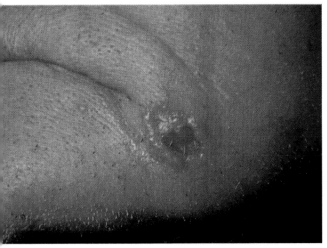

(B) Hemorrhagic lesion on helix of ear.

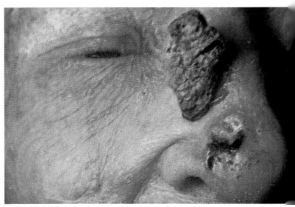

Ulcerated lesion on chin. (K.U.M.C.)

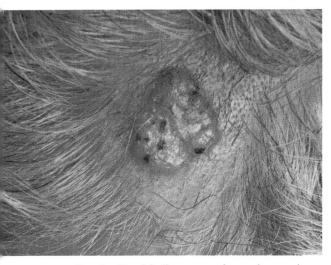

(C) Cutaneous horn with basal cell epitheliomatous degeneration of the base.

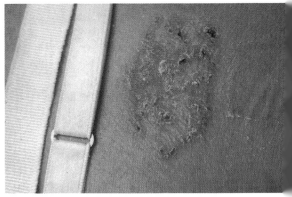

Basal cell epitheliomatous change in a syringo-cystadenoma papilliferum nevus on the scalp.

(D) Superficial basal cell epithelioma on posterior aspect of shoulder. Patient took arsenic (Fowler's solution) for 3 months 30 years previously for psoriasis.

Plate 55. Basal cell epitheliomas. (*Texas Pharmacal Co.*)

tient that a slight scar will result from the treatment.

2. If the diagnosis of the lesion is not definite clinically, a scissors biopsy, as described on page 11, may be done safely. Further treatment will depend on the laboratory report.

3. Surgical excision of a basal cell epithelioma is the only method of treatment that should be attempted by the physician who only occasionally is confronted with these tumors. (Some criticism will arise from this statement, but it is my belief that a great amount of experience is necessary to remove these tumors adequately by curettement, chemocautery, electrosurgery, radiation or any combination of these methods. If the operator feels that he is qualified in these procedures, then this statement is not meant for him.) To excise the lesion, anesthetize the area, make an elliptical incision with a scalpel to include a border of 3 to 4 mm. around the tumor, tag one side of the excised skin with a piece of suture, close the incision and submit the specimen for careful histologic examination. If the pathologist states that the tumor extends up to the edge of the excision, a further more radical excision should be performed.

4. Have the patient return for a check-up in 1 month, then 2, then 3, then 6 months, and then yearly for 3 to 5 years.

Treatment of deeply ulcerated, fibrosing or superficial basal cell epitheliomas should be in the domain of the competent dermatologist, surgeon or radiologist.

SQUAMOUS CELL CARCINOMA
(Plate 59)

This rather common skin malignancy can arise primarily or from a senile keratosis or leukoplakia. The grade of malignancy and metastasizing ability varies from Grade I (low) to Grade IV (high). Other terms for this tumor include prickle cell epithelioma and epidermoid carcinoma (Figs. 28-7 and 28-8).

Description. The commonest clinical picture is a rather rapidly growing nodule which soon develops a central ulcer and an indurated raised border with some surrounding redness. This type of lesion is

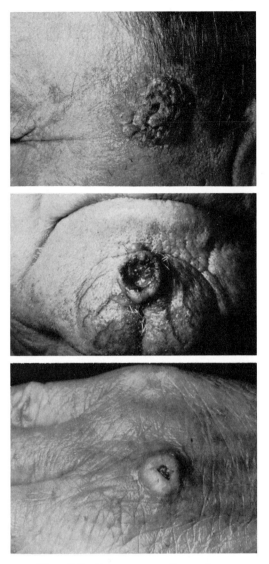

Fig. 28-7. **Squamous cell carcinoma.** (*Top*) On temple area. (*Center*) On chin with marked ulceration. (*Bottom*) On the dorsum of the hand.

the most malignant. The least malignant form has the clinical appearance of a warty, piled-up growth which may not ulcerate. However, it is important to realize that the grade of malignancy can vary in the same tumor from one section to another, particularly in the larger lesions. This variation demonstrates the value of multiple histologic sections.

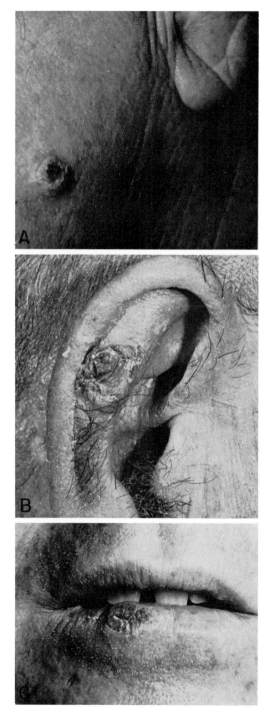

Fig. 28-8. Squamous cell carcinoma.
(*A*) On the cheek. (*B*) On the ear resembling a senile keratosis. (*K.C.G.H.*) (*C*) On the lower lip of a 36-year-old male.

Distribution. Can occur on any area of the skin and mucous membrane, but most commonly on the face, particularly lower lip and ears, tongue and dorsum of the hands. Chronic trauma associated with certain occupations can lead to formation of this cancer on unusual sites, such as mule skinners' cancer of the scrotum from machinery oils, chimney sweeps' cancer, etc.

Course. This varies with the grade of malignancy of the tumor. Lymph node metastases may occur early in the development of the tumor or never. The cure rate can be very high when the lesions are treated early and with the best indicated modality.

Etiology. As with basal cell epitheliomas, many factors contribute to provide the soil for growth of a squamous cell carcinoma. A simple listing of factors will be sufficient: hereditarily determined type of skin; age of patient; trauma from chemicals (tars, oils), heat, wind, sunlight, x-radiation and severe burns; skin diseases that form scars such as chronic discoid lupus erythematosus, lupus vulgaris and chronic ulcers; ingestion of inorganic arsenic; and in the natural course of xeroderma pigmentosum.

Age and Sex Incidence. Most usually seen in elderly males, but exceptions are not rare.

Differential Diagnosis. *Whenever the clinical appearance of a skin tumor suggests a squamous cell carcinoma, the lesion should be studied histologically.*

Basal Cell Epithelioma: see slower growth, pearly border with telangiectasis, less inflammation; biopsy may be necessary to differentiate (p. 267).

Senile or Actinic Keratosis: see slow-growing flat scaly lesions, no induration, little surrounding erythema (p. 264).

Pseudoepitheliomatous Hyperplasia: see primary chronic lesion, such as old stasis ulcer, bromoderma, deep mycotic infection, syphilitic gumma, lupus vulgaris, basal cell epithelioma and pyoderma gangrenosum; differentiation often impossible clinically and very difficult histologically.

Keratoacanthoma (Fig. 28-9): see very

Fig. 28-9. Keratoacanthomas. (*A*)
Single lesion on dorsum of the hand.

(*B*) Multiple lesions
on leg of 4 years' dura-
tion.

(*C*) Closeup of lesions
in B.

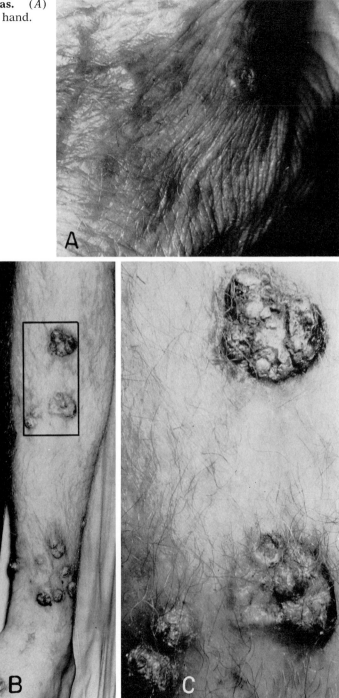

fast-growing single or, more rarely, multiple type of keratoacanthoma; clinically this is a firm, raised nodule with a central crater; it should be studied histologically; it may disappear spontaneously.

Treatment. Because of the invasive nature of squamous cell carcinomas, intensive surgical and/or radiation therapy is indicated. Such procedures are beyond the scope of this text.

HISTIOCYTOMA AND DERMATOFIBROMA

These are common, single, flat or very slightly elevated, tannish, reddish or brownish nodules, less than 1 cm. in size, that occur mainly on the anterior tibial area of the leg (Fig. 28-10). This tumor has a characteristic clinical appearance and firm buttonlike feel that establishes the diagnosis. It occurs in adults, and is nonsymptomatic and unchanging.

The histologic picture varies with the age of the lesion. The younger lesions are called histiocytomas, and the older ones dermatofibromas. If the nodule contains many blood vessels it is histologically labeled a *sclerosing hemangioma*.

Differential Diagnosis. *Fibrosarcoma:* see active growth with invasion of subcutaneous fat; any questionable lesion should be excised and examined histologically.

Treatment. None indicated. If there is any doubt as to the diagnosis, surgical excision and histologic examination are indicated.

KELOID
(Plate 3 B)

A keloid is a tumor resulting from an abnormal overgrowth of fibrous tissue following injury in certain predisposed individuals (Fig. 28-11). Very unusual configurations can occur, depending on the site, the extent and the variety of the trauma. This tendency occurs so commonly in Negroes that one should think twice before attempting a cosmetic procedure on a Negro or on any other person with a history of keloids. The face and

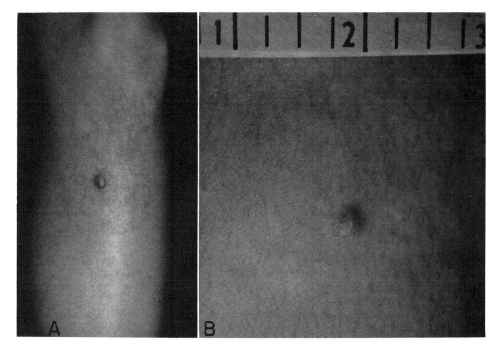

Fig. 28-10. Histiocytoma. (*A*) Of anterior tibial area of leg. (*B*) Closeup of another lesion on leg.

the upper chest areas are especially prone to this proliferation.

Treatment. Very unsatisfactory. Certain combined procedures utilizing excision, x-rays, intralesional corticosteroid and hyaluronidase injections have been used with varying success.

HEMANGIOMAS
(Plates 1 A and D and 58)

Hemangiomas are vascular abnormalities of the skin. Heredity is not a factor in the development of these lesions. There are 9 types of hemangiomas, which vary as to depth, clinical appearance and location.

1. Superficial hemangioma
2. Cavernous hemangioma
3. Mixed hemangioma (when both superficial and cavernous elements are present)
4. Spider hemangioma
5. Port-wine hemangioma
6. Nuchal hemangioma
7. Capillary hemangioma
8. Venous lake
9. Angiokeratoma

SUPERFICIAL AND CAVERNOUS HEMANGIOMAS
(Plate 58)

The familiar bright-red, raised "strawberry" tumor has been seen by all physicians (Fig. 28-12). Strawberries have to grow, and they start from a small beginning. The parents are usually the first to notice the small red, pinhead-sized, flat lesions. They are noticed at or soon after birth. These red tumors can occur on any area of the body and can begin as small lesions and stay that way, remaining as *superficial hemangiomas,* or they can enlarge and extend into the subcutaneous tissue, forming a *cavernous type.* The enlargement can occur rapidly or slowly. Occasionally there can be multiple lesions.

Two aspects of the larger hemangiomas can be disturbing. First, the mere presence of the lesion or lesions will cause concern to parents. If the lesion is on an exposed area of the body, this will cause additional concern and comment by relatives, neigh-

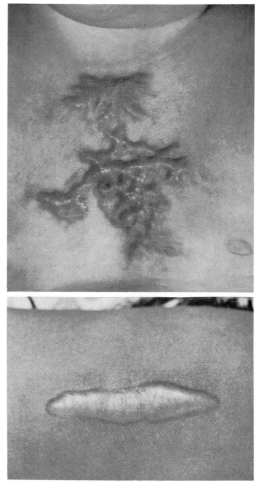

Fig. 28-11. Keloids. (*Top*) On the chest of a baby girl following a burn. (*Bottom*) On the forearm. (*K.C.G.H.*)

bors and other well-meaning individuals. This can be most disconcerting.

Secondly, if the lesion is large and near an eye, the nose or the mouth, it can by its physical size cause an obstructive problem. If this occurs, then appropriate surgical excision is usually indicated. However, even some massive hemangiomas in these areas can be left alone and will resolve amazingly over a period of several months.

Treatment. The treatment of hemangiomas that are not of the obstructive type has been the subject of considerable discussion. To begin with, the size, the depth

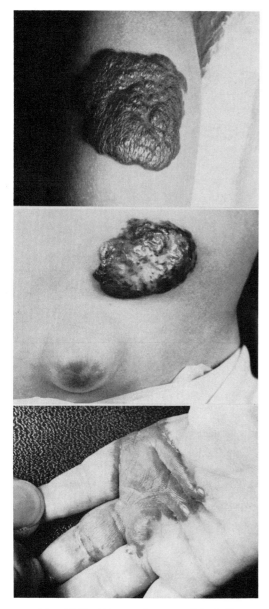

Fig. 28-12. Hemangiomas. (*Top*) Superficial hemangioma on calf of the leg of a child. (*Center*) Mixed hemangioma on the abdomen above an umbilical hernia. (See Color Plate 1.) (*Bottom*) Cavernous hemangioma on the palm of the hand.

and the location of the hemangiomas and, I might add, the pressure on the doctor from parents and relatives, are factors that must be considered for every case.

There are those who favor treating almost every superficial or cavernous hemangioma, and there are others who feel that all hemangiomas should be left alone to involute spontaneously. The latter group stand behind the studies of our English colleagues, Bowers, Simpson and others, who showed that around 85 percent of hemangiomas disappeared without any appreciable scar by the age of 7 years. They also found that the hemangiomas usually stopped growing by the age of 1 year. Personally, I advocate the treatment of some hemangiomas, and I leave others alone. Let me illustrate by 2 case histories.

A. Sarah Sue, age 6 weeks, is brought in by her parents. She has a 4 x 4 mm. slightly raised red lesion on her cheek. The parents first noticed it when she was 3 weeks of age, when it was of pinhead size.

MANAGEMENT

1. Reassure the parents that this birthmark is not hereditary, and that it will not turn into a cancer.
2. Inform them that you will treat this lesion because it probably will enlarge and could become quite a deformity. If you wish, you can explain that the lesion, if left alone, might or might not enlarge, and if it does enlarge will probably disappear without much of a mark in 5 to 7 years. However, state that you would suggest treatment now to possibly abort any further growth.
3. Apply a solid dry ice "pencil" directly to the lesion for 4 to 8 seconds with firm pressure. The "pencil" tip should be shaped to conform exactly to, or 1 millimeter larger than, the size of the tumor. Occasionally second and third treatments are necessary in 3 to 6 weeks. Tell the parents that a blister will form within 24 hours at the site of the treatment but, if left alone, it will heal in 6 to 14 days. If any infection develops, have them contact you.

Dry ice can be purchased in blocks from any ice cream manufacturer and shaped to fit the lesion, or it can be made in a Kidde Dry Ice Kit (see p. 46).

B. Mary Lou, age 8 months, is brought

in by her parents. They state that she has a birthmark on her cheek that began at the age of 3 weeks. Their physician was consulted and stated that the lesion should be watched since "a lot of them just go away."

At the age of 3 months, the lesion had grown further, but the doctor still advised them to wait and watch.

Now at the age of 8 months the red hemangioma measures 12 x 12 x 5 mm. and has a bluish mass at the base. It is a mixed hemangioma.

MANAGEMENT

1. Reassure the parents that the lesion is not hereditary and that it will not turn into a cancer.

2. Since the child is now 8 months of age and the lesion has in all probability reached its maximum growth, no treatment is indicated. The parents must be told in no uncertain terms *why* you are not going to treat the tumor. You should state that you feel it will not enlarge further and that you know from your experience, and that of others, that it will undoubtedly be gone by the age of 2 or 3 years and almost certainly by the age of 5 to 7. You can almost predict that the residual mark will be insignificant. However, if it doesn't disappear completely by that age, the remaining usually insignificant lesion can be excised.

To SUMMARIZE, the advantages of *early* treatment of *small* superficial or cavernous hemangiomas are as follows: (1) you eliminate the lesion completely or almost completely; (2) you do not leave to chance the fact that it might or might not enlarge considerably; (3) you put a halt to apprehension on the part of the parents and relatives regarding the course of the lesion; and (4) with properly applied dry-ice therapy you leave no mark or only a slight one that would be no worse than that resulting from leaving it alone.

The advantages of *not* treating one of these hemangiomas are as follows: (1) the residuum after 5 to 7 years may be better cosmetically than if the lesion had been treated with dry ice, or especially if

x-ray therapy was used; and (2) the cost of therapy will be saved.

SPIDER HEMANGIOMA
(Plate 56)

A spider hemangioma consists of a small pinpoint to pinhead-sized central red arteriole with radiating smaller vessels like the spokes of a wheel or the legs of a spider. These lesions develop for no apparent reason or may develop in association with pregnancy or chronic liver disease. The commonest location is on the face. The reason for removal is cosmetic.

Differential Diagnosis

Venous Stars: small bluish, telangiectatic veins, usually seen on the legs and the face but may appear anywhere on the body; these can be removed if desired by the same method as for spider hemangioma.

Hereditary Hemorrhagic Telangiectasis (Rendu-Osler-Weber): small red lesions on any organ of the body that can hemorrhage; get familial history.

Treatment of a spider hemangioma on the cheek of a young woman who is postpartum 6 months. This lesion developed during her pregnancy and has persisted unchanged.

Treat by electrosurgery. Use the fine epilating needle with either a very low coagulating sparking current or a low cutting current. Stick the needle into the central vessel and turn on the current for 1 or 2 seconds until the vessel blanches. No anesthetic is necessary in most patients. The area will form a scab and heal in about 4 days, leaving an imperceptible scar. Rarely, a second treatment is necessary to eliminate the central vessel. If the radiating vessels are large and persistent, they can be treated in the same manner as the central vessel.

PORT-WINE HEMANGIOMA
(Plate 56)

The port-wine hemangioma is commonly seen on the face as a reddish-purple, flat, disfiguring facial mark. It can occur elsewhere in a less extensive form. Faint

Two spider hemangiomas on the arm of a pregnant woman.

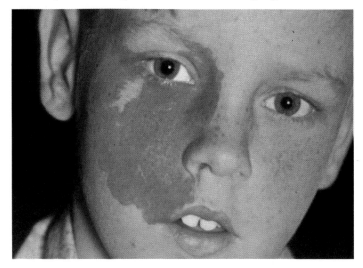

Port-wine stain on the face of a boy.

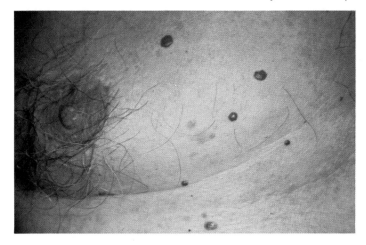

Capillary (senile) hemangiomas on the chest near the nipple.

Plate 56. Hemangiomas. (*Ortho Pharmaceutical Corporation*)

reddish lesions are often found on infants on the sides of the face, the forehead, the eyelids and the extremities. The color increases with crying and alarms the mother, but most of these faint lesions disappear shortly after birth.

Treatment of an extensive port-wine hemangioma on the left side of the face of an adult male.

1. There is no satisfactory treatment for this defect. Tattooing and dermabrasion have been used by some with minimal success.

2. Cosmetics, such as "Covermark" or any good pancake type of make-up, are effective to a certain degree.

NUCHAL HEMANGIOMA

This is a common, persistent, faint red patch on the posterior neck region at or below the scalp margin. It does not disappear with aging, and treatment is not effective or necessary. Since the posterior neck area is also the site of the common neurodermatitis, it is well to remember that following the cure of the neurodermatitis a redness that persists could be a nuchal hemangioma that was present for years and not noticed previously.

CAPILLARY HEMANGIOMA
(Plate 56)

These are also called *senile hemangiomas*, but this term obviously should not be used in discussing the lesion with the patient who is in the 30- to 60-year-old group. These pinhead or slightly larger, bright red, flat or raised tumors are present in many young adults and in practically all elderly persons. They cause no disability except when they are injured and bleed. Treatment is usually not desired but, if it is, light electrosurgery is effective.

VENOUS LAKE

Another vascular lesion that occurs in older persons is a *venous lake*. Clinically, it is a soft, compressible, flat or slightly elevated, bluish-red, 3 to 6 mm. sized lesion, usually located on the lips or the ears. Lack of induration and rapid growth distinguish it from a *melanoma*. Treat-

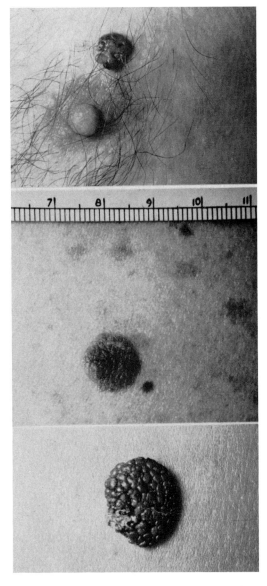

Fig. 28-13. Nevi. (*Top*) Compound nevus above the nipple. (*Center*) Compound nevus on the back. (*Bottom*) Verrucous compound nevus on the back.

ment is usually not desired, only reassurance concerning its nonmalignant nature.

ANGIOKERATOMAS

Three forms of this condition are known. The *Mibelli form* occurs on the dorsum of the fingers, the toes and the

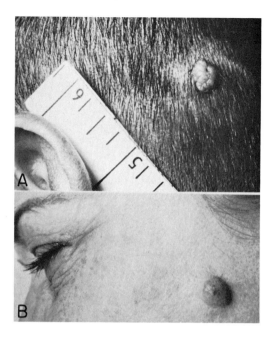

Fig. 28-14. Intradermal nevi. (*A*) On the scalp. (*B*) On the cheek.

knees; the *Fabry form* occurs over the entire trunk in an extensive pattern; and the *Fordyce form* occurs on the scrotum. The lesions are dark-red pinhead-sized papules with a somewhat warty appearance. Treatment is not indicated for the Mibelli and the Fordyce forms.

The Fabry form (angiokeratoma corporis diffusum), however, is the cutaneous manifestation of a systemic phospholipid storage disease in which phospholipids are deposited in the skin as well as in various internal organs. Death usually occurs in the 5th decade from the result of such deposits in the smooth muscles of the blood vessels, in the heart and in the kidneys.

NEVUS CELL TUMORS

CLASSIFICATION

I. Nevi
 1. Junction or active nevus
 2. Intradermal or resting nevus
II. Malignant Melanoma

NEVI
(Plates 58 and 59)

Nevi are pigmented or nonpigmented tumors of the skin that contain nevus cells (Figs. 28-13 and 28-14). Nevi are present on every adult, but some individuals have more than others. There are two main questions concerning nevi or moles. When and how should they be removed? What is the relationship between nevi and malignant melanomas?

Histologically, it is possible to divide nevi into *junction or active nevi* and *intradermal or resting nevi.* Combinations of these two forms commonly exist and are labeled *compound nevi.* Clinically, one never can be positive with which histopathologic type one is dealing, but certain criteria are helpful in establishing a differentiation between the two forms.

Description. Clinically, nevi can be pigmented or nonpigmented, flat or elevated, hairy or nonhairy, warty, papillomatous or pedunculated. They can have a small or a wide base. The brown or black pigmented, flat or slightly elevated, nonhairy nevi are usually *junction nevi.* The nonpigmented or pigmented, elevated, hairy nevi are more likely to be the *intradermal nevi.*

Distribution. Very prevalent on the head and the neck, but may be on any part of the body. The nevi on the palms, the soles and the genitalia are usually junction nevi.

Course. A baby is born with no, or relatively few, nevi; but with increasing age, particularly after puberty, nevi slowly become larger, can remain flat or become elevated, and may become hairy and darker. A change is also seen histologically with age. A junction-type active nevus, although it may remain as such throughout the life of the individual, more commonly changes slowly into an intradermal or resting nevus. Some nevi do not become evident until adult or later life, but the precursor cells for the nevus were present at birth. A malignant melanoma can originate in a junction nevus. Histologically, a benign junction nevus in a child can look like a malignant melanoma. This poses a difficult problem.

Histogenesis. The origin of the nevus cell is disputed, but the most commonly accepted theory is that it originates from cutaneous nerve cells.

Differential Diagnosis. IN CHILDHOOD, *warts:* flat or common warts not on the hands or the feet may be difficult to differentiate clinically; should see warty growth with black "seeds" (the capillary loops), rather acute onset and rapid growth (p. 152).

Freckles: see on exposed areas of the body, many lesions, faded in winter, not raised.

Lentigo (Fig. 28-15): see flat, tan or brown spot, usually on exposed skin surfaces; histologically, this is an early junction nevus.

Blue Nevus: see flat or elevated, soft, dark bluish or black nodule.

Granuloma Pyogenicum (Fig. 28-16): rapid onset of reddish or blackish vascular tumor, usually at site of injury.

Molluscum Contagiosum: see one, or usually more, crater-shaped, waxy tumors (p. 155).

Urticaria Pigmentosa: see single but more commonly multiple, slightly elevated, yellowish to brown papules, that urticate with trauma (p. 218).

IN ADULTHOOD, *warts:* usually rather obvious; see black "seeds" (p. 152).

Pedunculated Fibromas: see on neck and axillae (p. 260).

Histiocytoma: see on anterior tibial area of leg; flat, buttonlike in consistency (p. 272).

Other *epidermal and mesodermal tumors* are differentiated histologically.

IN OLDER ADULTS, *senile keratosis:* on exposed areas; scaly surrounding skin usually thin and dry; not a sharply demarcated lesion (p. 264).

Seborrheic Keratosis: see greasy, waxy, warty tumor, "stuck on" the skin; however, some are very difficult to differentiate clinically from nevus or malignant melanoma (p. 259).

Malignant Melanoma (Fig. 28-17 and Plate 59): seen at site of junction nevus or can arise from normal-appearing skin, shows a change in pigmentation either by

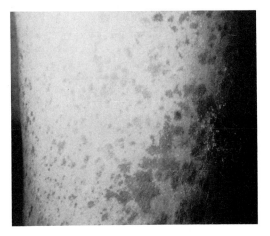

Fig. 28-15. Lentigines on the arm of the patient with the superficial melanoma in Figure 28-17 (*bottom*).

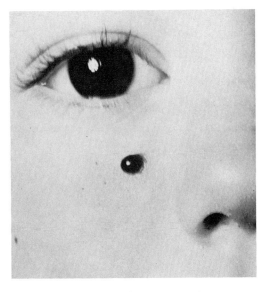

Fig. 28-16. Granuloma pyogenicum on the cheek of a 2-year-old boy.

spreading, becoming spotty or turning darker; may bleed, form a crust or ulcerate; partial or complete excision biopsy is indicated with more radical excision later if the histologic report is of a malignant melanoma.

Basal Cell Epitheliomas and Squamous Cell Carcinomas: if there is any question of malignancy, a biopsy is indicated (pp. 267 and 269).

Treatment

1. A mother comes into your office with her 5-year-old son, who has an 8 x 8 mm. flat brown nevus on the forehead. She wants to know if this "mole" is dangerous and if it should be removed.

A. Examine the lesion carefully. This lesion shows no sign of recent growth or change in pigmentation. (If it did, it should be excised and examined histologically.)

B. Reassure the mother that this mole does not appear to be dangerous and that it would be very unusual for it to become dangerous. If any change in the color or growth appears, the lesion should be examined again.

C. Tell the mother that it is best to leave this nevus alone at this time. The *only* treatment would be surgical excision, and you are quite sure that her boy would not sit tight for this procedure unless he was given a general anesthetic. When the boy is 16 years of age or older the lesion can be examined again and possibly removed at that time by a simpler method under local anesthesia.

2. A 25-year-old attractive female desires a brown raised hairy nevus on her upper lip removed. There has been no recent change in the tumor.

A. Examine the lesion carefully for induration, scaling, ulceration and bleeding. None of these signs is present. (If the diagnosis is not definite, a scissors biopsy may be performed safely, and the base gently coagulated by electrosurgery. Further treatment will depend on the biopsy report.)

B. Tell the patient that you can remove the mole safely, but that there will be a residual, very slightly depressed scar, and that probably the hairs will have to be removed separately after the first surgery has healed.

C. Surgical excision is the best method of removal. However, hairy raised pigmented nevi have been removed by electrosurgery for years with no real proof that this form of removal has caused a malignant melanoma. If a malignant melanoma becomes evident later, it undoubtedly was there prior to the treatment. Again, if there is any question of malignancy the lesion should be biopsied or excised!

Electrosurgery, following local anesthesia, can be performed with the coagulating or cutting current or with cautery. The site should not be covered and will heal in 7 to 14 days, depending on the size. If the hairs regrow they can be re-

---

DO'S AND DONT'S REGARDING NEVI

1. Don't remove a nevus in a child by electrosurgery; remove only by surgical excision.

2. Do remember that in a child a benign junction nevus may resemble a malignant melanoma histologically. Don't alarm the parents unnecessarily, since these nevi are usually no threat to life.

3. Don't remove a flat pigmented nevus, particularly on the palm, the sole or the genitalia by electrosurgery. These should be excised surgically if indicated.

4. Do tell the patient that a small slightly depressed scar will result from electrosurgery.

5. Don't remove a suspicious nevus by electrosurgery. Excise it and examine it histologically.

6. Don't perform a radical deforming surgical procedure on a possible malignant melanoma until the biopsy report has been returned. Many of these tumors will turn out to be seborrheic keratoses, granuloma pyogenicum, etc.

moved later by electrosurgical epilation (p. 45).

LYMPHOMAS

MYCOSIS FUNGOIDES
(Plate 50)

Also known as *lymphoma fungoides,* this polymorphous lymphoma involves the skin only, except in some rare cases that terminally invade the lymph nodes and the visceral organs. As is true with most lymphomas, the histology may change gradually to another form of lymphoma with progression of the disease. However, most cases of mycosis fungoides begin as such and terminate unchanged.

Description. The clinical picture of this disease is quite classic and is divided into 3 stages: the erythematous stage, the plaque stage and the tumor stage. The course usually proceeds in order, but all stages may be evident at the same time, or the first two stages may be by-passed.

Erythematous Stage: Commonly seen are scaly, red, rather sharply defined patches that resemble atopic eczema, psoriasis or parapsoriasis. The eruption may become diffuse as an exfoliative dermatitis. Itching is usually quite severe.

Plaque Stage: The red scaly patches develop induration and some elevation with central healing that results in ring-shaped lesions. This stage is to be differentiated from tertiary syphilis, psoriasis, erythema multiforme perstans, mycotic infections and other lymphomas.

Tumor Stage: This terminal stage is characterized by nodular and tumor growths of the plaques, often with ulceration and secondary bacterial infection. These tumors are to be differentiated from any of the granulomas (see Dictionary-Index).

Course. The early stages may progress slowly, with exacerbations and remissions over many years, or the disease may be rapidly fulminating. Once the tumor stage is reached, the eventual fatal outcome is imminent.

Treatment. The combined services of a dermatologist, a radiologist and an internist or a hematologist are required

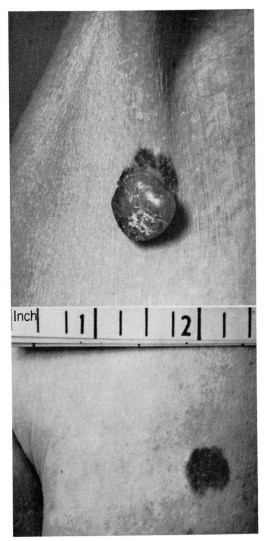

Fig. 28-17. Malignant melanomas. (*Top*) On posterior axillary fold. (*K.C.G.H.*) (*Bottom*) Superficial melanoma on the upper part of the arm of patient with lentigines. (Fig. 28-15).

for the management of this ultimately fatal disease. Corticosteroid therapy systemically is helpful during the early stages of the disease to relieve itching and scaling. The local application of a nitrogen mustard solution to the type of lesions seen in the first 2 stages of the disease, using the technic of Madison and Haserick,[3] has proved to be very effective

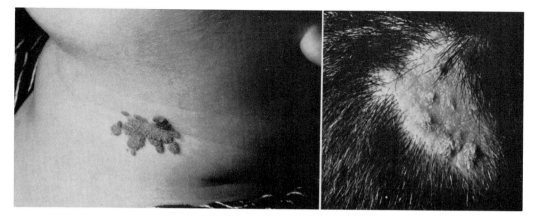

Fig. 28-18. Nevus verrucosus on the neck (*left*) **and on the scalp** (*right*).

in causing temporary resolution. X-ray therapy in small doses melts away the early lesions, but since the skin tolerance to radiation may be soon exceeded, it is advisable to withhold this form of therapy as long as possible. Nitrogen mustard and triethylenemelamine have been used systemically with some palliative effect. Antimony is of value in some cases.

COMPLETE HISTOLOGIC CLASSIFICATION

A complete histologic classification of tumors of the skin will be listed here. Those tumors discussed in the first part of this chapter are marked with an asterisk. The rarer tumors listed will be defined.

A. Epidermal tumors
  I. Tumors of the surface epidermis
    a. Nevoid tumors
      1. Nevus verrucosus (Fig. 28-18). A rather common tumor usually present at birth, consisting of single or multiple lesions in various forms that give rise to several clinical designations such as hard nevus, epidermal nevus, nevus unius lateralis, papilloma, ichthyosis hystrix, etc. No nevus cells are present.
      * 2. Seborrheic keratosis and dermatosis papulosa nigra
      * 3. Pedunculated fibromas
      4. Cysts

        * (a) Epidermal cyst
        * (b) Sebaceous cyst
        * (c) Milium
        * (d) Dermoid cyst
        * (e) Mucous retention cyst
      5. Clear cell acanthoma. A rare, usually single, slightly elevated, flat, pale red, scaling nodule less than 2 cm. in diameter, nearly always located on the lower extremities.
    b. Precancerous tumors
      * 1. Senile or actinic keratosis and cutaneous horn
      * 2. Arsenical keratosis
      * 3. Leukoplakia
      4. Warty dyskeratoma. A solitary warty lesion with a central keratotic plug most commonly seen on the scalp, face and neck.
    c. Epitheliomas and carcinomas
      * 1. Basal cell epithelioma
      * 2. Squamous cell carcinoma
      * 3. Keratoacanthoma
      4. Bowen's disease and erythroplasia of Queyrat. Bowen's disease is a single red scaly lesion with a sharp but irregular border that grows slowly by peripheral extension. Histologically it is an intra-epidermal squamous cell carcinoma (Fig. 28-6C). Erythroplasia of Queyrat (Plate 59) represents Bowen's disease of the mucous membranes and occurs

on the glans penis and rarely on the vulva. The lesion has a bright red velvety surface.

5. Paget's disease. (Plate 59) A unilateral scaly red lesion resembling a dermatitis, usually present on the female nipple. The early lesion is an intra-epidermal squamous cell carcinoma that also involves the mammary ducts and deeper connective tissue.

II. Tumors of the epidermal appendages
a. Nevoid tumors
1. Organic nevi or hamartomas
(a) Sebaceous nevi
(1) Nevus sebaceous (Jadassohn). Seen on the scalp or face as a single lesion present from birth, slightly raised, firm, yellowish, with furrowed surface.
(2) Adenoma sebaceum (Pringle). Part of a triad of epilepsy, mental deficiency and the skin lesions of adenoma sebaceum. The skin lesions occur on the face and consist of yellowish-brown papular nodular lesions with telangiectases.
(3) Senile sebaceous nevus or hyperplasia. Very common on the face in older persons and consists of one or several small yellowish translucent, slightly umbilicated, nodules.
(4) Fordyce disease (p. 237). A rather common condition of pinpoint-sized yellowish lesions of the vermilion border of the lips or the oral mucosa.
2. Adenomas or organoid hamartomas
(a) Sebaceous adenoma. A very rare solitary tumor of the face or the scalp, smooth, firm, elevated, often slightly pedunculated and measuring less than 1 cm. in diameter.
(b) Apocrine adenomas
(1) Syringocystadenoma

papilliferum. This adenoma of the apocrine ducts appears as a single verrucous plaque, usually seen on the scalp. Basal cell epitheliomatous change does occur.
(2) Hidradenoma papilliferum. This adenoma of the apocrine glands occurs almost exclusively on the labia majora and the perineum of women as a single intracutaneous tumor covered by normal epidermis.
3. Benign epitheliomas or suborganoid hamartomas
(a) Sebaceous epithelioma. A rare solitary, small nodule or plaque that has no characteristic clinical appearance.
(b) Apocrine epithelioma
(1) Syringoma. This is characterized by the appearance of pinhead-sized soft, yellowish nodules at the age of puberty in women, developing around the eyelids, the chest, the abdomen, and the anterior aspects of the thighs.
(2) Cylindroma. These appear as numerous, smooth, rounded tumors of various size on the scalp in adults and resemble bunches of grapes or tomatoes. These tumors may cover the entire scalp like a turban and are then referred to as turban tumors.
(3) Myoepithelioma. This occurs as a rare, moderately large, solitary, intracutaneous tumor. Mixed tumors of the salivary gland type clinically and histologically resemble myoepithelioma.
(c) Hair epitheliomas
(1) Trichoepithelioma. Also known as epithelioma adenoides cysticum and multiple benign cystic epithelioma. This begins at the age of puberty, frequently on a hereditary basis, and is charac-

terized by the presence of numerous, pinhead to pea-sized rounded yellowish or pink nodules on the face and occasionally on the upper trunk. Ulceration occurs when these lesions change into a basal cell epithelioma.

(2) Calcifying epithelioma (Malherbe). A rather rare solitary, hard, deep-seated nodule of the face or the upper extremities. Malignant degeneration does not occur.

(d) Eccrine epitheliomas

(1) Eccrine spiradenoma. A rare, usually solitary, intradermal firm tender nodule.

(2) Eccrine poroma. This occurs as an asymptomatic solitary tumor on the soles and the palms.

b. Carcinomas of sebaceous glands, and eccrine and apocrine sweat glands (rare)

III. Metastatic carcinoma of the skin. Occurs frequently from carcinoma of the breast, but rarely from other internal carcinomas.

Metastatic carcinoid nodules may appear in the skin as well as in lymph nodes and the liver. The primary tumor and the metastases produce excess 5-hydroxy-tryptamine (serotonin), which in turn produces attacks of flushing of the skin.

B. Mesodermal tumors

I. Tumors of fibrous tissue
* a. Histiocytoma and dermatofibroma
* b. Keloid
c. Fibrosarcoma
1. True fibrosarcoma. A rare tumor that starts most commonly in the subcutaneous fat, grows rapidly, causes the overlying skin to appear purplish and finally ulcerates.
2. Dermatofibrosarcoma protuberans. A small tumor that grows slowly in the corium and

spreads by the development of adjoining reddish or bluish nodules that may coalesce to form a plaque which can eventually ulcerate.

II. Tumors of mucoid tissue
a. Myxoma. Clinically seen as fairly well circumscribed, rather soft intracutaneous tumors with normal overlying epidermis.
b. Myxosarcoma. Subcutaneous tumors which eventually ulcerate the skin.
* c. Synovial cyst of the skin

III. Tumors of fatty tissue
a. Nevus lipomatosus superficialis. A rare, circumscribed nodular lesion, usually in the gluteal area.
b. Lipoma. A rather common tumor which may be multiple or single, lobulated, of varying size and in the subcutaneous tissue.
c. Hibernoma. A form of lipoma composed of embryonic type of fat cells.
d. Liposarcoma
e. Malignant hibernoma

IV. Tumors of nerve tissue and mesodermal-nerve sheath cells
a. Neuroma. Rare. Single or multiple small reddish or brown nodules that are usually tender as well as painful.
b. Neurofibromatosis (Fig. 21-5). Also known as von Recklinghausen's disease, this hereditary disease classically consists of pigmented patches, pedunculated skin tumors and nerve tumors. All of these lesions may not be present in a particular case.
c. Neurolemmoma
d. Granular cell schwannoma or myoblastoma. From neural sheath cells, this appears usually as a solitary tumor of the tongue, the skin or the subcutaneous tissue.
e. Malignant granular cell schwannoma or myoblastoma

V. Tumors of vascular tissue
* a. Hemangiomas
b. Granuloma pyogenicum. Also known as proud flesh, this is a rather common end-result of an in-

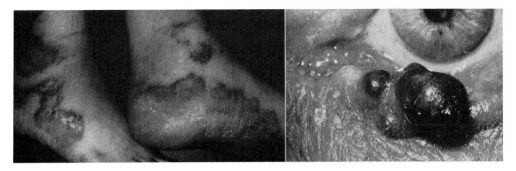

Fig. 28-19. Kaposi's sarcoma. (*Left*) Of feet (*Dr. David Morgan*). (*Right*) Of lower eyelid (*Drs. A. Lemoine and L. Calkins*).

jury to the skin which may or may not have been apparent. Vascular proliferation with or without infection produces a small red tumor that bleeds easily. It is to be differentiated from a malignant melanoma. Mild electrocoagulation is curative if the known cause is removed (Fig. 28-16).

c. Osler's disease. *See* Rendu-Osler-Weber disease in Dictionary-Index.

d. Lymphangioma. A superficial form, lymphangioma circumscriptum, appears as a group of thin-walled vesicles on the skin surface, whereas the deeper variety, lymphangioma cavernosum, causes a poorly defined enlargement of the affected area such as the lip or the tongue.

e. Glomus tumor. A rather unusual small, deep-seated, red or purplish nodule which is tender and may produce severe paroxysmal pains. The solitary lesion is usually seen under a nail plate, on the finger tips or elsewhere on the body.

f. Hemangiopericytoma

g. Kaposi's sarcoma (multiple idiopathic hemorrhagic sarcoma) (Fig. 28-19). Most commonly seen on the feet and the ankles as multiple bluish-red or dark brown nodules and plaques associated with visceral lesions. Sarcomatous malignant degeneration can occur.

h. Hemangio-endothelioma

i. Postmastectomy lymphangiosarcoma

VI. Tumors of muscular tissue

a. Leiomyoma. Solitary leiomyomas may be found on the extremities and on the scrotum, whereas multiple leiomyomas occur on the back and elsewhere as pinhead to pea-sized, brown or bluish firm elevated nodules. Both forms are painful and sensitive to pressure, particularly as they enlarge.

b. Leiomyosarcoma. Very rare.

VII. Tumors of osseous tissue

a. Osteoma cutis

1. Primary. The primary form of osteoma cutis develops from embryonal cell rests. These may be single or multiple.

2. Secondary. Secondary bone formation may occur as a form of tissue degeneration in tumors, in scar tissue, in scleroderma lesions, and in various granulomas.

VIII. Tumors of cartilaginous tissue

a. Nodular chondrodermatitis of the ear. A painful, hyperkeratotic nodule usually on the helix of the ear of elderly males.

C. Nevus cell tumors

I. Nevi

* a. Junction (active) nevus

* b. Intradermal (resting) nevus

c. Lentigines. These represent early junction nevi which are to be differ-

entiated from freckles (ephelides). A freckle histologically shows hyperpigmentation of the basal layer but no elongation of the rete pegs and no increase in the number of clear cells and dendritic cells. *Juvenile lentigines* begin to appear in childhood and occur on all parts of the body. *Senile lentigines* (Plate 59), also known as "liver spots," occur in elderly persons on the dorsum of the hands, the forearms and the face. *Lentigo maligna* (Plate 59) is a dark brown or black macular lesion, usually on the face of elderly persons, that is relatively benign. It may arise from a senile lentigo.
d. Mongolian spot (Plate 57). These are seen chiefly in Oriental or Negro babies, usually around the buttocks. They disappear spontaneously during childhood.

Related bluish patchy lesions are the *nevus of Ota,* seen on the side of the face, and the *nevus of Ito* located in the supraclavicular, scapular and deltoid regions.
e. Blue nevus. Clinically, the blue nevus appears as a slate-blue or bluish-black sharply circumscribed, flat or slightly elevated nodule occurring on any area of the body.
* II. Malignant melanoma
D. Lymphomas
I. Monomorphous group. This includes stem-cell lymphoma, reticulum-cell lymphoma, lymphoblastic lymphoma, lymphocytic lymphoma and follicular lymphoma. Lymphomas may have specific skin lesions containing the lymphomatous infiltrate, or nonspecific lesions may be seen. These latter consist of macules, papules, purpuric lesions, blisters, eczematous lesions, exfoliative dermatitis, and secondar-

ily infected excoriations that are a part of severe itching. Synonyms for follicular lymphoma include Brill-Symmers disease, giant follicular lymphoblastoma and the localized variety of Spiegler-Fendt sarcoid. The disseminate variety of Spiegler-Fendt sarcoid is now classified as a reticulum cell lymphoma.
II. Polymorphous group
a. Hodgkin's disease. Specific lesions are very rare, but nonspecific dermatoses are rather commonly seen.
* b. Mycosis fungoides
Sézary's syndrome. This is a very rare form of exfoliative dermatitis that occurs at an early stage of a lymphoma. It is diagnosed by finding unusually large monocytoid cells (so-called Sézary cells) in the blood. See chapter on Exfoliative Dermatitis. Another name for this is malignant reticulemic erythroderma.

E. Myelosis
I. Leukemia. Refers to circulating abnormal blood cells. May be seen along with lymphomas, but it is almost always associated with myelosis, such as myeloid leukemia. Cutaneous lesions are quite uncommon but may be specific or nonspecific.

BIBLIOGRAPHY

Allen, A. C.: The Skin: A Clinicopathologic Treatise, ed. 2. New York, Grune & Stratton, 1967.

Bowers, R. E., Graham, E. A., and Tomlinson, K. M.: The natural history of the strawberry nevus. Arch. Dermat., *82:*667, 1960.

Lever, W. F.: Histopathology of the Skin, ed. 4. Philadelphia, J. B. Lippincott, 1967.

Madison, J. F., and Haserick, J. R.: Mycosis fungoides topically treated with mechlorethamine. Derm. Digest, *3:*31, 1964.

Simpson, J. R.: Natural history of cavernous hemangiomata. Lancet, *2:*1057, 1959.

29

Pediatric Dermatology

The skin and the skin problems of infants and children are different enough from adult skin and skin problems to warrant special consideration of the subject of pediatric dermatology (Figs. 29-1 and 29-2).

Certain skin problems are seen **only** in infants and children (i.e. cradle cap and diaper dermatitis). Other dermatoses are seen in both children and in adults, but in children these dermatoses clinically appear different from the adult counterpart (i.e. the infantile form of atopic eczema).

Pediatric dermatology can be divided

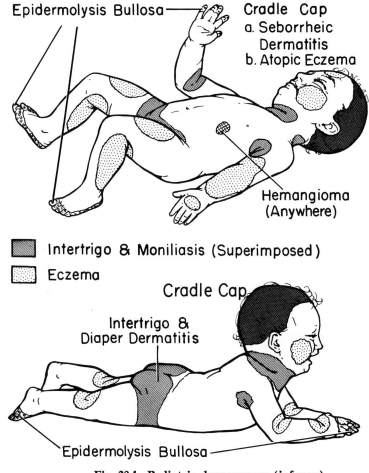

Fig. 29-1. Pediatric dermograms (infancy).

287

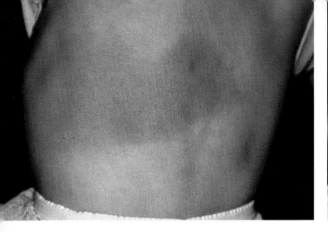
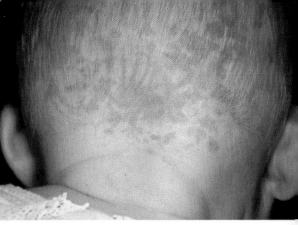

(A) Mongolian spot on back   (B) Nuchal hemangioma

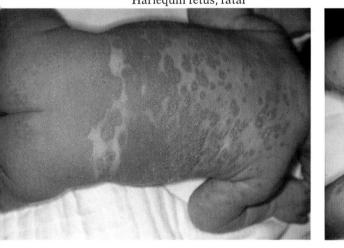
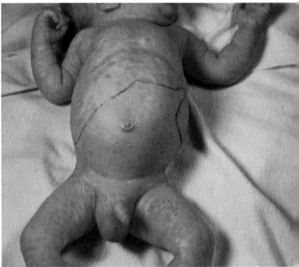

(C) Ichthyosiform erythroderma or   (D) Congenital syphilis with hepatomegaly
    Harlequin fetus, fatal   and splenomegaly

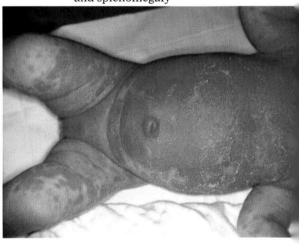

(E & F) Generalized moniliasis in 5-week-old child from diabetic family

Plate 57. Dermatoses of Newborns and Infants.

288

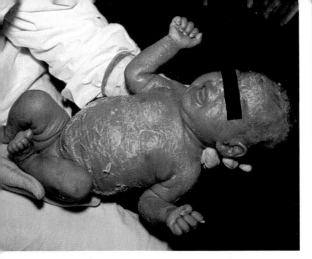
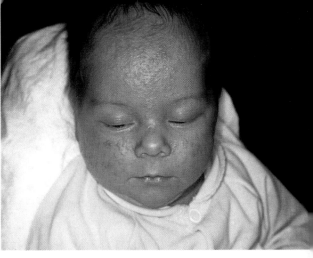

(G) Bullous impetigo or Ritter's disease; no thymus on autopsy

(H) Prickly heat, age 3 wks.

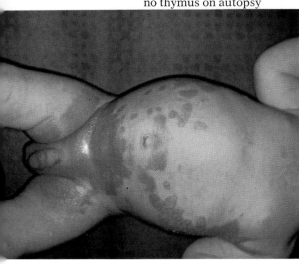
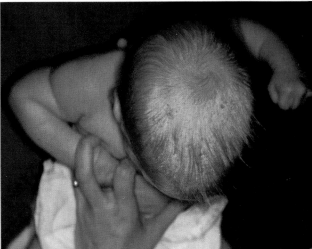

(I & J) Psoriasis of 2½-month-old child of body and scalp that began in diaper area

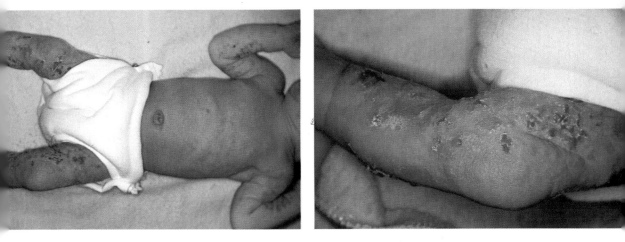

(K & L) Incontinentia pigmenti of 1-month-old girl in vesicular and warty stage, with (F) closeup

Plate 57. Dermatoses of Newborns and Infants (*Continued*)

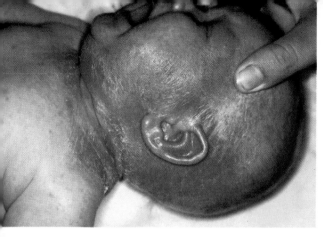

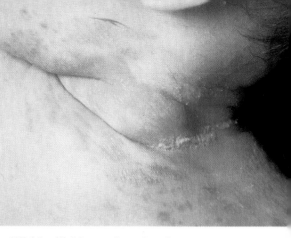

(*M*) Bacterial intertrigo and seborrheic dermatitis

(*N*) Monilial intertrigo of neck

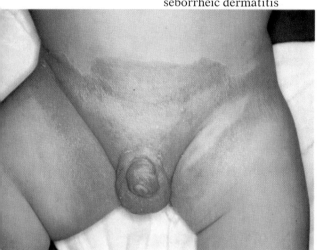

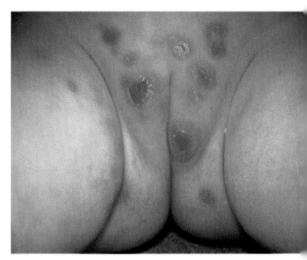

(*O*) Diaper dermatitis due to seborrhea

(*P*) Diaper erythema of Jacquet

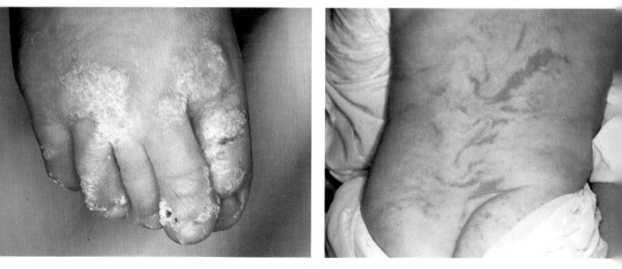

(*Q*) Incontinentia pigmenti of foot in warty stage at age 2 mo.; (*R*) of back in pigmented stage at age 14 mo. in same girl

Plate 57. Dermatoses of Newborns and Infants (*Continued*)

Fig. 29-2. Pediatric dermograms (childhood).

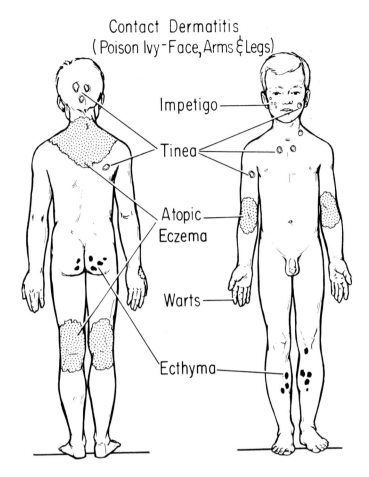

Contact Dermatitis
(Poison Ivy - Face, Arms & Legs)

Impetigo

Tinea

Atopic
Eczema

Warts

Ecthyma

into the dermatoses at birth, dermatoses of infancy, and dermatoses of childhood.

DERMATOSES AT BIRTH
(Plate 57)

There are really very few problems found on the skin at birth. The phrase "babies' skin" conveys an image and sensation of smooth, soft skin.

Of the many so-called **"birthmarks"**, only the superficial erythematous *hemangiomas* at the nape of the neck (*nuchal*) and center of the brow (*glabellar*) are commonly seen at birth. Most of the glabellar hemangiomas disappear in later childhood, while the nuchal ones can persist. The disfiguring *port-wine type of hemangioma* may also be present at birth, but it is a rare defect. The well known *strawberry* and *cavernous hemangiomas* usually are noticed at birth as only a small

red spot on the skin surface, and do not appear as obvious skin defects until the age of 3 or 4 weeks.

Neonatal erythema is quite common but rather unimportant. At birth, but more frequently a few days after birth, a blotchy macular erythema with minute pustules can arise most profusely on the trunk. Rarely papules or hives are seen. These lesions fade without treatment in 2 to 3 days. The cause is unknown.

Mongolian spots on the buttocks and sacral area are also commonly seen in yellow and black races.

Neonatal jaundice, from several causes, is very commonly seen, and can prove to be a diagnostic problem.

A few **growths,** such as *linear epidermal hamartomas,* are present on the skin at birth, but the more common true *cellular nevi* or "moles" found on the skin of

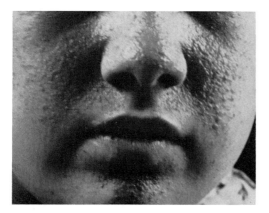

Fig. 29-3. Adenoma sebaceum with epiloia. (*Dr. A. Theodore Steegmann*)

almost every adult are rarely seen at birth. An exception is the *bathing trunk nevus* which fortunately is extremely rare.

A true **dermatitis** is rarely seen at birth; even *cradle cap* takes a few days after birth to develop.

Of the **infections**, moniliasis, syphilis and viral herpetic lesions are rarely seen at birth. Pyodermas usually are not present at birth but begin in the nursery.

Acne and *milia* can be present at birth. The acne, as small comedones or pustules, may be related to the administration of progesterone to the pregnant mother.

The remaining list of the dermatoses present at birth consists of a very rare group of **congenital** and/or **hereditary defects** of the skin, such as *ichthyosis* in several forms, *congenital aplasias* (absence of nails, hair, glands, or areas of skin), *congenital ectodermal dysplasias, incontinentia pigmenti* in the blister stage, and *epidermolysis bullosa.*

Thus, while the only **common** defects of the skin at birth are the flat superficial nuchal and glabellar hemangiomas, neonatal jaundice, neonatal erythema, and Mongolian spots, there are quite a number of **rarer** abnormalities that can be present on the skin at birth.

For completeness sake, the following dermatoses are listed as being present at birth.

Neonatal erythema is common. See above.

Infectious dermatoses

Moniliasis (p. 175 and Plate 57) clinically is an intertriginous eruption with small red pustule-like lesions.

Syphilis (p. 134 and Plate 57) can mimic almost any dermatosis with macules to papules to bullae. Rare.

Herpes simplex (p. 145) seen usually as vesicles in clusters. Rare.

Rubella syndrome. Very rare. There can be purpuric lesions of the skin along with other defects. Purpura can also be due to several other causes.

Neonatal acne and milia are rather commonly seen.

Psoriasis and chronic discoid lupus erythematosus have been reported only rarely at birth.

Bullous dermatoses

Epidermolysis bullosa (p. 254 and Plate 53) is seen mainly as denuded bullae on toes, fingers, elbows or entire body in the severe forms (dystrophic and letalis). All forms are rare.

Incontinentia pigmenti (p. 218 and Plate 57) is seen in the first stage with red-based vesicles or bullae most commonly on the dorsum of the hands and feet. Rare.

Pigmentary changes

Albinism, very rare, with entire loss of pigment.

Piebaldism, very rare, with patchy loss of pigment.

Neurofibromatosis (von Recklinghausen's syndrome) (Fig. 21-5 and Plate 58) can be anticipated if macular café-au-lait spots are found.

Adenoma sebaceum (Fig. 29-3 and Plate 53) can also be diagnosed at birth if there is depigmentation in an ash leaf configuration.

Mongolian spots (Plate 57) are common in certain races.

Jaundice is commonly seen at birth and can be due to several causes.

Congenital ectodermal dysplasias or defects (Plate 58). The extent and involvement of the defects of the skin and/or glands, and/or nails and/or hair accounts for the existence of a multiplicity of complicated syndromes. These are rare.

Ichthyosis, p. 250. The 2 vulgaris types (Plate 53 and Fig. 27-1) are not present at birth but the rarer lamellar form and the erythroderma forms are present at birth. The Harlequin fetus (Plate 57) is a severe lethal type of the erythroderma form. Rarely palmar and plantar keratodermas occur.

New Growths

Hemangiomas (see above)
Superficial flat type of neck (nuchal) (Plate 57) or brow (glabella) are common (p. 277).
Port-wine type (p. 275).
Superficial strawberry or cavernous types (Fig. 28-12, Plate 58 and p. 273).
Epidermal tumors (p. 282). Linear warty growths (hamartomas) or pigmented non-cellular nevi are rarely seen. Bathing trunk nevi cover large areas.

DERMATOSES OF INFANCY (BIRTH TO 2 YEARS)

From the protected, quite sterile, temperature and humidity controlled environment of the uterus, the baby is launched into a less protected, contaminated, 30 to 40 degree cooler, and much dryer environment. That the body, and the skin in particular, can adjust so rapidly and without apparent abnormal reaction is a miracle. There is some toll, however.

The newborn infant is usually washed gently with a mild soap and then oiled daily. A skin problem can develop if the mother is too fastidious and bathes the skin *excessively*. This can cause *dry skin* (*xerosis*) or even a *contact dermatitis*. If there is a familial tendency toward *atopic eczema* (Plates 9 and 10), then excess and too frequent bathing, especially in the winter, is definitely very harmful. For the atopic child, the lanolin in baby oils can also be irritating, and a switch should be made to non-lanolin oils such as Allercreme Special Formula Body Lotion or Syntex Lotion. Other management tech-

niques for atopic eczema are listed on p. 56.

A problem from *lack* of daily bathing and adequate drying of the skin is that debris can accumulate in the intertriginous areas of the neck, axilla and groin. This can lead to a *bacterial* or *monilial intertrigo* (Plate 58). The fatter the child, the greater this problem. (See pages 129 and 178.)

Cradle cap (Plate 19) is a yellowish, greasy and crusted collection of vernix caseosa and shedding skin caught around the hairs of the scalp. If the inherited tendency for the child is to have a seborrheic or atopic diathesis, this also contributes to the mess. But another more common contributing factor is the tendency on the part of the mother to want to avoid damage to the "soft spot" on the scalp, so that she avoids adequate cleansing of it. When the baby's body skin is oiled, the scalp is oiled also, and this adds to the accumulation of the debris. Thus, many factors lead to the development of cradle cap.

Treatment consists of explaining to the mother the causative factors, prescribing a corticosteroid cream twice a day to cut down on inflammation and epidermal shedding, and the use of a mild shampoo 2 to 3 times a week followed by gentle physical removal of the scaling with a comb.

Neonatal erythema, seen at birth, is more commonly seen 2 to 3 days later. (See p. 291.)

Diaper area dermatitis (Plate 57) can be caused by many factors also. It can be a manifestation of a *contact dermatitis* from too enthusiastic bathing of the diaper area with inadequate rinsing of the soap, or, conversely, it can be an *intertrigo* caused by accumulation of debris because of too little bathing, inadequate cleansing of the skin folds and infrequent changing of soiled diapers. By proper questioning, a physician can determine which of these divergent factors apply to a given case of diaper area irritation.

Seborrheic dermatitis (Plates 19 and 57), and rarely *psoriasis* (Plate 57), can be found in infants, usually as an intertriginous type of dermatitis.

Prickly heat (Plate 57) is another one of the problems caused by the wrong environment, in this case too many clothes and/or too warm a room. One sees small pinpoint sized vesicles or pustules localized in the intertriginous areas or even quite generalized. Treatment consists of removing the cause (less clothes or lower room temperature) and application of a zinc oxide-talc lotion (p. 37) 3 or 4 times a day.

In summary, the following is a list of the **common** dermatoses of infants. Consult the Dictionary-Index for additional page references on these conditions.

Neonatal erythema
Cradle cap dermatitis
   Greasy and scaly debris
   Seborrheic dermatitis
   Atopic eczema
Dry skin (xerosis)
Contact dermatitis
Atopic eczema
Intertrigo
   Bacterial
   Monilial
Diaper area dermatitis
   Contact dermatitis
   Intertrigo
   Erythema of Jacquet is an uncommon form of diaper dermatitis characterized by discrete papuloerosive lesions (Plate 57).
Seborrheic dermatitis
Prickly heat
New growths
   Hemangiomas, strawberry and cavernous types
Exanthems
   Roseola
Chickenpox

Some **less common** skin problems of infants include:
Burns (p. 242)
Pyodermas
   Furuncles (boils) (p. 120 and Plate 32). These can develop as a nursery epidemic.
   Impetigo (p. 114). A more severe form with large bullae quite extensive on the body is called *bullous impetigo* or *Ritter's disease* (Plates 32 and 57).
Fungal infections (p. 159)

Insect bites and stings (p. 317). Also can see *papular urticaria* (p. 318).
Pediculosis (p. 183)
Scabies (p. 182)
Icthyosis, and congenital and hereditary defects as listed on p. 253 and Plate 53.
Other exanthems (p. 157)

Rare diseases of infants from birth to 2 years of age include:
Generalized Erythrodermas
   The following conditions can be difficult to differentiate, and prolonged observation is helpful in ascertaining the final diagnosis. Most of these conditions are rare.

Atopic eczema as an erythroderma is rare, but can occur in the first few weeks of life. With the passage of time it assumes the more typical pattern of eczema. (See p. 56)

Monilial erythroderma is rare but can spread out from the intertriginous areas (Plate 57).

Leiner's disease. A severe form of generalized exfoliative dermatitis of infants presents in different cases varying degrees of atopy, seborrhea and perhaps infectious eczematization. It is accompanied by a peculiar systemic reaction which is most evident in its gastro-intestinal manifestations. Secondary infection results in mortality in over 10% of cases.

Ritter's disease is another name for *bullous impetigo* of the infant that has become generalized (Plate 57).

Toxic epidermal necrolysis (*Lyell*) or *scalded skin syndrome* is a rare severe problem where large bullae form and the skin peels off in sheets. It occurs predominantly in infants and children and occasionally in adults. The cause is usually not ascertained or has been attributed to drugs such as sulfa, barbiturates or phenylbutazone, or to trauma, or to infections with *staphylococcus* or to *E. Coli.* Treatment is supportive with antibiotics and corticosteroids as the severity warrants.

Lamellar desquamation or *collodion baby.* This is a syndrome of generalized erythema, scaling, peeling and cracking of the skin. Mild physiological cases are transitory. Severe forms are seen as the early stage of *lamellar ichthyosis, bullous* and *non-bullous ichthyosiform erythroderma,* and *sex-linked ichthyosis.* These conditions are discussed on p. 250.

Disorders of the subcutaneous fat

Neonatal cold injury is relatively frequently seen in babies born at home and exposed to cold temperature. The skin is pallid, cool to touch, edematous and immobile. The hands, feet and cheeks are red. Sclerema or hardening may occur on the limbs and cheeks. Most cases recover with careful rewarming.

Sclerema is an extremely rare condition of premature or debilitated infants affected by a pre-existing respiratory or gastro-intestinal infection. Progressive hardening, spreading from the buttocks and thighs, occurs. The mortality is around 50%.

Fat necrosis in the newborn. A benign, self-limited localized process occurring over the bony prominences in infants born after a difficult labor. Nodular thickening of the subcutaneous tissue is detected usually in the second or third week of life. The nodules may coalesce to form large plaques. In a few months they disappear but some lesions may become calcified.

Scleredema and *scleroderma* are rare in children and not related to the above conditions.

Localized scleroderma or *morphea* develops frequently in older children.

Acrodermatitis enteropathica. A rare disease of infants, usually fatal, characterized by pustular and psoriasiform lesions around body orifices, on the face, the perineum and also on the limbs. It is associated with recurrent episodes of diarrhea. Diodoquin and sulfamethazine are sometimes effective.

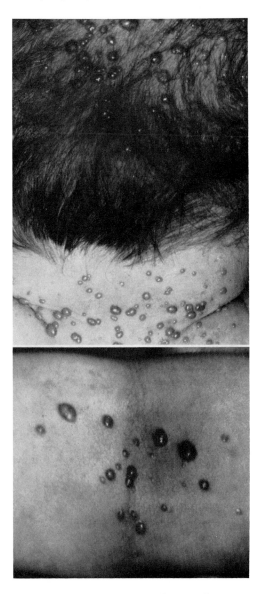

Fig. 29-4. Tumors. Xanthogranuloma. (*Top*) Back of head and neck of child. (*Bottom*) Arm of same child. (*Dr. David Morgan*)

Acrodynia. A rare disease due to hypersensitivity to mercury characterized by weight loss, anorexia and painful hands and feet. Death can occur from secondary infection.

Duke's disease. A mild exanthem occurring usually in the spring or summer months, with an incubation period of from 9 to 21 days. The eruption becomes generalized within a few hours, is bright red in color and is accompanied by a low-grade fever.

Granulosis rubra nasi. A chronic rare disease characterized by increased sweating of the nose and surrounding skin with development of reddish maculopapular lesions.

Lichen striatus. A rare skin condition of infants and children, characterized by acute onset of linear bands of papular and lichenified lesions which usually do not itch. This occurs mainly on the arms or the legs and disappears spontaneously in a few months. It is to be differentiated from *lichen planus* and *nevus unius lateris.*

Xanthogranuloma (Fig. 29-4). This rather frightening condition consists of small discrete, yellowish-tan papules that can cover the body. They develop in the first year of life, and without therapy disappear by the age of 5 or so.

DERMATOSES OF CHILDREN
(Plate 58)

Children seem to fall heir to most of the skin diseases of their adult counterparts, especially those problems that also affect their parents or other relatives. A discussion of the skin diseases of children aged 2 to 12 years would really cover the majority of all dermatologic ills in this book.

Here is a list of the commonest children's skin problems along with a short note about pertinent points. For more complete coverage in this book refer to the chapters and pages listed.

Chapter 7. Dermatologic Allergy
Contact dermatitis.
Very commonly see *poison ivy dermatitis* (p. 52 and Plate 6)
Atopic eczema (Plates 9, 10 and 58)
In children, see especially eczema of the feet or toes, and depigmented scaly eczema lesions on the cheeks and arms (pityriasis simplex type)
Drug Eruption
Not too common (Plate 14).

Chapter 9. Vascular Dermatoses
Urticaria
See especially a *papular urticaria* often due to bites (p. 318).
Erythema multiforme of Hebra type. Rather rare.
Granuloma annulare. A chronic inflammatory dermatosis, characterized by reddish papules that spread peripherally leaving a normal appearing center. It is moderately common, the cause is unknown and it disappears spontaneously in months or years.

Chapter 10. Seborrheic Dermatitis and Acne. Both are seen as child approaches puberty. Comedones are early signs of acne.

Chapter 11. Papulosquamous Dermatoses
Psoriasis.
Not uncommon, but a special type, the *guttate form* (Plate 58), is seen quite frequently and usually follows a streptococcal infection of the tonsils or throat.
Pityriasis rosea.
In children, it is common to have unusual variations of pityriasis rosea, such as lesions on the face and large irregular lesions on body.
Tinea versicolor.
A 9-year-old girl patient had been told she had *vitiligo* on her chest and that there was no cure. In reality she had tinea versicolor, and the scaly depigmented areas cleared with Selsun treatment in 2 weeks. Be sure of your diagnosis, especially when you give a label of one that has a poor prognosis.

Chapter 12. Dermatologic Bacteriology
Impetigo
Ecthyma
Furuncle

Chapter 14. Dermatologic Virology
Herpes simplex
Kaposi's varicelliform eruption
Chickenpox
Warts
These can prove to be the bane of a dermatologist's existence.
Molluscum contagiosum
Also know as "water warts" because of appearance. These can also occur

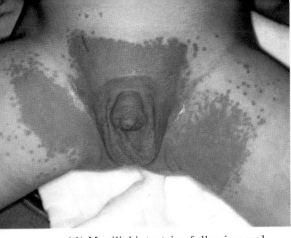
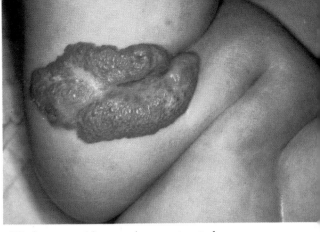

(A) Monilial intertrigo following oral
antibiotics, age 1 yr.

(B) Compound hemangioma untreated
of the crural area, age 4 mo.

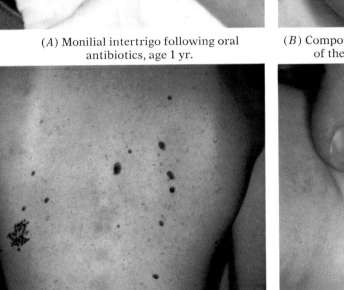
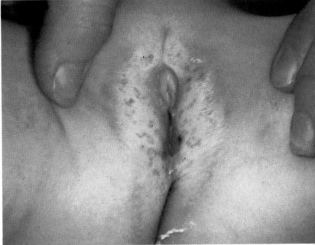

(C) Junction nevi of the back, age 16 yrs.

(D) Lichen sclerosis et atrophicus
of labia of 3-yr.-old girl

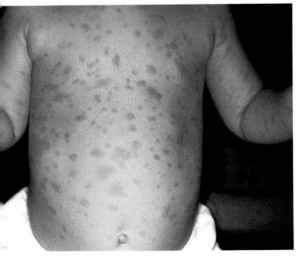
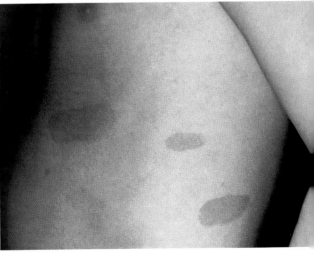

(E) Urticaria pigmentosa of chest, age 2 yrs.
(Note the red urticating lesion)

(F) Neurofibromatosis with early oval
café-au-lait lesions, age 5 yrs.

Plate 58. Dermatoses of Children.

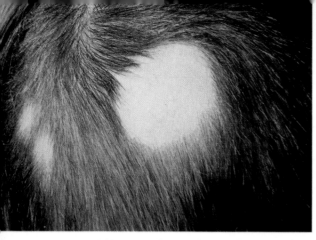

(G) Tinea of scalp due to *M. audouini*

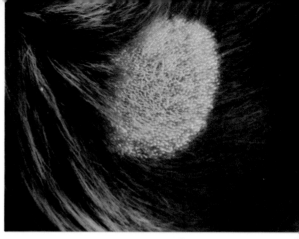

(H) Tinea hairs fluorescing under
Wood's light

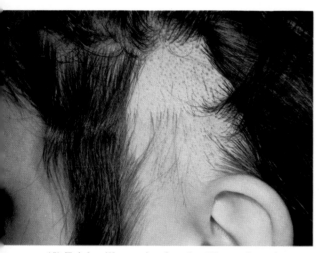

(I) Trichotillomania of scalp. (Note: there is no
complete baldness in area as in alopecia areata.)

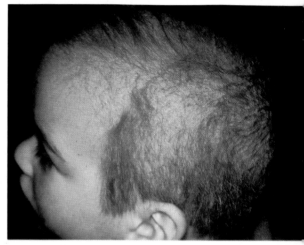

(J) Diffuse alopecia with general
ectodermal defect, age 3 yrs.

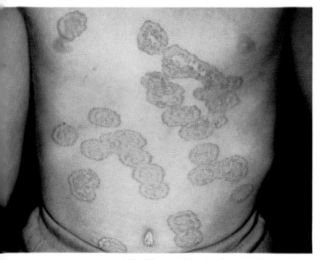

(K) Tinea of body due to *M. canis*

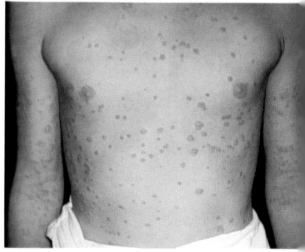

(L) Guttate psoriasis following
streptococcus throat infection

Plate 58. Dermatoses of Children (*Continued*)

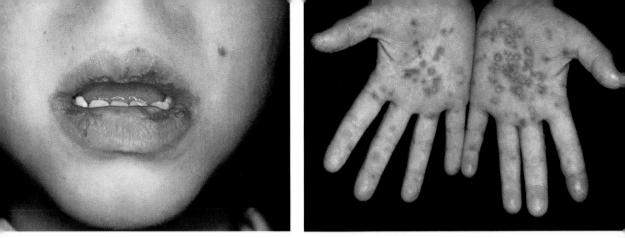

(M) Viral exanthem with erosions of lips and (N) hemorrhagic blisters in palms

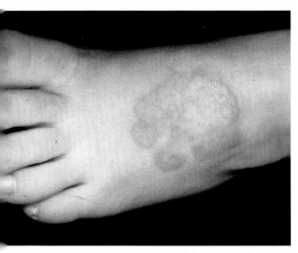

(O) Granuloma annulare of dorsum of foot

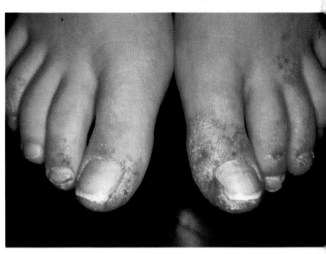

(P) Atopic eczema of toes

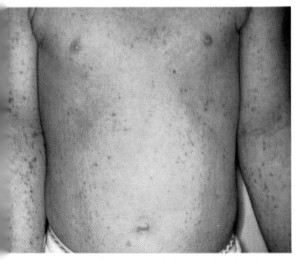

(Q) Atopic eczema of chest and cubital
fossae, age 9 yrs.

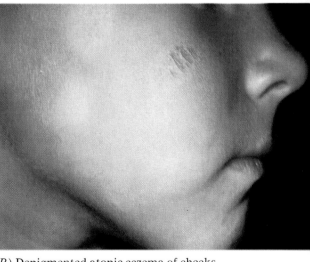

(R) Depigmented atopic eczema of cheeks
(pityriasis simplex faciei), age 5 yrs.

Plate 58. Dermatoses of Children (*Continued*)

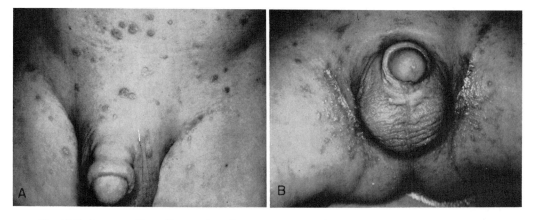

Fig. 29-5. Letterer-Siwe disease in a 7-month-old boy. (*A*) Abdominal lesions. (*B*) Crural lesions.

in the excoriated patches of *atopic eczema.*

Measles

German measles

Erythema infectiosum

Other viral exanthems (Plate 58)

Chapter 15. Dermatologic Mycology

Tinea of the feet

The most common foot dermatitis in children is *atopic eczema.*

Tinea of the groin

Differentiate this from *monilial intertrigo.* The treatment is very different.

Tinea of smooth skin (Plate 58)

Quite common, from kittens and puppies and other children. Usually see round, not oval lesions.

Tinea of the scalp (Plate 58)

Fortunately the epidemic *M. Audouini* type is becoming more rare.

Moniliasis (Plate 58)

In children, see mainly involvement of the crural area. Differentiate from the sharply bordered *tinea eruption.*

Sporotrichosis

A chancriform disease usually seen in farm children or those having played in hay.

Chapter 16. Dermatologic Parasitology

Scabies

Not common, but must be considered when you see generalized excoriated skin lesions.

Pediculosis

Uncommon, but your index of suspicion must be high.

Chapter 17. Bullous Dermatoses

Dermatitis herpetiformis

Rare in children, but easily missed unless one is alert. Distribution of vesicles or excoriations on scapulae, buttocks and elbows is typical.

Chapter 19. Pigmentary Dermatoses

Vitiligo

Early lesions can begin on ankles and wrists. Do not confuse with the depigmentation seen in *tinea versicolor* (p. 107) or *pityriasis simplex variety of atopic eczema* occurring on the cheeks and arms (p. 56).

Chapter 21. The Skin and Internal Disease

Puberty state

Letterer-Siwe disease (Fig. 29-5)

Rare, but can look like *seborrhea* of the groin area.

Neuroses

Neurotic nail biting

Trichotillomania

Quite a common problem involving the scalp and eyelashes. Can be related to chronic television watching or other stressful situations.

Urticaria pigmentosa (Plate 58)

Mastocytosis, while rare, is seen more frequently in children than adults.

The flat tan lesions urticate on stroking, or there can be a somewhat frightening generalized erythematous flush.

Incontinentia pigmenti (Plate 57)

Rare. After the vesicles and wart-like lesions of infancy quiet down, the whorls of hyperpigmentation and other ectodermal defects become manifest.

Neurofibromatosis (Plate 58)

These lesions usually begin in childhood as small soft tumors and pigmented patches.

Chapter 22. Diseases Affecting the Hair

Alopecia areata

This condition in children has a more severe prognosis for chronicity than when it occurs in adults.

Tinea of scalp (see above, p. 170 and Plate 58)

Trichotillomania (see above. p. 217 and Plate 58)

Congenital and hereditary hair defects (Plate 58)

Chapter 23. Diseases Affecting the Nails (Plate 51)

Nail-biting (see above)

Warts around the nails

A difficult therapeutic problem.

Atopic eczema can affect the nails secondarily

Other nail defects

Chapters 25 and 26. Dermatoses Due to Physical Agents and Photosensitivity Dermatoses

Sunburn

Tanning is so much to be desired that kids have a tendency to go overboard the first sunny days.

Hydroa aestivale

Rare, but one should know about this photosensitivity eruption of butterfly area of face.

Chapter 27. Genodermatoses (Plate 53)

Ichthyosis

The dominant vulgaris type and the x-linked type develop in early childhood.

Keratosis pilaris. A common mild hereditary dermatosis characterized by accumulation of horny material at the hair follicle openings producing a nutmeg-graterlike sensation. It is worse in the winter and is most marked on the extensor surfaces of the legs and the arms. Similar lesions are seen from vitamin A deficiency.

Chapter 28. Tumors of the Skin

Hemangiomas

Nuchal and brow hemangiomas

Some may have faded by childhood but many persist.

Superficial strawberry and cavernous hemangioma (Plate 58)

Approximately 90% of these disappear without treatment by the ages of 5 to 7.

Port-wine hemangioma

Persists in spite of time and treatment.

Granuloma pyogenicum

A bright red papule that bleeds easily. Arises from trauma ("proud flesh") or spontaneously.

Nevus Cell Tumors

Junction and Intradermal Nevi (Plate 58)

Nevi or moles usually begin to become obvious after the age of 6 or so. Around puberty they become most conspicuous in numbers and in size. It is common for a parent to suddenly notice their presence, and come in to the physician claiming they have all come at once. Of course, this is not true; they grew gradually and became more pigmented.

Some junction nevi of children on histopathologic examination can appear very "active" with immature cells. These are not malignant and are called *benign juvenile melanomas*.

Another disturbing change noticed rarely around nevi in older children is the development of a white or depigmented halo. This is called a *halo nevus* or *leucoderma acquisitum centrifigum*. There is nothing sinister about this change. No therapy is indicated. The patient or family can be reassured that the halo and also the nevus will probably disappear with time. Some cases, however, are an early manifestation of *vitiligo*.

Nevi in children, if they are to be removed should be cut out by excisional surgery and examined histopathologically.

Freckles (ephelides)

Rarer tumors of children:

Nevus verrucosus (a hamartoma)

This is more common on the scalp or neck, but can be on any body area. Usually warty, tannish, and in a linear configuration.

Adenoma sebaceum (Fig. 29-3 and Plate 53)

Acne-like solid papules on the butterfly area of face as part of *epilepsy* and *mental deficiency* (*epiloia*).

Chapter 31. Geographic Skin Diseases

Chigger bites (Fig. 31-3)

Children can get many bites all over the body and this extensiveness can be confusing. When they occur on the scalp, the excoriations can become infected and develop into *impetigo*.

Creeping eruption

The South, barefeet and this disease go hand in hand (or foot in foot).

BIBLIOGRAPHY

Korting, G. W. translated by Curth, W., and Curth, H.: Diseases of the Skin in Children and Adolescents. Philadelphia, W. B. Saunders, 1970. This is an excellent atlas, but nothing on treatment.

Leider, M.: Practical Pediatric Dermatology. ed. 2. St. Louis, C. V. Mosby, 1961.

Solomon, L. and Esterly, N. B.: Neonatal Dermatology. Philadelphia, W. B. Saunders, 1972.

30

Geriatric Dermatology

Man ages gradually. While the entire body changes gradually with advancing years, skin aging is most readily visible and most readily noticed by both men and women. If the sale of cosmetics (moisturizing creams, "age-spot" removers, wrinkle creams, wigs, hair dyes for men and women, etc.) is any sign, it would seem obvious that the constant search for the "elixir of youth" is mainly directed toward maintaining a youthful looking skin.

For the trained and careful observer, the elderly patient with even a so-called "normal skin" presents a wealth of skin changes, some obvious and others less obvious (Fig. 30-1).

Some of the earliest signs of aging of the skin are the development of the hyperpigmented macular lesions known as *freckles* and *lentigines* (Plate 59). These can begin in the forties. They develop most commonly on the dorsum of the hands and on the face in direct proportion to the fair complexion of the individual and the dosage of sun gained through the earlier years of life.

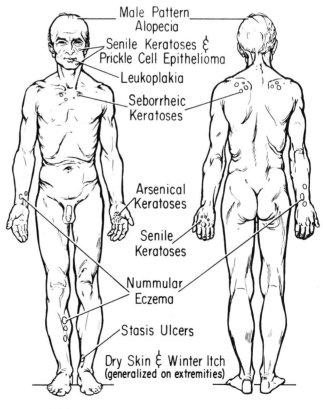

Fig. 30-1. Geriatric dermograms.

303

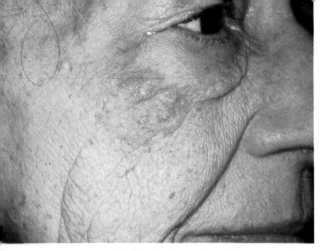 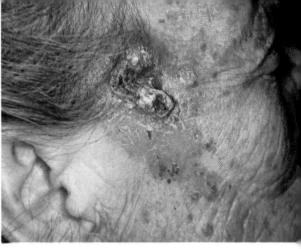

(A) Senile elastosis with cysts and comedones of cheek

(B) Squamous cell epithelioma and keratoses on aged skin

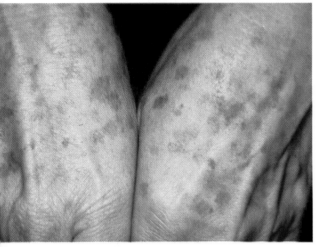 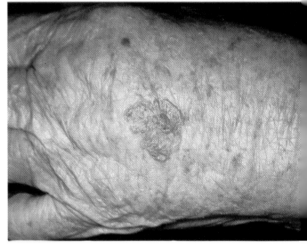

(C) Senile freckles on dorsum of hands

(D) Basal cell epithelioma and wrinkling of hand

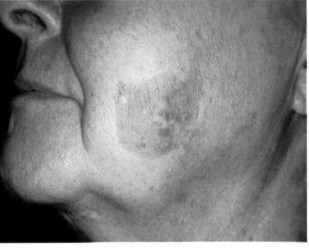 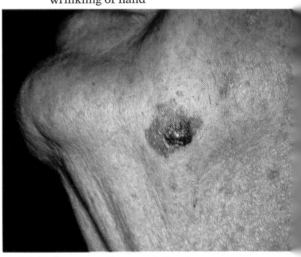

(E) Lentigo on cheek

(F) Malignant melanoma in lentigo on jaw area

Plate 59. Geriatric Dermatoses.

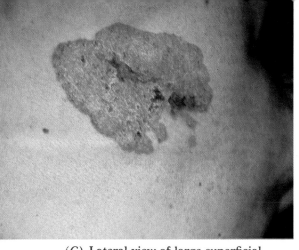

(G) Lateral view of large superficial basal cell epithelioma on back

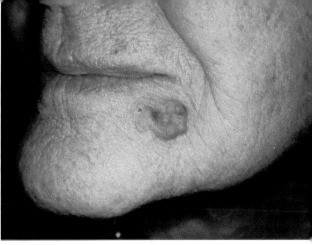

(H) Basal cell epithelioma on chin

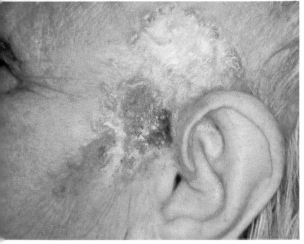

(I) Extensive basal cell epithelioma, age 79

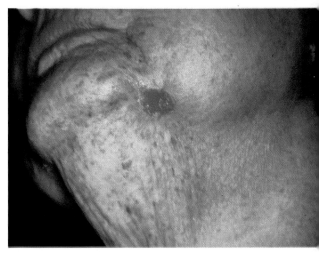

(J) Squamous cell epithelioma in area of chronic radiodermatitis for hypertrichosis of skin

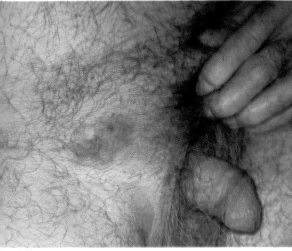

(K) Paget's disease of crural area

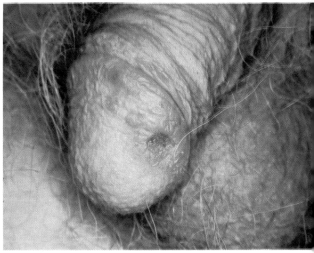

(L) Erythroplasia of Queyrat on penis

Plate 59. Geriatric Dermatoses (*Continued*)

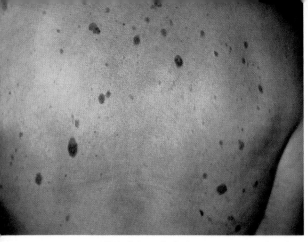

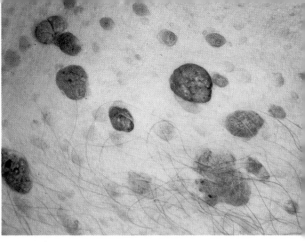

(M) Seborrheic keratoses over back of 71-yr.-old male

(N) Seborrheic keratoses closeup

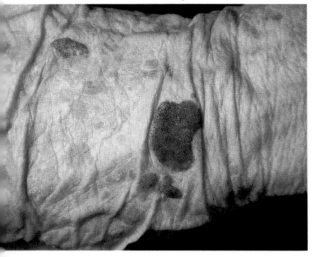

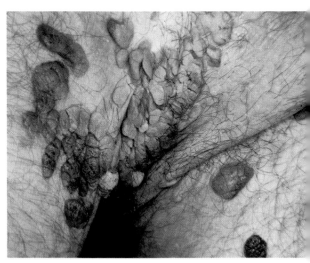

(O) Large seborrheic keratosis on hand in 84-yr.-old woman

(P) Multiple seborrheic keratoses of crural area

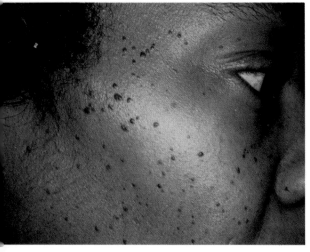

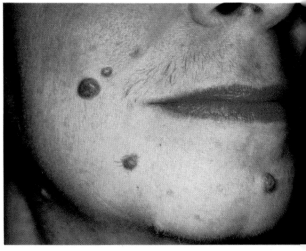

(Q) Seborrheic keratoses or dermatosis papulosa nigri on face

(R) Compound nevi on face

Plate 59. Geriatric Dermatoses (*Continued*)

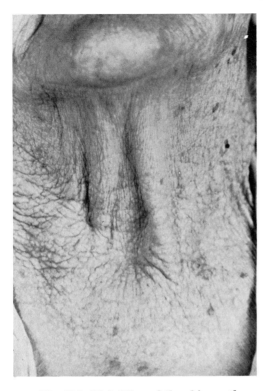

Fig. 30-2. Wrinkling of the skin on the front of the neck.

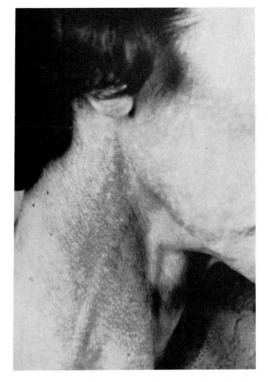

Fig. 30-3. Poikiloderma of Civatte. Very common red-brown discoloration on sides of neck.

On the face, and to a lesser extent on the rest of the body, *wrinkling* of the skin also progresses with age (Fig. 30-2).

Diffuse hyperpigmentation of the face and hands, again in the sun exposed areas, becomes more definite with age. The quite common hyperpigmentation on the side of the neck, which is a combination of brown and red discoloration and is seen particularly in women, is called *poikiloderma of Civatte* (Fig. 30-3).

Actinic keratoses (Plate 54) obviously have a definite predilection for the sun exposed areas of the body, and also are related to the genetically determined complexion of the individual and the environmental sun exposure.

The very common *seborrheic keratoses* (Plate 59) can also be on the face but are most commonly seen on the neck, back, chest and even on the crural area. These lesions can be so black and angry looking as to make one believe that they are dealing with a *malignant melanoma*.

Another manifestation of aging is the development of *comedones* on the face lateral to the orbicular area. (Plate 59).

Pedunculated fibromas and *pedunculated seborrheic keratoses* are extremely common on the neck and axilla. These can begin in the forties and fifties.

Moving down to the trunk, practically every elderly individual has small bright red *capillary hemangiomas* (Plate 45). These are of no clinical significance but can sometimes be disturbing for some vain individuals.

On the legs, and to a lesser extent on the arms and body, it is very common to see *dry skin* or *xerosis* (Plate 60). Most individuals are not aware of the fact that as they age they need to cut down on their frequency of bathing, especially in the wintertime. *Winter itch* is quite common

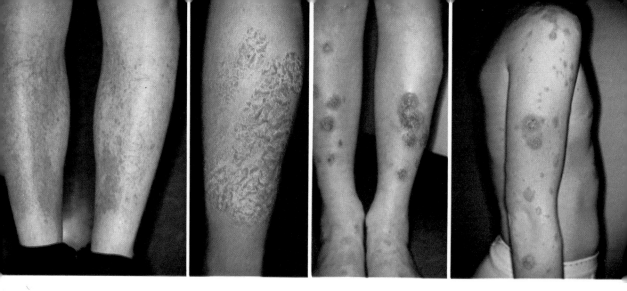

(A) Redness of winter
itch on legs

(B) Xerosis with secondary
infection on legs

(C) Nummular eczema of legs and
(D) of arm of same patient

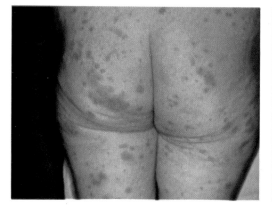

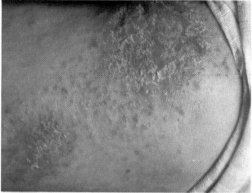

(E) Nummular eczema of buttocks

(F) Closeup showing oozing in nummular
eczema of leg

Plate 60. Geriatric Dermatoses (*Johnson & Johnson*)

(G) Stasis dermatitis
of leg aggravated
by contact allergy
to neomycin

(H) Stasis ulcer of leg
with varicose veins

(I) Senile pruritis
in 74-yr.-old woman

(J) Drug eruption
from phenacetin

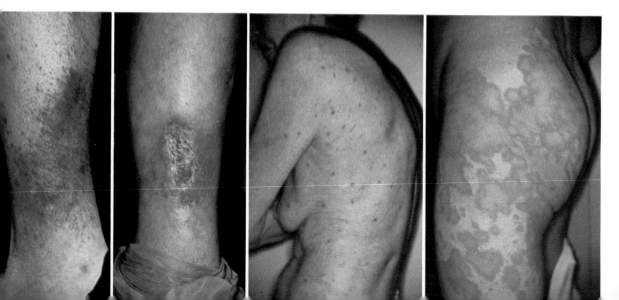

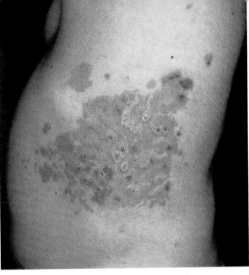

(K) Fixed bullous drug eruption
due to tetracycline

(L) Pemphigoid on lateral abdominal area

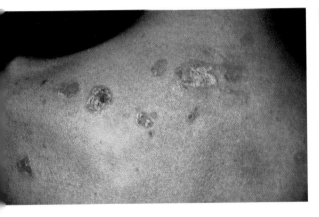

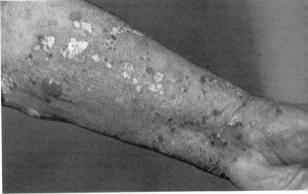

(M) Pemphigus vulgaris of upper back area

(N) Pemphigus vulgaris of forearm

Plate 60. Geriatric Dermatoses (*Continued*)

(O) Benign mucosal
pemphigoid of vulva
showing erosions

(P) Lichen sclerosis et
atrophicus of vulva
(*not* leukoplakia)

(Q) Herpes zoster of
shoulder and neck

(R) Chronic discoid lupus
erythematosus of cheek in
77-yr.-old woman

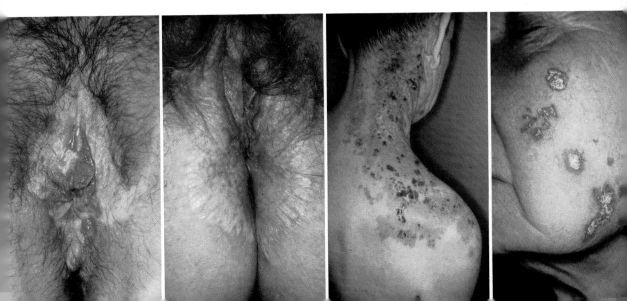

on the legs and can make the patient miserable. Yet the treatment is simple with less frequent bathing and a corticosteroid ointment.

Bruising occurs much more frequently in the aged skin and is most commonly seen on the extremities.

Generally speaking the *color* of the entire skin becomes pale and opaque.

The **appendages** of the skin change also. The most obvious and common changes are in the scalp where the **hair** develops varying shades from *grayness* to *pure white color* in certain individuals.

The *male pattern alopecia*, which can begin in the late teens becomes more progressive through life. For the elderly patient though, who has not had this hereditary balding problem, another form of hair loss, manifested as a diffuse thinning of the scalp hair, can develop. This *senile alopecia* can occur in both males and in females. Diffuse hair loss is also obvious in the axillae and the pubic area.

Excess facial hair (Fig. 22-1) is quite commonly seen in the elderly woman and can require shaving.

The **nails** do not change tremendously with age but there is an increase in the longitudinal ridging.

The **sebaceous glands** and **sweat glands** become less active in the older individual. For the unfortunate individuals who have had *acne* for years, age can be pleasant for them with a clearing of this problem. If an individual does present with a complaint of the recent development of acne, question carefully regarding the administration of *testosterone* either orally or by injection.

The decrease in the secretion of oil and sweat glands contributes directly to the development of the *dry skin* or *xerosis* mentioned earlier.

The **mucous membranes** become drier. Patients complain of dry lips and tongue. The mucous membranes of the vaginal orifice also become dry, atrophic and fragile.

Thus, essentially every elderly person has some evidence, however mild, of a skin problem.

INCIDENCE OF GERIATRIC SKIN DISEASES

For a study of the incidence of true skin diseases in a group of geriatric patients, here is a summary of a report by Gip and Molin.

They studied 286 patients over the age of 60 who were hospitalized in a Swedish geriatric clinic. The skin of each patient was examined carefully. Histopathological, bacteriological or mycological examinations were undertaken in some cases.

In the 107 males there were 231 skin diagnoses (2.2 per person) and in the 179 females 372 skin diagnoses were found (2.1 per person). The number of skin diagnoses per person ranged from 1 to 5. No skin diagnoses were registered in 22 cases (only 8%), 5 males and 17 females.

All of the skin diagnoses were recorded. The following list contains the 10 most frequent dermatological disorders registered.

Pigmented nevus	143
Discoloration of the toenails	133
Seborrheic keratosis	84
Plantar hyperkeratosis	36
Stasis dermatitis of the legs	31
Seborrheic dermatitis	27
Dermatitis of the legs (unspecified)	23
Marked atrophy of the skin	19
Xanthelasma	12
Capillary hemangiomas	10

The numbers of cases refer to the total number of dermatologic disorders found in the 286 males and females examined.

They attributed the majority of the cases of discoloration of the nails as being due to bacterial and fungal infections, or related to air content of the nail plate, or due to hemmorhage.

MANAGEMENT OF GERIATRIC SKIN PROBLEMS

Nowhere is the broadness of the term "management" more meaningful than when it is used in reference to the handling of a skin problem for an elderly patient. "Management" implies the imparting of much more information and instruction than the simple prescribing of "treatment."

The dermatologic management of an elderly patient is considerably complicated, however, by the physical and mental inability to understand and carry out instructions. The correct application of wet dressings, the lack of ease of tub bathing, and even the simple application of creams and ointments are more complex processes for the elderly. And as age progresses and debility increases, this care is further complicated by having to be administered by another person such as a family member or nurse; this additionally has esthetic and economic limitations.

Most elderly patients can be treated at home, but some of the more severe skin problems are seen in institutionalized persons. Depending on the care available and the extent of the dermatosis, hospitalization may be necessary. The role of both corticosteroids and antibiotics in decreasing the number of elderly patients needing hospitalization is enormous and is most fortuitous.

CLASSIFICATION OF GERIATRIC DERMATOSES

The elderly patient is subject to the majority of skin ills. But, as with the other age extreme, the child, there can be a different reaction by the aged skin to a given skin problem by virtue of the presence of fragility, dryness and atrophy.

It would be unusual to see certain skin problems in the aged, such as *atopic eczema, acne, pityriasis rosea, impetigo, primary and secondary syphilis, herpes simplex, warts, exanthems, chloasma* and *sunburn.*

A compilation of the more common problems of the geriatric patient is as follows, listed according to chapter groupings:

Chapter 7. Dermatologic Allergy

Contact dermatitis. For the geriatric patient this commonly is a dermatitis caused by the use of too harsh a local medication. This is seen quite frequently where too strong a salve is used in the treatment of itching legs.

Nummular eczema (Plate 60). This is quite a common problem, seen particularly in the wintertime and characterized clinically by coin-shaped vesicular areas on the arms, the legs and, less frequently, the buttocks.

Drug eruptions (Plates 14 and 60). Not too common, but can be seen as a *photosensitivity type* dermatitis when the patient is on a diuretic or a phenothiazine type tranquilizer, or as an *acne-like picture* due to the administration of testosterone.

Chapter 8. Pruritic Dermatoses

Generalized pruritus.

This is quite common and can defy adequate therapy. Careful examination of the patient is necessary to rule out any internal cause of the generalized pruritus. Rather frequently and rather unfortunately no apparent cause is ascertainable. Scalp and face itching can be a real problem.

Xerosis (Plate 60) as a cause of the generalized itching in the wintertime is rather easily managed by decreasing bathing and applying an emollient lotion or even a mild corticosteroid cream. See p. 71 for a more detailed discussion of this common problem in the elderly patient.

Localized pruritic dermatoses. Not as common as the more generalized pruritus.

Chapter 9. Vascular Dermatoses

Urticaria is not commonly seen.

Stasis dermatitis (Plate 60). This is rather commonly seen in the elderly patient and is almost always associated with venous insufficiency due to varicose veins or other circulatory problem (p. 82.) It is important to stress that circulatory support is indicated on a *continuing* basis after the dermatitis has responded to therapy. This can prevent the development of *stasis ulcers.*

Chapter 10. Seborrheic Dermatitis, Acne and Rosacea

Seborrheic dermatitis becomes less bothersome with age, but can recur following a cerebral vascular accident or stroke.

Acne. Rarely seen in the elderly patient.

Testosterone and related drugs can produce an acnelike picture, so be sure to ascertain whether such drugs are being administered.

Chapter 11. Papulo-Squamous Dermatoses

Psoriasis (Plate 46). It is rare to see psoriasis develop as a new problem in an elderly individual. Thus most elderly persons who have psoriasis have learned to exist with the disease.

Chapter 12. Dermatologic Bacteriology

Furuncles and carbuncles are not too commonly seen.

Secondary bacterial infections. *Stasis ulcers* (Plate 60) are the cause of marked disability in the elderly patient. The ulcers heal slowly and can be very painful. The care required to heal these ulcers, or even prevent them from spreading, can be considerable. More often than not other members of the family or nursing personnel must take over the management of these chronic sores.

Chapter 13. Syphilology

Tertiary syphilis of the skin or other organs is now rarely seen. The commonest problem seen in the elderly patient in relation to syphilis is the persistently positive serology following adequate therapy. Some syphilologists are alarmed that dormant but persistent spirochetal infections can become clinically significant with involvement of the eye and central nervous system.

Chapter 15. Dermatologic Mycology

Monilial infections are the most common mycological infections seen in the elderly patient particularly if the patient is obese. Lack of bathing and cleansing of the individual is a major factor.

Chapter 17. Bullous Dermatoses

Pemphigoid (Plate 60) is probably the most common bullous condition seen in the elderly patient.

Dermatitis herpetiformis in the elderly should prompt a careful work-up to rule out an *internal malignancy*.

Chapter 18. Exfoliative Dermatitis

Exfoliative dermatitis (Plate 46) is a miserable disease, and the etiology can be difficult to ascertain. An axiom is that 50% of the patients over the age of 50 with an exfoliative dermatitis have a *lymphoma*.

Chapter 19. Pigmentary Dermatoses

Hyperpigmentation or hypopigmentation of the skin can occur in the elderly from many causes. Aside from a simple change in pigmentation of the skin due to age, other pigmentary problems are uncommon.

Chapter 20. Collagen Diseases

Chronic discoid lupus erythematosus can begin in old age (Plate 47).

Chapter 21. The Skin and Internal Disease

Diabetes mellitus causes a degeneration of the vascular supply, and skin changes in the diabetic are progressive with age. *Ulcers, gangrene* of the digits and *ulcerations of the mal-perforans-type* are most commonly seen (Plate 49).

Chapter 22. Diseases Affecting the Hair

Graying of the hair and thinning of the hair have been discussed earlier.

Hypertrichosis or excessive growth of hair is common on the face of women (Fig. 22-1).

Chapter 23. Diseases Affecting the Nails

Other than the development of increased ridging of the nail plates and the discoloration of the toenails mentioned earlier, there are no major nail changes in the aged individual.

Chapter 24. Diseases of the Mucous Membranes

The mucous membranes become dry and fragile with age (Plate 60).

Chapter 25. Dermatoses Due to Physical Agents

Sunlight effects on the skin are extremely common and can result in simple hyperpigmentation and atrophy of the skin, or can produce *actinic keratoses* (Plate 54) that can eventuate as *squamous cell epitheliomas*.

Chapter 26. Photosensitivity Dermatoses
Photosensitivity problems are rarely seen unless triggered by drugs.

Chapter 27. Genodermatoses
The genetic inheritance of the individual has considerable influence on the aging of the skin, including wrinkling, the effect of sunlight, the activity of the oil and sweat glands and the hair changes.

Chapter 28. Tumors of the Skin
Seborrheic keratoses (Plate 59), as mentioned earlier, are very common and seen in almost every elderly person. The number of these lesions is genetically determined.

Pedunculated fibromas of the neck and axilla are quite common, and again there is a familial tendency for these to develop.

Precancerous tumors, such as *senile* or *actinic keratoses*, develop in relation to earlier sun exposure and the genetic make-up of the skin complexion.

Squamous cell carcinoma can develop by itself or from degeneration of actinic keratoses.

Basal cell epitheliomas (Plate 55) are the most common malignancy of the skin in the elderly patient. These are characterized by waxy nodular lesions with or without ulceration in the center.

Hemangiomas of the lips are not uncommon, and frighten the patient into thinking that he has a *melanoma*.

Capillary hemangiomas (Plate 56) on the chest and back are present in almost every elderly person.

Nevi mature with age and many seem to disappear. Junctional elements are rarely seen in nevi in the geriatric patient.

Malignant melanoma. This is a rare malignancy, but it can develop in the brownish black flat lesion known as *lentigo maligna* (Plate 59).

BIBLIOGRAPHY

Gip, L., and Molin, L.: Skin Diseases in Geriatrics. Cutis, 6:771, 1970.

Rossman, I., (Ed.): Clinical Geriatrics. Philadelphia, J. B. Lippincott, 1971. Chapter 11 on "Skin Disease" by Dr. A. W. Young, Jr. is an excellent detailed presentation. Chapter 1 on "The Anatomy of Aging" is also most fascinating and contains much interesting material on skin aging.

Tindall, J. P., and Smith, J. G.: Skin lesions of the aged and their association with internal changes J.A.M.A., *186*:1039, 1963.

31

Geographic Skin Diseases

Geographic Skin Diseases of North America

Most common skin diseases of North America are universal in geographic distribution, but a few are confined to, or more prevalent in, certain sections of the country. In my attempt to cover completely the common skin diseases, I have called upon other dermatologists from representative areas of the United States (including Alaska and Hawaii) and Canada to list their geographic skin diseases (Fig. 31-1). A list of the dermatologists consulted follows. I am taking the liberty of quoting certain parts of their letters because they add interest to this question of geographic dermatoses.

CANADA

Vancouver, British Columbia—Dr. Stuart Maddin. "It was quite generally agreed that we did not have any important or common dermatologic problem out here that was unusual due to our geographic location."

Winnipeg, Manitoba—Dr. Saul Berger. "We do have a fungus condition here which is called *suppurative ringworm*. It is contracted from cattle and is a common infection in rural Manitoba." Dr. Berger enclosed a reprint of an article on the subject by A. R. Birt and J. C. Wilt (A.M.A. Arch. Dermat. and Syph., 69: 441, 1954). They concluded that the majority of cases of *suppurative ringworm* seen in rural areas of Manitoba are due to *Trichophyton faviforme*.

UNITED STATES

Anchorage, Alaska—Dr. Thomas McGowan. In a long informative letter Dr. McGowan stated that the data he had gathered in Alaska had not yet been completely tabulated or evaluated and should be considered as his personal clinical impression based on examination and interviews of several thousand natives. ". . . these impressions actually apply only to the Aleuts, resident in the Aleutian Islands and Alaska Peninsula, and to the Indians resident in Southeastern Alaska. Among these two groups I found that the only skin diseases seen with any frequency were impetigo, scabies, pediculosis capitis, and pruritus ani associated with pinworms, and all of these were almost completely limited to children. Acne vulgaris was quite common in the Indian but very rare in the Aleut. Very rare in both groups were allergic infantile eczema, vesicular eczematoid dermatoses of the hands, and fungus infections of the nails and of the scalp. I found no cases of fungus infection of the skin, of psoriasis, of skin malignancy or of tuberculosis cutis (other than old healed scars of scrofuloderma), nor did I find any active venereal disease. One condition of interest, common among children of both groups in the springtime, was an acute *dermatitis venenata*, similar to poison ivy, occurring on the face and hands after contact with the juice of the outer skin of the local 'wild celery.'"

Seattle, Washington—Dr. Harvey Roys. "I know of no skin disease that is peculiar to the Northwest."

Milwaukee, Wisconsin—Dr. Daniel Hackbarth. "*Swimmer's itch* is seen occasionally and possibly you could also list *milker's nodules*."

New York, New York—Dr. A. I. Weidman. ". . . there is no specific regional dermatologic condition present in New York City. Perhaps conditions having their origin primarily in tension could be listed." (From my limited experience in New York City I feel that *exudative discoid and lichenoid chronic dermatosis* should be listed. This will be discussed later in this chapter.)

Hanover, New Hampshire—Dr. Otis Jillson. "I am sure that we see quite a bit more of what we call 'barn itch,' the suppurative ringworm from cattle, because we are practicing here in the country."

Los Angeles, California—Dr. Samuel Ayres, III. In addition to *human flea bites* which will be discussed more fully later, Dr. Ayres listed *actinic keratoses* and *skin cancers*, and, as an uncommon condition, *coccidioidomycosis* of the San Joaquin Valley. "On the negative side, we do not have *chiggers, chilblains,* or *miliaria.*"

Water skiers, skin divers, waders and swimmers in Southern California waters are frequently bitten by the crustaceans of the *Cymothoid* suborder. This has been called *sea louse dermatitis.* The small punctate bites heal in 5 to 6 days time.

Salt Lake City, Utah—Dr. Arthur M. Burton. "The exanthem of Rocky Mountain spotted fever is characteristic and well documented. The tick bite itself, however, does not leave a characteristic cutaneous lesion. This I have observed from personal observation on myself. The tick burrows into the skin with its head, engorges itself with blood, then withdraws and drops off the body. There is actually very little if any evidence remaining at the site of the tick bite."

Kansas City, Missouri—Author. The two commonest geographic dermatoses of the Midwest are *chigger bites* and *prickly heat.* These will be referred to later in the chapter. *Milker's nodules, grain itch, bites from the brown spider* (Figs. 31-2 C and 31-3), *tick bites and tick bite granulomas* are peculiar to this area but not common.

Cleveland, Ohio—Dr. George H. Curtis. "I know of no common skin disease endemic to this area." Dr. Curtis proceeded to list the most common skin conditions seen and treated at the Cleveland Clinic. At the top of the list were neurodermatitis circumscripta (including pruritus ani), superficial fungal infections and pyogenic infections.

Tucson, Arizona—Dr. Otis Miller. I requested information concerning *atopic eczema,* since so many of these patients improve when in Tucson or Phoenix. Dr. Miller's reply was, "There is little question that the warm climate of Arizona is beneficial to many, but not all, cases of atopic dermatitis. In the acute and angry stage, sunlight and heat make the condition considerably worse. There are many children who are born in Arizona with familial histories of allergies, who deveop atopic dermatitis right here in Tucson. Many of these are highly allergic to pollens which are peculiar to this neck-of-the-woods. One of the most common troublemakers is Bermuda grass."

He continued with a discussion of *cactus granuloma.* "This is a tissue reaction which is found principally on the exposed areas of the body, due to the penetration of the sticker-weed into the skin. It's conceivable that the same type of reaction is produced by small thorns found on various cacti.

"*Coccidioidomycosis* is of more vital concern to Arizonians. This respiratory disease occurs with varying degrees of severity in humans and about 20% of cases require the services of a physician. Nearly every long-time resident of the southwestern region is exposed to this disease. It also occurs in desert rodents, sheep, cattle and most severely in dogs. As far as the skin manifestations of this disease, contrary to what is written in the textbooks, erythema multiforme is much more commonly seen than erythema nodosum. The primary involvement of the skin is an extremely rare condition.

"I think the frequency of *vitiligo* is higher here in the land of the sun than elsewhere. I don't believe that there is actually a greater frequency, but I do believe that it is more apparent here because of the fact that sun exposure magnifies the difference between the normal skin and that which is involved by the vitiligo."

McAllen, Texas—Dr. Ivan Kuhl. Dr. Kuhl listed *tinea capitis* due to *T. tonsurans, keratoses* and *skin cancers, leprosy, contact dermatitis* due to Mango fruit, *moniliasis* of all forms and *fleabites.* "Tineas and other fungus infections plus keratoses and skin cancers probably constitute about 60% of my practice. The biggest single problem is the tinea capitis due to *T. tonsurans* and *T. violaceum.*"

Galveston, Texas—Dr. J. Fred Mullins. "Fortunately we have very few *fire ants* in this area."

It would seem that *larvae migrans* (*creeping eruption*) is going to be effectively controlled and treated by the utilization of thiabendazole. (See p. 320.)

"We see a new case of *tinea nigra* every 2 to 3 months. I think the most important thing to emphasize is that you must be cognizant of such an entity and not to interpret it as a junctional nevus and proceed with excision. Almost any topical fungicide is effective in the treatment of this problem."

New Orleans, Louisiana—Dr. Vincent J. Derbes. "In our area we see a great deal of *moniliasis* in the form of onychomycosis, erosio interdigitalis, and candidiasis of such areas as the groin, axillae, and areas under the breasts of fat women. We of course have a great deal of trouble from *fire ant bites* and some, but not a great deal, of *creeping eruption.* On the active service at Charity Hospital we have perhaps two, or at the most, three cases of *tinea nigra palmaris* annually. Perhaps the most important change in skin disease in our area in the past few years has been the increasing prevalence of *T. tonsurans* as a cause of tinea capitis. It now accounts for about 60 per cent of our cases."

Miami, Florida—Dr. Harvey Blank. Dr. Blank listed *creeping eruption, cutaneous moniliasis, Portuguese Man-of-War stings, contact dermatitis* due to various members of the Anacardiaceae, not only Rhus, but Mango, Cashew, Poison wood (*Metopium toxiferum*) and Brazilian pepper tree (*Schinus terebinthifolius*), *eczema solare, berlock dermatitis* due to lime oil and *actinic skin with keratoses and carcinomas.*

Honolulu, Hawaii—Dr. Harry Arnold, Jr. "There is no basis at all for the prevailing impression that exotic tropical diseases are commoner in Hawaii than on the North American continent; only *leprosy*, of them all, is endemic in Hawaii, and its incidence is now down to around 2 cases per 100,000 population per year —with one of these being imported, usually from the Far East.

"Of perhaps greatest interest is the negative difference between Hawaii and the 'mainland' U.S.A. In Hawaii, not a single case of *sarcoidosis* has as yet been encountered; not a single case of *tinea capitis* due to *Microsporon audouini;* not a single case of *larva migrans*, or *chiggers*, or *coccidioidomycosis*, or *blastomycosis.*

"A few diseases familiar in other tropical or subtropical areas do occur here. Leprosy has been mentioned. *Stings* produced by marine hydroids—*Halecium beani, Physalia* (the Portuguese Man-of-War), *Syncoryne mirabilis* and others— occur occasionally. The Australian bottlebrush or *kahili* flower, *Grevillea banksii,* produces an occasional case of *dermatitis venenata* (the leaf of the plant, uniquely, is harmless), and visitors (but almost never natives, even as in Mexico and Cuba) may sometimes get a rash from handling or eating mangoes.

"Unique in Hawaii, and happily infrequent even here, are two disorders: a *chronic cutaneous granuloma* caused by *Mycobacterium balnei,* and a *dermatitis escharotica* produced by contact with a common seaweed, a blue-green marina alga, *Lyngbya majuscula.*

"The Hawaiian version of the swimming-pool granuloma is clinically unlike the usual one: an arcuate verrucous plaque, usually on knee, ankle, or elbow, slowly enlarging over a period of as long as 15 or 20 years to a maximum diameter of 7 to 10 cm. Histologically it shows diffuse lymphocytic infiltration and marked epidermal hyperplasia, with only an occasional tubercle, and never the sarcoidlike picture usually seen in swimming-pool granuloma. Infections have occasionally been traced tentatively to irrigation ditches and reservoirs, espe-

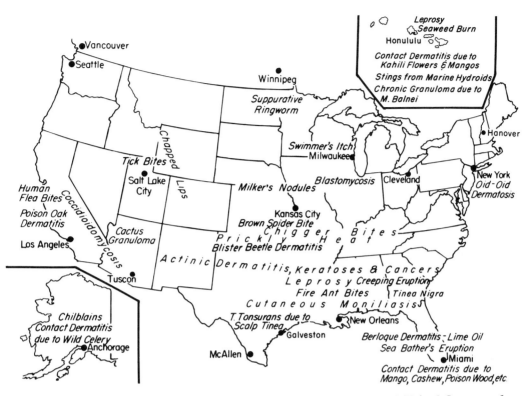

Fig. 31-1. Predominant localization of geographic dermatoses of United States and Canada.

cially on the island of Maui. Swimming pools have never been implicated. *M. balnei* has been positively identified by Walker and his associates in 8 cases.

"The *'seaweed burn'* reported by Grauer and Arnold in 1962 is an acute chemical burn produced by contact of the most dependent portion of the scrotum or the perianal area with fragments of the threadlike blue-green alga, *Lyngbya majuscula*, broken up by heavy surf on swimming beaches, and held against the skin by the wet swimming suit for some minutes after the victim emerges from the water. Prompt removal of the suit, and thorough bathing, effectively prevent it. Several score cases have been encountered, every one from a swimming beach on the northeast or windward shore of the island of Oahu—though the offending seaweed is found on all the beaches in the state and indeed throughout the world."

These letters corroborated my feeling that in addition to certain skin diseases we as dermatologists know to be endemic to a particular area, such as swimmer's itch in Wisconsin and creeping eruption in the Gulf States, there are a few other common but less well-known geographic dermatoses.

The accompanying map (Fig. 31-1) lists these geographic skin diseases. A few will be discussed in greater detail.

BITES DUE TO THE HUMAN FLEA

The following is quoted from Dr. Ayres's letter regarding dermatoses localized to the California area, "I would first list human fleabites, that is, those due to *Pulex irritans*. These seem to be more or less limited to the Pacific coast and more particularly to San Francisco. They are not to be confused with dog or cat fleas which may occasionally bite humans but

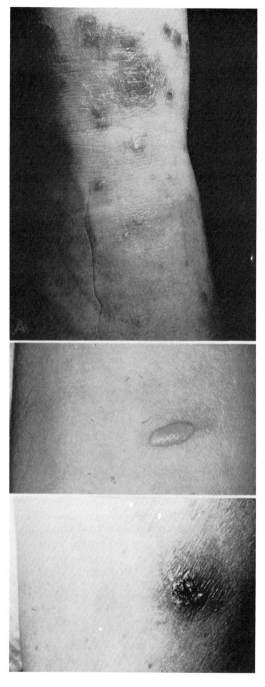

prefer their natural hosts. Inhabitants of the area frequently are immune to the effect of the bites so that only newcomers are aware of the infestation. Interestingly enough this was my own experience when I went to medical school in San Francisco (Stanford). I had grown up in Southern California and had never known anything about human fleabites but I was nearly eaten alive by them during my years in San Francisco, while those of my fellow students who were native San Franciscans had no trouble at all. This is a widely recognized phenomenon in these areas. The manifestations are typically grouped, highly pruritic papules with central punctae, more prevalent over the covered portion of the body."

Certain cases of *papular urticaria* have been found to be due to the bites of insects such as fleas, bedbugs, chiggers (a mite larva), flies and mosquitoes. This form of urticaria represents an allergic reaction to such bites which develops in children who have not been previously sensitized.

Treatment of fleabites consists of preventive measures to destroy the insects. This is done best by spraying the home environment with an insecticide. Some insecticide powders can also be used directly on the patient and his clothing.

CHIGGER BITES

Chigger bites, or trombidiosis, is a very common summer eruption of inhabitants of the southern United States (Figs. 31-2 and 31-3). The small urticarial papule is caused by the bite of the larva of the Chigger. The larva does not burrow into the skin, but drops off after engorging itself on blood. Due to its almost microscopic size it is rarely seen on the skin.

Clinically, the markedly pruritic papules occur where the larva meets resistance as it climbs up the legs, such as around the tops of the socks, the beltline and the neckband area. Excoriation of the lesions leads to secondary infection. An allergic papulovesicular eruption is seen occasionally in sensitive individuals following extensive generalized chigger bites. Papular urticaria has been mentioned above.

Fig. 31-2. Geographic dermatoses of the Midwestern and Southern states. (*A, top*) Excoriated chigger bites on the dorsum of the ankle. (*B, center*) Blister bettle vesicle on the arm. (*C, bottom*) Brown spider bite on leg. (*Dr. Thomas Burns*)

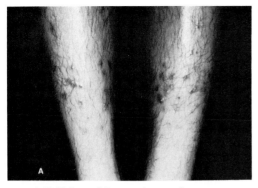

(*A*) Chigger bites on legs at boot-tops

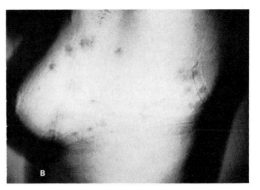

(*B*) Chigger bites on chest under bra

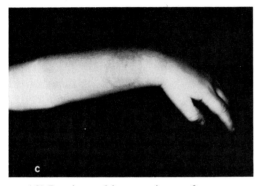

(*C*) Persistent bite reaction on forearm, probably from mosquito, in 4-year-old

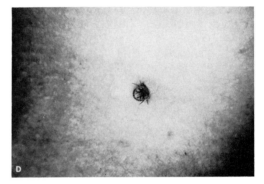

(*D*) Tick imbedded in skin mistaken by patient for a tumor

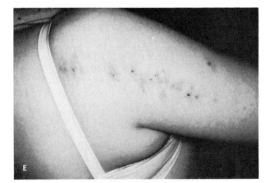

(*E*) Bedbug bites on arm in typical linear pattern

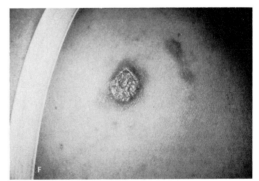

(*F*) Brown recluse spider bite necrosis on shoulder

Fig. 31-3. Bites on the skin.

In children particularly, chigger bites are a common cause of *secondary impetigo*, especially in the scalp. For the first two summers that we lived in Kansas City my two youngest children developed recurrent crops of impetiginous lesions on the scalp from the chigger bites. It was difficult to eradicate the lesions because of continued reinfestation and recurrent secondary infection. In recent summers the bites have been milder. This may be another example of the development of immunity following repeated exposure, similar to that seen from the fleabites of the San Francisco area.

Treatment. Preventive measures that are partially successful consist of applying Flowers of Sulfur powder to the feet and the stockings, and, if desired, spraying the infested lawn with insecticide. Active therapy includes the use of the alcoholic white shake lotion for the pruritus (see Formulary p. 37), with the addition of sulfur (3%), or Aureomycin 250 mg. per ounce if secondary infection is present. For infected scalp lesions, sulfur (5%) in an antibiotic ointment is beneficial.

SWIMMER'S ITCH

Bathers in the fresh-water lakes of Wisconsin, Michigan and Minnesota are prone to periodic attacks of inflammatory papular, urticarial and vesicular eruptions on the uncovered areas of the body, mainly the legs. This pruritic eruption, which usually subsides within a week, is caused by the invasion of the skin by the cercariae of the schistosomes of ducks and mammals. The life cycle of these various species of schistosomes includes the snail as an intermediate host. Upon invasion of the abnormal definitive host, the human skin, the cercariae dies, and the resulting skin eruption is the skin's reaction in ridding itself of the foreign bodies. Repeated attacks are met with stronger resistance, and the dermatitis becomes increasingly more severe. Secondary infection, edema and lymphangitis can occur.

Seabather's eruption is a similar clinical entity but of unknown etiology. Two main differences separate it from swimmer's itch: the predominance of the seabather's eruption on the bathing suit area and the limitation of this dermatosis to saltwater areas, particularly around the Florida coast.

Treatment. Prevention of swimmer's itch is accomplished best by destruction of the snails through careful addition to the lake water of a combination of copper sulfate and hydrated lime. Rapid drying of the swimmer with a towel apparently prevents penetration of the cercariae.

Active therapy is directed toward the relief of the itching and secondary infection.

CREEPING ERUPTION

Larva migrans is a dermatosis of the southeastern United States characterized by the presence of a serpiginous, advancing, ridge overlying the tunnel of a migrating *Ancylostoma* larva. The advancing ridge is slightly behind the larva and is the skin's reaction to the foreign body. Itching and secondary infection are common.

The larva most commonly is derived from the roundworms of the genus *Ancylostoma* but occasionally from various species of botflies. The natural reservoir of the *Ancylostoma* hookworm is the intestines of dogs and cats. Infected feces on sand provide an excellent source for the passage of the larvae to the unsuspecting sunbather or barefoot child. Man is not the natural host, so the parasite remains in the skin until destroyed.

Treatment. Thiabendazole effectively controls and treats creeping eruption. One routine is 50 mg. per kilogram of body weight in a single oral dose, which may be repeated 24 to 48 hours later. The pruritus begins to subside within 4 to 6 hours. Rarely, side-effects of nausea and dizziness have been observed.

PRICKLY HEAT
(Plate 57)

Prickly heat, or miliaria rubra, is a common disease of hot and humid climates. The physiologic pathology of the disease is the constant maceration of the skin which leads to a blockage of the sweat duct opening. Continued exercise and further maceration of the skin results in dilatation of the epidermal portion of the sweat duct and rupture into the mid-epidermis. The result is a tiny vesicular papule that itches and burns. Pustular and deep forms of miliaria are observed mainly in the tropics and in particularly susceptible individuals.

The distribution of the eruption is predominantly on the neck, the back, the chest, the sides of the trunk, the abdomen and the folds of the body. Babies commonly show prickly heat confined to the diaper area. The eruption under adhesive tape is a form of localized miliaria due to blockage of the sweat pores.

Treatment. Prevention is of paramount importance. If the cycle of maceration and heat can be broken for a few hours out of each day, the eruption will not develop. Rest under fans or air-conditioning for some hours of the day or the night is of great value. When these conditions are not available, application of a mild lotion or powder gives relief from the itching and may eliminate some of the skin maceration. A good example is:

Alcoholic white shake lotion q.s. 120.0 (see Formulary p. 37).

EXUDATIVE DISCOID AND LICHENOID CHRONIC DERMATOSIS

Oid-oid disease of Sulzberger and Garbe is probably a variant of atopic eczema, but with several important additional characteristics. It is seen predominantly among Jewish males in the New York City area and is a very chronic, disabling, markedly pruritic, lichenoid and exudative dermatitis. Characteristic penile lesions are a diagnostic feature.

Treatment. Similar to that for a severe case of atopic eczema. A vacation or permanent removal of the patient to the southwestern part of the United States is quite often beneficial.

Geographic Skin Diseases of Central and South America

Central and South America have extremes of climate and a mixture of ethnic groups that combine to produce some exotic and unique geographic skin diseases (Figs. 31-4 and 31-5).

As with the North American section of this chapter, representative dermatolo-

gists of Central and South America were consulted for information on geographical skin diseases of these areas. Fortunately, the task of compilation of such information did not need to be done by me, since it had already been done for a pioneer series of papers on this subject by Dr.

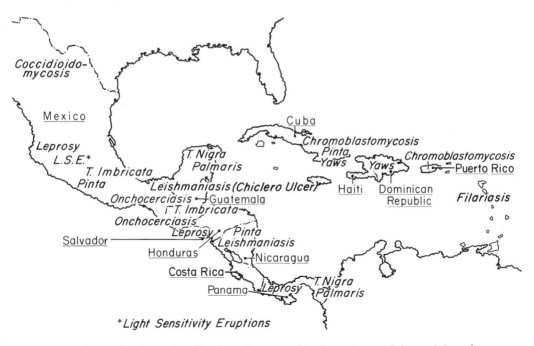

Fig. 31-4. Predominant localization of geographic dermatoses of Central America.

Orlando Canizares. I therefore asked Dr. Canizares to submit material on this subject for this section and also maps of the two areas. He graciously complied, and I am greatly indebted to him.

For the more detailed information on the various diseases which is presented at the end of this chapter, the papers of Dr. Canizares and Dr. Pardo-Castello were consulted along with others listed in the bibliography.

It is my hope that those who are interested in these areas or these geographical diseases will contact me regarding changes, so that future editions can be kept up to date. This request applies especially to the readers of the Spanish edition of this book.

FACTORS INFLUENCING EPIDEMIOLOGY*

The factors that influence the epidemiology of skin diseases in Central and South America can be roughly divided, following the concepts of John Paul, into two types: the macroclimate and the microclimate. The macroclimate is the climate in its geographic sense and refers to temperature, humidity, rainfall, etc.

* This section was contributed by Dr. Orlando Canizares.

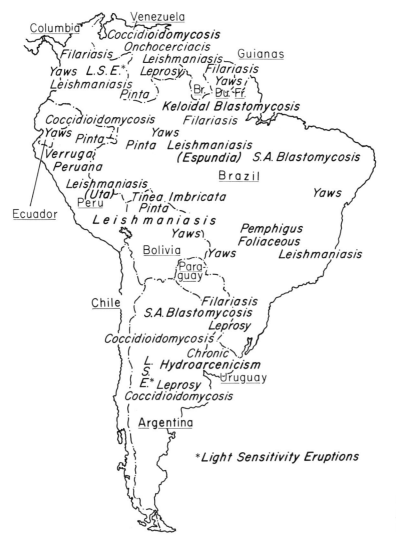

Fig. 31-5. Predominant localization of geographic dermatoses of South America.

The microclimate refers to the environment and to the sum of conditions that affect the individual, his origin, his socioeconomic status, his occupation, his home, his diet, etc.

Macroclimate of Skin Diseases in Central and South America. One of the most important physical characteristics affecting the pattern of diseases in Central and South America is the *altitude*. Within the tropical belt, between sea level and about 2,000 feet of altitude, the warm weather and the high humidity predispose to *pyogenic* and *fungal infections, moniliasis* and *tinea versicolor*. Between 2,000 and 5,000 feet, the pattern of diseases encountered changes. Fungal and pyogenic infections, although present, are not as frequent as at lower altitudes. This elevation is within the flying range of the phlebotomus and the simulium, the former transmitting *leishmaniasis* and *verruga peruana*, and the latter *onchocerciasis*. *Deep mycoses* are more common at this elevation.

At higher altitudes the climate is colder, regardless of the distance from the equator. Large cities, such as Mexico City. Bogotá, Quito and La Paz, are on elevated plateaus, where *light-sensitivity eruptions, "winter eczemas"* and other conditions encountered in colder Nordic climates are common.

THE SOIL is another factor in the epidemiology of skin diseases. In the northern deserts of Mexico, *coccidioidomycosis* is abundant. The high content of arsenic in the drinking water near Cordoba, Argentina, causes the skin changes characteristic of *chronic arsenic ingestion*.

THE FAUNA is important and varies in the different regions. Insect bites are common during the rainy season, causing a variety of *zoonoses*. *Tunga penetrans*, spiders, etc., may cause severe local or systemic reactions.

THE FLORA is an important factor in the epidemiology of skin diseases. *Contact dermatitis* is caused by plants, their leaves or fruits, and the causative agents vary in different regions.

Microclimate: Man and His Environment. One of the main characteristics of

the population of Central and South America is its racial and cultural diversity. At present, more than half the population is of mixed ancestry. The role of race in the development of skin diseases is extremely difficult to determine. *Psoriasis* has been found to be absent in some pure-blooded Indians. *Actinic keratosis* and other actinic changes appear to be less common in those presenting hyperpigmented skin. Some diseases are probably more common in the native Indians due to their lower socio-economic status and therefore greater exposure to infections.

DIET plays an important role, since the great bulk of the population of Central and South America is in a chronic state of malnutrition. The basic diet of the working class is corn, yucca, rice and beans, which are starches with very little protein.

HOUSING is an evidence of the socioeconomic status of the individual. The housing of the farmer and worker usually lacks the most elementary hygienic requirements. Construction in the country is usually of wood or adobe which harbors many insects that cause and transmit diseases.

OCCUPATION plays an important role in the development of diseases. The increased industrialization of Central and South America has resulted in a noticeable increase in *occupational dermatoses*. The farmers also develop dermatoses related to their work, such as *leishmaniasis* in woodcutters, *onchocerciasis* in the workers of the coffee plantation, and *sporotrichosis* in carpenters and packers.

EPIDEMIOLOGY OF SKIN DISEASES IN
CENTRAL AMERICA ON A REGIONAL
BASIS*

Region I—Middle America, Mexico and Central America. Mexico City is located on a plateau at 10,000 feet above sea level and presents the characteristic metropolitan high-altitude type of skin pathology. Some sections of Guatemala and Costa Rica, also at high altitudes, present a similar pattern of skin diseases. Bands of

* This section was contributed by Dr. Orlando Canizares.

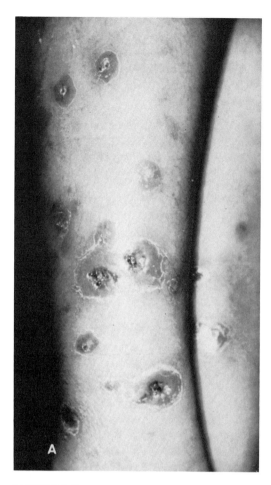

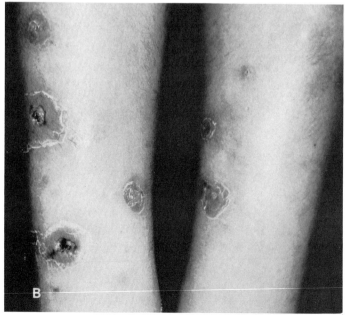

lowlands cut across with the typical hot and humid type of pathology. *Pinta* prevails at the basin of the river Balsas in Mexico. There are foci of *rhinoscleroma* and *onchocerciasis*. *Leishmaniasis* predominates in Yucatan and in some countries of Central America. There is a high incidence of deep mycosis, especially *mycetomas* and *sporotrichosis*.

Region II—The Caribbean Islands. The islands of the Caribbean include the Greater Antilles, the Lesser Antilles and the Bahamas. In all, the climate is warm with rather high humidity.

The characteristic of this region is a negative one. It is the absence of many serious skin diseases affecting the continent. Leishmaniasis, cutaneous tuberculosis, onchocerciasis and deep mycoses, with the exception of *chromoblastomycosis*, are absent. *Pinta* is rare. *Yaws*, previously exceedingly common in Haiti and parts of Cuba and Jamaica, has been almost entirely eradicated.

Region III—Caribbean South America. This region includes Colombia, Venezuela and the Guianas. The Caribbean coast of this region is the heat belt of South America, with the highest temperature and humidity. In the northern cities of

Fig. 31-6. Bacterial ulcers of legs of Mexican girl.

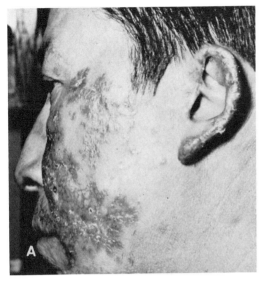

(*A*) Lepromatous form on face

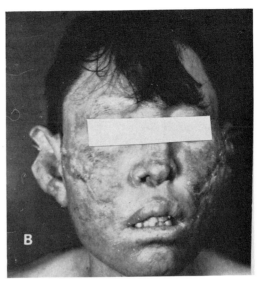

(*B*) Lepromatous form on face

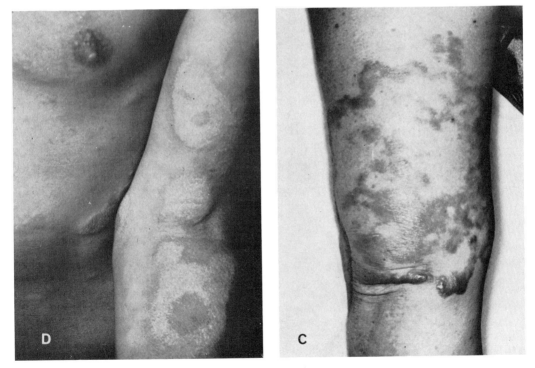

(*C*) Lepromatous form on leg

(*D*) Tuberculoid form on arm and chest

Fig. 31-7. Leprosy. (*A, B* and *D—Dr. A. Gonzalez-Ochoa, Mexico*) (*C—Dr. D. Grinspan, Argentina*)

Colombia, in the Maracaibo lowlands of Venezuela and along the coast of the Guianas, we find the diseases common to this type of climate.

It has already been shown that Colombia is an excellent example of vertical zonation in dermatology. In the regions of the interior, west of the Andes, *leishmaniasis* is highly endemic. Recently, foci of *rhinoscleroma* and *onchocerciasis* have been isolated in Venezuela.

Region IV—Eastern South America: Brazil. In the jungles of the Amazon and in the northeast, *yaws, filariasis, keloidal blastomycosis of Lobe,* and *leishmaniasis* are frequent. Due to an effective campaign, the incidence of yaws is being greatly reduced.

The large cities of Rio de Janeiro, Belo Horizonte and São Paulo present a metropolitan type of skin pathology with a noticeable increase in *industrial dermatoses.*

Endemic pemphigus foliaceus, (fogo selvagem) a typical Brazilian skin disease, has its highest prevalence in the subtropical region of central Brazil, primarily at an altitude of 1,500 feet.

In Brazil, as in most regions of Central and South America, *sarcoidosis* and *lymphoblastomas* are exceedingly rare.

Region V—Interior South America: Bolivia and Paraguay. Bolivia and Paraguay share the common handicap of isolation from the sea. La Paz, the highest capital in the world, lies at an altitude of over 12,000 feet, showing the characteristics of a high-altitude type of cutaneous pathology. *Leishmaniasis* and *yaws* predominate in the plains of the Gran Chaco, and occasional foci of *pinta* are found.

Region VI—Pacific South America: Ecuador, Peru and Chile. The high mountains of the Andes form the backbone of these countries. In the canyons of these high mountains, isolated foci of the typical Peruvian disease, *verruga peruana,* exist.

Chile, a long ribbon along the Pacific, has its population concentrated in the center. It has a mild-climate, low-altitude type of skin pathology. As if walled off by the Andes, Chile is free of most of the

serious diseases affecting its neighbors, including *leprosy.*

Region VII—Southeastern South America: Argentina and Uruguay. This region, with a middle altitude climate, is geographically and ethnologically uniform. Its dermatologic pathology, because of the European origin of the population and the moderate climate, is similar to that of northern United States or Continental Europe. In the northern region, the Chaco, some of the characteristic cutaneous pathology of warm and humid climate is seen. The city of Mendoza, at the foot of the Andes, shows evidence of the higher altitude pattern of diseases. In the Cordoba region, a peculiar characteristic of the soil makes the drinking water high in arsenic content. This is called by Argentinean dermatologists "regional, chronic, endemic, *hydroarsenicism"* and causes melanodermia, keratoses and multiple carcinomas.

SPECIFIC SKIN DISEASES

The various geographic skin diseases can be grouped into bacterial infections, fungal infections, protozoal diseases, helminthic diseases, spirochetal diseases and miscellaneous conditions. They are elaborated on in the sections that follow.

BACTERIAL INFECTIONS

Warm weather, high humidity and poor hygiene predispose the skin to many of the pyodermas such as impetigo, ecthyma, furunculosis, abcesses, ulcers and secondary infection of other skin diseases.

Ulcers of the legs (Fig. 31-6) are especially common and prove resistant to therapy. The causative factors are usually multiple and include trauma, malnutrition and poor hygiene. A severe type with a rather distinct clinical pattern is the *tropical phagedenic ulcer.*

Management of tropical pyodermas is in general the same as that for the pyodermas discussed in Chapter 12. But, in addition, greater stress must be made toward improvement of general hygiene and diet.

Leprosy (Fig. 31-7) is quite common in Mexico, especially in an area on the central

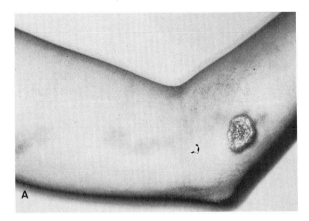

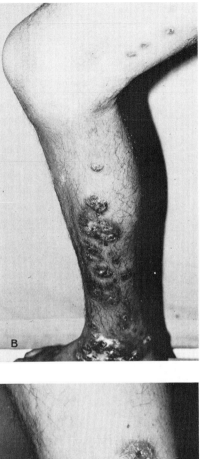

Fig. 31-8. Sporotrichosis. (*A*) Chancre on forearm with lymphatic spread. (*B*) Secondary nodules on leg.

(*C*) Verrucous primary lesion on foot. (*D*) Chancre on ankle. (*B, C* and *D—Dr. A. Gonzalez-Ochoa, Mexico*)

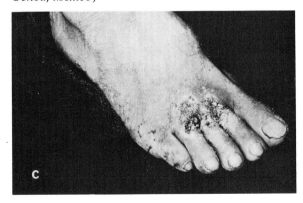

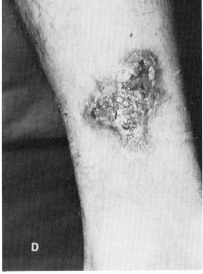

west coast. The distribution of cases of leprosy in Mexico apparently has no relationship to climate, latitude, humidity or altitude. *Diffuse lepromatosis* (Lucio's leprosy) is a form of lepromatous leprosy with rather definite characteristics of a diffuse, non-nodular generalized skin infiltration and a necrotic lepra reaction. This variant is especially common in the Mexican state of Sinaloa.

More information on leprosy appears on page 132.

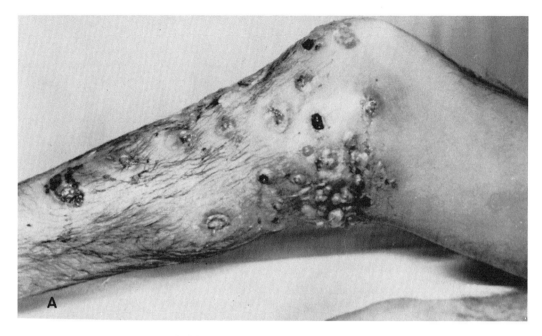

(*A*) Draining ulcers of leg and thigh.

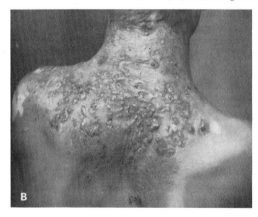

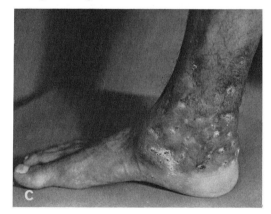

(*B*) Ulcers and nodules of back　　　　　　(*C*) Ulcers of foot

Fig. 31-9. Mycetoma due to *N. brasiliensis*. (*Dr. A. Gonzalez-Ochoa, Mexico*)

FUNGAL INFECTIONS

Superficial fungal infections and monilial infections are very common in a humid climate.

Tinea imbricata is a unique superficial fungal infection of the smooth skin caused by *T. concentricum*. It occurs primarily in Brazil, Colombia, Guatemala, and the state of Puebla, Mexico. Clinically, it is characterized by concentric rings of overlapping scales. It is ex-tremely pruritic. Treatment with oral griseofulvin is apparently successful.

Deep fungal infections are relatively frequent in Central and South America.

Sporotrichosis (Fig. 31-8 and 15-8) is one of the most common deep mycotic diseases, and is seen especially among workers in the sugar cane fields and coffee plantations. Facial primary lesions are not uncommon and occur especially frequently in children. (See p. 180.)

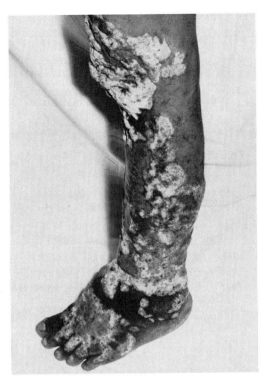

(A) Cauliflower-like leg lesions

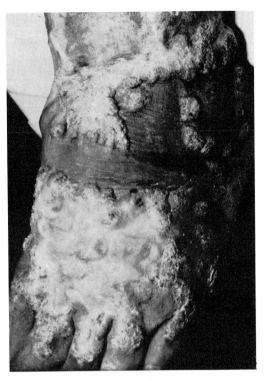

(B) Closeup of foot

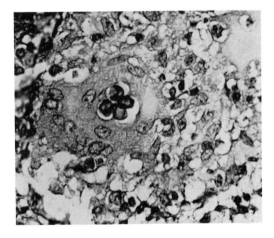

Fig. 31-10. Chromoblastomycosis. (*Drs. William Schorr* and *F. Kerdel-Vegas*)

(C) Copper penny-like yeast cells with 4 buds inside giant cell

Mycetomas (Fig. 31-9) have been reported as being the commonest deep mycotic infection in Central America. Clinically, one sees granulomatous nodules, pustules, ulcers and sinuses of the feet with destruction of the bones in severe cases. The infection is caused by several species of *Actinomycetes* (*Nocardia* or *Streptomyces*) and fungi (*Madurella* species). The latter type of infection is called *maduromycosis*. Cases due to *Actinomycetes* respond to streptomycin therapy.

Chromoblastomycosis (Fig. 31-10) is frequently seen in Panama, Costa Rica

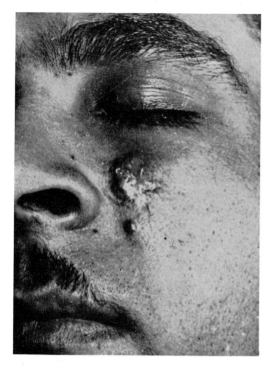

Fig. 31-11. South American Blastomycosis. Granulomatous nodule on the cheek. (*Dr. D. Grinspan, Argentina*)

and, less frequently, in other Central and South American countries. It is characterized by warty nodules or ulcers, primarily of the lower extremities, that can coalesce to form large cauliflowerlike masses. Internal involvement has not been reported. The causative organisms are *Hormodendrum pedrosoi, H. compactum* and *Phialophora verrucosa*. Therapy with oral potassium iodide is effective in some cases. For early cases, curettage and electrodesiccation are successful.

Coccidioidomycosis, caused by *Coccidioides immitis,* is as common in the arid and desert areas of northern Mexico as it is in the southwestern part of the United States. Primary and secondary lesions can involve the skin. Systemic involvement is usually mild, but the disease can be fatal in rare instances.

South American blastomycosis, or *paracoccidioidal granuloma,* (Fig. 31-11) is a rare fungal disease, mainly of Brazilian farmers, caused by *Paracoccidioides brasiliensis*. Primary granulomatous lesions appear in or around the mouth, with secondary ulcers and nodules occurring around the face and the neck along with a massive lymphadenopathy of the neck. It is fatal in a few months.

PROTOZOAL DISEASES

Leishmaniasis (Fig. 31-12) is a protozoal infection of the reticuloendothelial cells of the viscera and the skin. The vectors are sandflies of the genus *Phlebotomus;* man and dogs serve as the reservoir. The disease occurs in 3 forms, caused by 3 species of *Leishmania* which produce overlapping clinical pictures.

The visceral form, *kala-azar,* occurs in Paraguay, Argentina and Brazil. A post-kala-azar dermal leishmaniasis characterized by depigmentation and nodules in the skin can occur some 2 years after the onset of the disease.

The cutaneous form is known as *oriental sore* and occurs in the tropical areas of Central and South America.

The mucocutaneous form is very common in Central and South America. The causative protozoa is *Leishmania brasiliensis*. At least 3 clinical forms of this disease exist.

ESPUNDIA is characterized by deep and destructive lesions of the nose and the mouth and is found mainly in Brazil and other South American countries.

UTA is a form that affects the skin and only rarely the mucous membranes. Discrete ulcerating lesions occur usually on the face but can occur on any exposed area of the body. Verrucous lesions can develop. This form is endemic in the Andes.

CHICLERO ULCERS occur commonly in the chicle gatherers of Mexico and Central America. The lesion begins as a painful nodule of the ear which can ulcerate and destroy all of the cartilage. There are no generalized symptoms.

Therapy of these mucocutaneous forms of leishmaniasis is disappointing. Amphotericin B has been used with some success.

Trypanosomiasis is a protozoal disease occurring in 2 forms: the African form

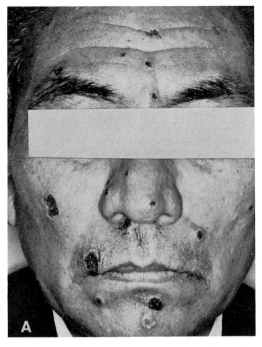

(A) Cutaneous leishmaniasis (oriental sore).

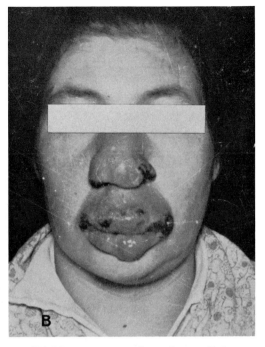

(B) Mucocutaneous form (espundia).

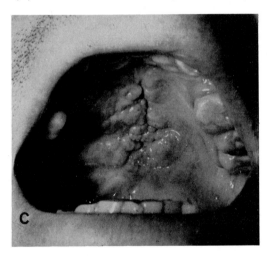

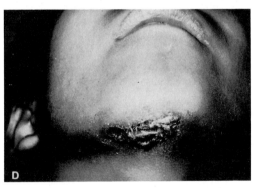

(D) Mucocutaneous lesion on chin.

(C) Mucocutaneous form, roof of mouth.

(E) Mucocutaneous chiclero ulcer of ear.

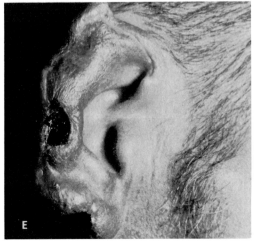

Fig. 31-12. Leishmaniasis. (*A, B* and *C—Dr. D. Grinspan, Argentina*) (*D* and *E—Dr. A. Gonzalez-Ochoa, Mexico*)

331

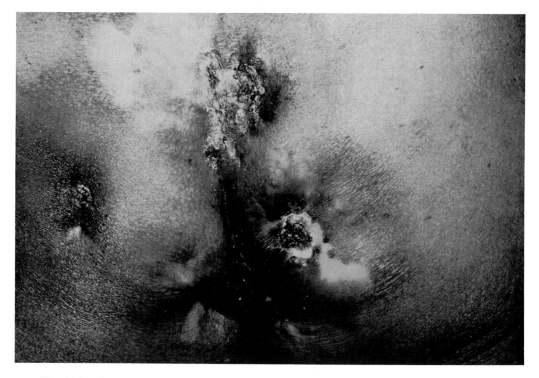

Fig. 31-13. Cutaneous amoebiasis. Deep ulcers of the buttocks caused by direct extension following amoebic dysentery. (*Dr. A. Gonzalez-Ochoa, Mexico*)

(sleeping sickness) and the American form (Chagas' disease).

Chagas' disease is widely distributed in Argentina, Brazil and other South American countries, but is seen less frequently in Central America. It is caused by the protozoa *Trypanosoma cruzi* and is transmitted from man to man or animal to man by the reduviid or "kissing" bugs.

Dermatologically, an early sign of the disease is a unilateral edema of an eyelid called Romaña's sign. Nonspecific eruptions of an urticarial or morbilliform nature can occur in the course of this severe systemic disease. There is no uniformly successful therapy.

Cutaneous amoebiasis (Fig. 31-13). Amoebic dysentery caused by *Entamoeba histolytica* is a very common intestinal disease in Central and South America.

Skin lesions are less common, but, unless diagnosed early, the prognosis is very poor.

The ulcers or ulcerated granulomas usually seen in a serpiginous configuration are not characteristic. Examination of fresh tissue in saline reveals the amoeba.

Lesions develop (1) from direct extension from the bowel, (2) from direct extension from an hepatic abscess, (3) after surgery in an infected individual or (4) from direct contact inoculation.

Treatment with 10 daily injections of emetine is quite effective.

Helminthic Diseases

Filariasis bancrofti, caused by the presence of adult *Wuchereria bancrofti* in the lymphatic system or the connective tissues of man, is characterized clinically by several conditions related to the lymphatic system. The disease is present in Cuba and other West Indian islands, Colombia, Venezuela, Panama and coastal areas of the Guianas and Brazil. Mosquitos of several species act as vectors and bite man.

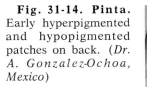

Fig. 31-14. Pinta. Early hyperpigmented and hypopigmented patches on back. (*Dr. A. Gonzalez-Ochoa, Mexico*)

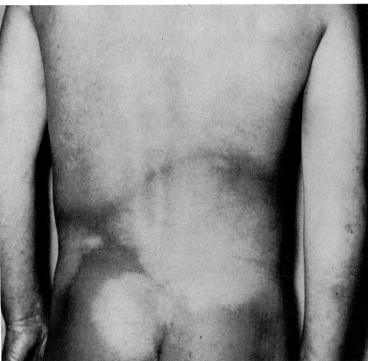

Clinically, a phase of inflammation of the lymphatic system is followed by an obstructive phase which is marked by the eventual development of elephantiasis of the leg, the scrotum, the arm or the breasts. Early treatment with diethylcarbamazine (Hetrazan) is quite successful.

Onchocerciasis is another form of filarial infection, but it is confined to the southern states of Mexico and Guatemala. In these areas of coffee plantations, the disease is very common. The adult parasite, *Onchocerca volvulus*, is introduced into man by the bite of species of *Simulium*, or black or coffee flies. Clinically, one sees subcutaneous nodules on the scalp and the face caused by the migration or the disintegration of the microfilariae or the death of the adult worms. Other skin changes include facial redness and edema and severe pruritus of any of the body areas infected with the microfilariae. Involvement of the eye can lead to blindness. Early therapy with diethylcarbamazine kills the microfilaria, and intravenous

administration of antrypol kills the adult worm.

SPIROCHETAL DISEASES

Pinta, mal del Pinto, or carate, (Fig. 31-14) is a nonvenereal treponemal infection caused by *Treponema carateum* that exists rather commonly in the West Indian islands and Mexico. Since the advent of penicillin therapy the incidence of the disease has decreased considerably. Primary lesions are not observed clinically, but the secondary lesions, or pintids, begin as scaly papules on a red base. These areas progress to form bilateral and symmetrical areas of hyperpigmented and hypopigmented patches, usually on the palms, the soles and the face. Hyperkeratotic lesions may also develop. Penicillin is curative, but the depigmented areas may not return to normal.

Yaws, caused by *Treponema pertenue*, has been successfully treated with penicillin in the areas in the West Indies, Mexico and Central America where it was once prevalent. Some cases still exist in isolated areas of tropical South America. The primary lesion, or "mother yaw," is frequently found in children. Secondary skin lesions can appear in crops up to 5 years after the initial papule. These secondary skin lesions can be wartlike or papular with ulceration, and appear in many configurations. The third-stage lesions are very destructive gummatous nodules or hyperkeratotic lesions of the palms and the soles. Bone lesions are common. Penicillin is curative, but the destructive changes are permanent.

Miscellaneous Conditions

Verruga peruana is the chronic dermatologic phase of *bartonellosis*. This disease is endemic along the steep valley slopes of Peru, Colombia and Ecuador. The organism, *Bartonella bacilliformis*, is transmitted to man by the bite of infected *Phlebotomus* sandflies.

The acute severe phase of the disease, Oroya fever, is characterized by high fever and a rapidly developing, often fatal, anemia. The cutaneous phase of bartonellosis, verruga peruana, can develop in the patient who survives Oroya fever, or it can develop as an initial manifestation of the disease. Verruga peruana is characterized by an eruption of hemangiomatous papules or nodules varying in size from 0.1 to 2 cm. The larger nodules can ulcerate and hemorrhage severely and can last for several years before healing. There is no specific therapy for verruga peruana, but the morality is very low.

Pemphigus foliaceus, or fogo selvagem, is an endemic form of pemphigus that occurs in the tropical regions of Brazil and possibly in Honduras. Family groups can be affected with this disease. The initial lesions are flaccid bullae which usually spread over the entire body, forming a generalized moist exfoliation. The course is chronic for several years, with death usually inevitable from intercurrent infection. Oral corticosteroids are beneficial. For a general discussion of pemphigus see page 187.

Rhinoscleroma is present in areas of higher altitude of Guatemala, Salvador and Venezuela, especially in persons with poor personal hygiene. The etiologic agent is thought to be *Klebsiella rhinoscleromatis*, but some believe it to be caused by a filtrable virus. Rhinoscleroma passes through 3 clinical stages, from a period of rhinitis, to a stage of plaques and masses on the septum, the lower part of the nostrils and the larynx, to a final stage with large nodules and tumors. Treatment with chloromycetin is partially effective.

BIBLIOGRAPHY

Cahill, K. M.: Tropical Diseases in Temperate Climates. Philadelphia, J. B. Lippincott, 1964.

Canizares, Orlando: Geographic Dermatology: Mexico and Central America. Arch. Derm. *82*:870, 1960. A very comprehensive article with communications from leading dermatologists of the area.

———: Epidemiology of Cutaneous Diseases According to Geographic Locale: Latin America. Proceedings of the XII International Congress of Dermatology, Vol. 2, p. 1153. Amsterdam, Excerpta Medica Foundation, 1963.

———: Role of Altitude in Dermatology, Presented at the V° Congreso Ibero-Latino-americano de Dermatologia, Buenos Aires, Argentina.

Dermatologia Tropica. Official Organ of the International Society of Tropical Dermatology, published quarterly. Philadelphia, J. B. Lippincott. Contains many articles relating to geographic distribution of diseases.

Pardo-Castello, V.: Dermatoses of the Americas. Derm. Tropica, *2*:232, 1963.

32

Basic Dermatologic Equipment

Those of us engaged in the practice of medicine can well recall the opening of our first office and the many decisions that had to be made concerning purchase of equipment. Certain mistakes were made; some were avoidable. I can remember wishing that I had a list of necessary materials to guide me in making my selection. With this in mind, the following is a compilation of basic equipment used in my office. This is not the most complete list, and some will find that they can perform with less. For the physician already in practice much of this equipment, particularly that in the Biopsy Set-up, will be on hand, but the list can serve as a guide for organization and completeness in treating dermatologic patients.

The use of a definite manufacturer's name has been done for only one rea-

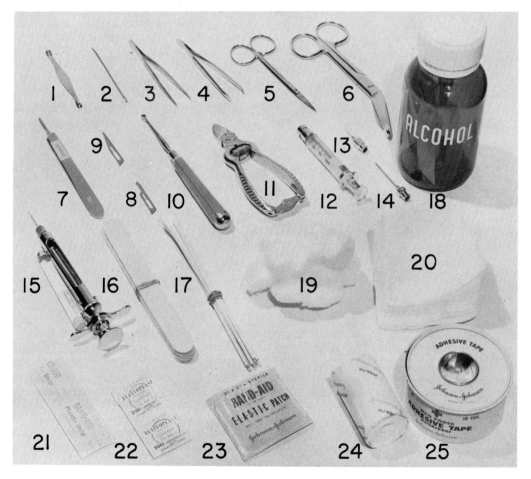

Fig. 32-1. Basic dermatologic tray.

son—to aid you and your supply dealer in the selection of the equipment. I have been told that almost every dealer has these manufacturers' catalogs on hand and therefore can supply their equipment or similar equipment from any of the many other reliable surgical supply manufacturers. The manufacturers mentioned on the following list are not necessarily those used in my office.

I am indebted to Mr. Robert Goetze for providing the catalog numbers which we hope will be available for reference at your dealer.

BASIC DERMATOLOGIC TRAY
(Fig. 32-1)
(Numbers in Parentheses Refer
to the Illustration)

(1)   1—Comedone extractor, Sklar, #115-52
(2)   1—Hagedorn needle, straight, cutting edge, flat body, 3 in., Torrington #719 (can use eye end as comedone extractor)
(3)   1—Splinter forceps, 4 in., Sklar, #160-115
(4)   1—Tweezers, eyebrow, sharp points, 3½ in., Sklar, #320-65
(5)   1—Scissors, iris, straight S/S, 4½ in., Sklar, #320-415
(6)   1—Scissors, bandage, 5½ in., Sklar, #130-05
(7)   1—Knife handle, Bard-Parker, #3
(8)   2—Knife blades, Bard-Parker, #15
(9)   2—Knife blades, Bard-Parker, #11 (to obtain skin scrapings for fungus culture)
(10) 1—Piffard dermal curette, #2 size, Kny-Scheerer, #46-161
(11) 1—Nail clipper, Sklar, #430-100
(12) 1—2 cc. syringe, Becton-Dickinson, #2YL, Luer-Lok
       1—Olsen-Hegar needle holder and scissor combination, 5½ in., Sklar, #170-53
(13) 2—Hypodermic needles, #25, ⅜ in., Becton-Dickinson, #LNR
(14) 2—Hypodermic needles, #21, 1¼ in., Becton-Dickinson, #LNR
(15) A good substitute for the above syringe and needles is the following: Cook-Waite Carpule Syringe, with carpules of Ravocaine 0.4%,

Novocain 2%, and Levophed 1:30,000, 2.2 ml., with 26 gauge dental needles, 1⅝ in.
      1—25% Podophyllum resin in alcohol, 30 ml.
      1—Saturated soln. trichloracetic acid, 30 ml.
      1—Powdered soda bicarbonate, 30 Gm. (to neutralize locally applied acids)
      1—20% Potassium hydroxide soln., 30 ml. (for mycologic slide preparations)
      1—Cover slips, box, 22 mm. square, #1 thickness
      1—Microscopic slides, box, 1 in. x 3 in.
      1—Zephirin Solution diluted 1:1,000, with 16 Anti-rust Tablets, one gallon
      1—9 in. x 5 in. x 2 in. tray with lid, stainless steel (for cold sterilizing liquid in which the above surgical instruments should be placed)
(16) 12—Tongue blades, adult
(17) 12—Cotton-tipped applicators, 6 in.
(18) 1—Alcohol dispenser, Menda, #608
(19) 24—Cotton balls, Johnson and Johnson, medium
(20) 12—3 in. x 3 in., 12-ply gauze sponges, Johnson and Johnson
(21) 12—Band-aid sheer strips, 1 in. x 3 in., Johnson and Johnson #4644
(22) 12—Elastoplast Coverlets, Duke, 1 in. round, #302
(23) 12—Band-aid 2 in. x 2 in. elastic patch, Duke #320
      100—Elastopatch, large, Duke #71 (for patch tests)
      1—Gauze roll, 1 in wide
      1—Gauze roll, 2 in. wide
      1—Tape roll, ½ in. wide
      1—Tape roll, 1 in. wide
      1—Tape roll, 3 in. wide

SKIN BIOPSY SET-UP
(Fig. 32-2)
(Numbers in Parentheses Refer
to the Illustration)

A. *Sterilized in Wrapper:*
(1)   1—Thumb forceps, delicate pattern, 5 in., Sklar, #160-05

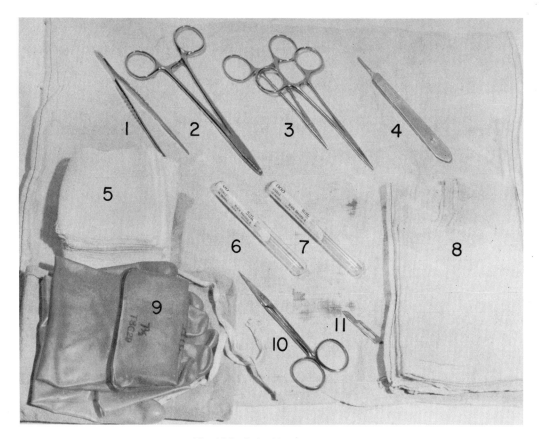

Fig. 32-2. Skin biopsy setup.

(2) 1—Needle holder, Mayo-Hegar, 6 in., Sklar, #170-30

(3) 2—Halsted mosquito hemostats, straight, 5 in., Sklar, #150-70

(4) 1—Bard-Parker #3 knife handle

(5) 10—Gauze sponges, 3 in. x 3 in., 12 ply, Johnson and Johnson

(6) 1—Cuticular silk suture, with cutting needle, 00, Ethicon, 685-G

(7) 1—Cuticular silk suture, with cutting needle, 000, Ethicon, 684-G

(8) 1—12 in. x 12 in. piece of cloth with square 3 in. x 3 in. hole in center

(9) B. *Rubber Gloves, Powdered, Sterilized in Separate Wrapper.*

  C. *In Cold Sterilizing Liquid:*

(10) 1—Scissors, iris, 4½ in., Sklar, #320-415

(11) 2—Bard-Parker knife blades, #15

  1—Biopsy punch, sizes 2, 4, 6, and 8. Keyes, Sklar, #115-60

After use, remove the scissors, the blades and the biopsy punches from the dirty set-up, clean them and put them back in the cold sterilizing liquid. This prevents rusting.

OPTIONAL EQUIPMENT

Wood's light, Burton Fluorescing Ultra-Violet Light, #9100, around $37.00 (for diagnosing tinea of the scalp)

Dry Ice Kit, Kidde Manufacturing Company, Bloomfield, N. J., #5605125, around $50.00 (for treating small hemangiomas, warts, seborrheic keratoses and other superficial growths)

Liquid nitrogen and container. See p. 46.

Moto-Tool Hand Drill, Dremel Manufacturing Company, Racine, Wisconsin, Model 1, around $13, with steel carving cutters #HS-413 and HS-89 (for debriding tinea of nails)

33

Where To Look for More Information About a Skin Disease

"Doctor, I saw a patient yesterday who was diagnosed as having epidermolysis bullosa. Where can I read more about this disease? Where would I find the latest papers on this subject?"

These are questions frequently asked of any teaching dermatologist. First, I would suggest that the inquiring student or doctor read what he can about the disease in any of the larger dermatologic texts.

The following comprehensive texts are suggested:

Demis, D. J., Crounse, R. G., Dobson, R. I., and McGuire, J.: Clinical Dermatology (Looseleaf). Hagerstown, Harper and Row, 1972.

Domonkos, A. N.: Andrew's Diseases of the Skin. ed. 6. Philadelphia, W. B. Saunders, 1971.

Fitzpatrick, T. B., Arndt, K. A., Clark, W. H., Jr., Eisen, A. Z., Van Scott, E. J., and Vaughan, J. H.: Dermatology in General Practice. N.Y., McGraw-Hill, 1971.

Rook, A., Wilkinson, D. S., and Ebling, F. J. G.: Textbook of Dermatology. 2 vol. Philadelphia, Davis, 1968.

Two excellent books fall into the category of color atlases:

Burckhardt, W.: Atlas and Manual of Dermatology and Venereology. ed. 2. Translated and edited by Epstein, S. Baltimore, Williams & Wilkins, 1963.

deGraciansky, P., and Boulle, S.: Color Atlas of Dermatology. English-language adaptation by Sulzberger, M. B., and Dobkevitch-Morrill, S., 4 volumes. Chicago, Year Book Publishers, 1955.

After these larger texts are consulted, then I would suggest that the most recent information about the skin disease be sought in the following publications and indexes:

Archives of Dermatology, a monthly journal published by the American Medical Association, Chicago. It is indexed in both the June and the December issues.

Cutis, a monthly magazine for the general practitioner published by Dun-Donnelley Publications, New York—10017.

Dermatology Digest, a monthly summary of the dermatology literature of the world, published by Dermatology Digest, Inc., Northfield, Illinois—60093.

Index Medicus, published monthly by the National Library of Medicine, and the *Cumulated Index Medicus* published annually by the American Medical Association, Chicago. These contain current references to published paper and books listed according to subject.

Index of Dermatology, National Institutes of Health, U. S. Govt. Printing Office, Washington, D.C. 20402.

Journal of Investigative Dermatology, a monthly journal published by the Society of Investigative Dermatology, Baltimore, Maryland—21202.

MEDLARS (MEDical Literature Analysis and Retrieval System). Provides free of charge machine-produced literature searches using Index Medicus from 1964 to present. Available without charge from NLM is a 16 page Guide to MEDLARS Services. Write to: Assistant to the Director, National Library of Medicine, 8600 Rockville Pike, Bethesda, Maryland—20014.

Year Book of Dermatology, edited by F. D. Malkinson and R. W. Pearson, and published annually by the Year Book Publishers, Chicago. The *Year Book* contains abstracts of the majority of important articles related to dermatology.

There are also many excellent foreign journals. Ones in English include *Acta Dermato-venereologica*, Stockholm, and the *British Journal of Dermatology*, London.

SPECIALIZED TEXTS

If information on a special subject is desired, the following list of texts or the Bibliography at the end of the appropriate chapters in this book should be helpful. Some of these texts are out-of-print, but, as classics, they can and should be consulted in your medical library.

ANATOMY

Montagna, W.: The Structure and Function of Skin. ed. 2. New York, Academic Press, 1962.

Zelickson, A. S.: Ultrastructure of Normal and Abnormal Skin. Philadelphia, Lea & Febiger, 1967.

BACTERIOLOGY

Dubos, R. J., and Hirsch, J. G.: Bacterial and Mycotic Infections of Man. ed. 4. Philadelphia, J. B. Lippincott, 1965.

CANCER OF THE SKIN

Urbach, F. (ed.): Conference on Biology of Cutaneous Cancer. Washington, D.C., U.S. Gov't. Printing Office, 1963.

HAIR AND SCALP

Behrman, H. T.: The Scalp in Health and Disease. St. Louis, C. V. Mosby, 1952.

Savill, A. and Warren, C.: The Hair and Scalp. ed. 5. Baltimore, Williams & Wilkins, 1962.

HEREDITARY DERMATOSES

Butterworth, T., and Strean, L. P.: Clinical Genodermatology. Baltimore, Williams & Wilkins, 1962.

HISTORY OF DERMATOLOGY

Pusey, W. A.: The History of Dermatology. Springfield, Charles C Thomas, 1933.

Shelley, W. G., and Crissey, J. T.: Classics in Clinical Dermatology. Springfield, Charles C Thomas, 1953.

Syntex Laboratories, Palo Alto, California —94304, has published several small volumes on historical "Leaders in Dermatology."

MYCOLOGY

Hildick-Smith, G., Blank, H., and Sarkany, I: Fungus Diseases and Their Treatment. Boston, Little, Brown & Co., 1965.

Wilson, J. W., and Plunkett, O. A.: The Fungous Diseases of Man. Los Angeles, University of California, 1966.

NAILS

Pardo-Castello, V., and Pardo, O. A.: Diseases of the Nails. ed. 3. Springfield, Charles C Thomas, 1960.

Samman, P. D.: The Nails in Disease. ed. 2. Springfield, Charles C Thomas, 1972.

OCCUPATIONAL DERMATOSES

Adams, R. M.: Occupational Contact Dermatitis. Philadelphia, J. B. Lippincott, 1969.

Schwartz, L., Tulipan, L., and Birmingham, D. J.: Occupational Diseases of the Skin. ed. 3. Philadelphia, Lea & Febiger, 1957.

PEDIATRIC DERMATOSES

Leider, M.: Practical Pediatric Dermatology. ed. 2. St. Louis, C. V. Mosby, 1961.

PATHOLOGY

Lever, W. F.: Histopathology of the Skin. ed. 4. Philadelphia, J. B. Lippincott, 1967.

PHYSIOLOGY

Rothman, S.: Physiology and Biochemistry of the Skin. Chicago, University of Chicago Press, 1954.

SKIN AND INTERNAL DISEASES

Braverman, I. M.: Skin Signs of Systemic Disease. Philadelphia, W. B. Saunders, 1970.

Johnson, S. A. M., (ed.): The Skin and Internal Disease. New York, McGraw-Hill, 1967.

Weiner, K.: Systemic Associations and Treatment of Skin Diseases, St. Louis, C. V. Mosby, 1955.
———: Skin Manifestations of Internal Disorders. St. Louis, C. V. Mosby, 1947.

SURGERY

Epstein, E.: Skin Surgery. ed. 3. Springfield, Charles C Thomas, 1970.

SYPHILIS

Stokes, J. H.: Beerman, H., and Ingraham, N. R.: Modern Clinical Syphilology. ed. 3. Philadelphia, W. B. Saunders, 1944. A classic text.
Youmans, J. B., (Ed.). Syphilis and Other Venereal Diseases. Med. Clinics N. Am., Vol. 48, No. 3. Philadelphia, W. B. Saunders, 1964.

THERAPY

Lerner, M. R., and Lerner, A. B.: Dermatologic Medications. Chicago, Year Book Publishers, 1960.
Maddin, S., (Ed.): Current Dermatologic Management, St. Louis, C. V. Mosby, 1970.
Physicians' Desk Reference. Oradell, N.J. —07649, Medical Economics, annually.

VETERINARY DERMATOLOGY

Kral, F. and Schwartzman, R. M.: Veterinary and Comparative Dermatology. Philadelphia, J. B. Lippincott, 1964.

VIROLOGY

Blank, H., and Rake, G.: Virus and Rickettsial Diseases of the Skin. New York, Little, Brown & Co., 1955.
Horsfall, F. L., Jr., and Tamm, Igor: Viral and Rickettsial Infections of Man. ed 4. Philadelphia, J. B. Lippincott, 1965.

X-RAYS AND RADIUM

Cipollaro, A. C., and Crossland, P. M.: X-rays and Radium in the Treatment of Diseases of the Skin. ed. 5. Philadelphia, Lea & Febiger, 1967.
Wansker, B. A.: X-ray and Radium in Dermatology. Springfield, Charles C Thomas, 1959.

Finally, a unique publication is *A Dictionary of Dermatological Words, Terms and Phrases* by Leider and Rosenblum. It is published by McGraw-Hill, New York, 1968. Any interested student or physician will enjoy and profit by perusing this dictionary.

Dictionary-Index

The purpose of this section is to add to the usefulness of the book by defining and classifying some of the rarer dermatologic terms not covered in the main section. Some very rare or unimportant terms have purposely been omitted, but undoubtedly some terms that are *not* rare and *are* important have also been omitted. Most of the histopathologic terms have been defined. Suggestions or corrections from the reader will be appreciated.

Boldface numbers refer to the main discussion.

Italicized numbers refer to important illustrations.

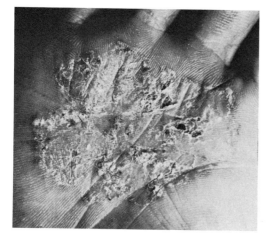

Fig. I-1. Acrodermatitis perstans.

Amyloidosis (*continued*)
B. Secondary amyloidosis. Secondary amyloid deposits are very rare in the skin, but are less rare in the liver, the spleen and the kidney, where they occur as a result of certain chronic infectious diseases, and in association with multiple myeloma.
C. Primary systemic amyloidosis, 256. This peculiar and serious form of amyloidosis commonly involves the skin along with the tongue, the heart, and the musculature of the viscera. The skin lesions appear as transparent-looking, yellowish papules or nodules which are occasionally hemorrhagic. This form is familial.
Anatomy of skin, 1
Anchorage, Alaska, 314
Angioid streaks of retina, 218
Angiokeratomas, 254, 277
Angiomatosis, encephalo-trigeminal, 254
Angioma serpiginosum. Characterized by multiple telangiectases which may start from a congenital vascular nevus but often arise spontaneously. This rare vascular condition is to be differentiated from *Schamberg's disease, Majocchi's disease* and *pigmented purpuric dermatitis (Gougerot and Blum)*.
Angioneurotic edema, 78
Anhidrosis. The partial or complete absence of sweating, seen in ichthyosis, extensive psoriasis, scleroderma, prickly heat, vitamin A deficiency and other diseases. Partial anhidrosis is produced by many antiperspirants.
Anhidrotic asthenia, tropical. Described in the South Pacific and in the desert in World War II. Soldiers showed increased sweating of neck and face and anhidrosis (lack of sweating) below the neck. It was accompanied by weakness, headaches and subjective warmth and was considered as a chronic phase of prickly heat.
Anthralin. A proprietary name for dihydroxy-anthranol, which is a strong reducing agent useful in the treatment of chronic cases of psoriasis. Its action is similar to chrysarobin.

Anthrax. A primary chancre-type disease caused by *Bacillus anthracis*, occurring in people who work with the hides and the hair of infected sheep, horses or cattle. A pulmonary form is known.
Antimalarial agents. Dermatologically active agents include quinacrine (Atabrine), chloroquine (Aralen) and hydroxychloroquine (Plaquenil). Their mode of action is unknown, but these agents are used in the treatment of chronic discoid lupus erthematosus and the polymorphic actinic dermatoses. (See p. 205.)
Aphthous stomatitis, 236
Apocrinitis, 121
Argyll Robertson pupils. Small irregular pupils that fail to react to light but react to accommodation. This is a late manifestation of neurosyphilis, particularly tabes.
Argyria, 201
Arnold, Dr. Harry, 316
Arsenic. Inorganic arsenic preparations include Fowler's solution and Asiatic pills and are used in the treatment of resistant cases of psoriasis but can cause arsenical pigmentation and keratoses. Organic arsenic agents include neoarsphenamine and Mapharsen, used formerly in the treatment of syphilis.
Arsenical keratosis, 266
pigmentation, 201
Arthritis, rheumatoid, 208
Arthropod dermatoses, 182
Arthus phenomenon. Characterized by local anaphylaxis in a site that has been injected repeatedly with a foreign protein.
Athlete's feet, 161
Atopic eczema. *See* Eczema, atopic, 56
Atrophies of the skin
A. Congenital atrophies. Associated with other congenital ectodermal defects.
B. Acquired atrophies
  1. Noninflammatory.
    a. *Senile atrophy*. Often associated with senile pruritus and winter itch.
    b. *Linear atrophy* (*striae albicantes or distensae*). On abdomen, thighs and breasts associated with pregnancy and obesity.
    c. *Secondary atrophy* from sunlight x-radiation, injury, and nerve diseases.
    d. *Macular atrophy* (*anetoderma of Schweninger-Buzzi*). Characterized by the presence of small, oval, whitish depressions or slightly elevated papules which can be pressed back into the underlying tissue. This may be an early form of von Recklinghausen's disease.
  2. Inflammatory.
    a. *Acrodermatitis chronica atrophicans.* A moderately rare idiopathic atrophy in older adults, particularly females, characterized by the presence of thickened skin at the onset, with ulnar bands on the forearm, changing into atrophy of the legs below the knee and of the forearms. In the early stages this is to be differentiated from scleroderma. High doses of penicillin may be effective.
    b. *Folliculitis ulerythematosa reticulata.* A very rare reticulated atrophic condition localized to the cheeks of the face; seen mainly in young adults.

Fig. I-2. Basal cell nevus syndrome. Back lesions. The patient also had x-ray evidence of bone cysts in the mandible.

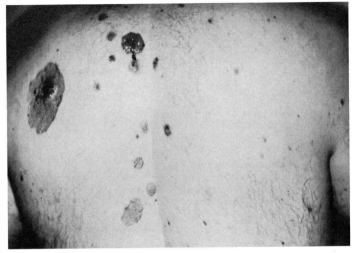

Atrophies of the skin, acquired atrophies, inflammatory (*continued*)

c. *Ulerythema ophryogenes.* A rare atrophic dermatitis that affects the outer part of the eyebrows, resulting in redness, scaling, and permanent loss of the involved hair.

d. *Macular atrophy (anetoderma of Jadassohn).* A very rare condition characterized by the appearance of circumscribed reddish macules which develop an atrophic center that progresses toward the edge of the lesion, seen mainly on the extremities.

e. *Lichen sclerosus et atrophicus (kraurosis vulvae, kraurosis penis and balanitis xerotica obliterans)* 208, 266. An uncommon atrophic process, mainly of women, which begins as a small whitish lesion that contains a central hyperkeratotic pinpoint-sized dell. These 0.5 cm. size or less whitish macules commonly coalesce to form whitish atrophic plaques. The commonest localizations are on the neck, shoulders, arms, axillae, vulva, and perineum. Many consider kraurosis vulvae, kraurosis penis and balanitis xerotica obliterans to be variants of this condition.

f. *Poikiloderma atrophicans vasculare (Jacobi).* This rare atrophic process of adults is characterized by the development of patches of telangiectasia, atrophy and mottled pigmentation on any area of the body. This resembles chronic radiodermatitis clinically and may be associated with dermatomyositis or scleroderma. May precede the development of a lymphoma.

g. *Hemiatrophy.* May be localized to one side of the face or may cover the entire half of the body. Vascular and neurogenic etiologies have been propounded, but most cases appear to be a form of localized scleroderma.

Atrophies of the skin, acquired atrophies, inflammatory (*continued*)

h. *Atrophie blanche en plaque.* A rare form of cutaneous atrophy characterized by scarlike plaques with a border of telangiectasia and hyperpigmentation that cover large areas of the legs and the ankles, mainly of middle-aged or older women.

i. *Secondary atrophy.* From inflammatory diseases such as syphilis, chronic discoid lupus erythematosus, leprosy, tuberculosis, scleroderma, etc.

Atrophoderma idiopathic, 208

Autoeczematization. See Id reaction

Autohemotherapy. A form of nonspecific protein therapy, administered by removing 10 cc. of venous blood from the arm and then immediately injecting that blood intramuscularly into the buttocks. It has been shown to produce a fall in circulating eosinophils presumably due to a mild increase in the adrenal steroid hormones.

Ayres, Dr. Samuel, III, 315

Babinski's reflex. Extension of the toes instead of flexion following stimulation of the sole of the foot, due to lesions of the pyramidal tract from syphilis infection or other causes.

Bacterial infection, 114
  in Latin America, 326
  scalp, 226

Bacterid, pustular, 163, 165

Bacteriologic dermatoses, 114

Balanitis, fusospirochetal, 238

Balanitis xerotica obliterans, 238

Barber's itch, 119

Bartonellosis, 334

Basal cell nevus syndrome. (Figure I-2) This is a rare hereditary affliction characterized primarily by multiple genetically determined basal cell epitheliomas, cysts of the jaws, peculiar pits of the hands and the feet, and developmental anomalies of the ribs, the spine and the skull.

Baths, 35

Bazin's disease. Erythema induratum. *See* Tuberculosis, 131

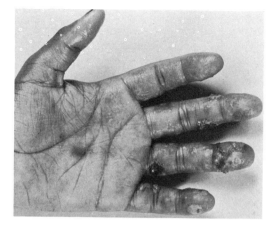

Fig. I-3. Dyshidrosis with secondary infection in a Negro.

Dermatolysis. Also known as *cutis laxa*. This is a rare condition where the skin is abnormally loose and hangs in folds. It is most often associated with *Ehlers-Danlos syndrome.*

Dermatomycosis. Signifies all cutaneous infections due to fungi.

Dermatomyositis, 209, 247

Dermatophytid, 174

Dermatophytosis. A term applicable to superficial fungus infection.

Dermatosis, exudative discoid and lichenoid chronic, 315, 321

Dermatosis, subcorneal pustular, 192

Dermatosis papulosa nigra, 259

Dermis, 1

Dermogram, geriatric, *303*
    Negro, *26, 27*
    pediatric, *287, 291*

Dermographism, 78
    black, 201

Diabetes mellitus, plate 49, 213

Diagnosis, by location, 21
    diseases of the back, *20*
    palmar dermatoses, *23*
    penile dermatoses, *22*
    plantar dermatoses, *24*
    skin diseases, 21

Diaper rash, 129, 293

Diphtheria, cutaneous. The skin ulcer due to *Corynebacterium diphtheriae* has a characteristic rolled firm border and a grayish membrane that progresses to a black eschar with surrounding inflammation, vesicles and anesthesia.

Dog-faced boys, 220

Donovan bodies, 130

Dopa, 4

Drill, 337

Drug eruptions, plate 14, 60, 199

Drugs, internal, 43
    local, 31
    office, 41

Dry ice, 46

Dry ice kit, 337

Duhring's disease, 189, *See* Dermatitis herpetiformis.

Duke's disease, 295

Dyshidrosis (Fig. I-3), 165. A syndrome characterized by blisters on the palms of hands and feet. If the cause is known, this term should not be used. The common causes of dyshidrosis, or *pompholyx*, are mycotic, contact dematitis, drugs, and associated as a manifestation of a generalized skin disease.

Dyskeratoma, warty, 282

Dyskeratosis, benign. A histopathologic finding of faulty keratinization of individual epidermal cells with formation of corps ronds and grains. Seen in Darier's disease and occasionally in familial benign chronic pemphigus.

Dyskeratosis congenita. With pigmentation, dystrophia unguis and leukokeratosis oris, this is a rare syndrome characterized by a reticulated pigmentation, particularly of the neck, dystrophy of the nails, and a leukoplakialike condition of the oral mucosa. Increased sweating and thickening of palms and soles may occur.

Dyskeratosis, malignant. A histopathologic finding in Bowen's disease and also in prickle cell epithelioma and senile keratosis where premature and typical keratinization of individual cells is seen.

Ear fungus, 74, 160

Ear-piercing, 121

Ecchymoses. *See* Purpura, 84

Eccrine tumors, 284

ECHO virus infection, 158

Ecthyma, 116

Ectoderma defect, congenital. *See* Congenital ectoderma defect

Ectodermosis erosiva pluriorificialis. A synonym for Stevens-Johnson form of erythema multiforme.

Eczema, atopic, plate 8, 9, 10 & 11, **56**, 217, 255, 293, 315
    in Arizona, 315
    infantile, 57
    nummular, plate 13, 60

Ehlers-Danlos syndrome, 254

Elastosis perforans serpiginosa. A rare asymptomatic disease where keratotic papules occur in a circinate arrangement around a slightly atrophic patch usually on the neck.

Electrolysis, 46

Electrosurgery, 45

Elephantiasis, 332
    from radiation, 242
    nostras, 125

Embolic nodules, 82. Emboli can come from a left atrial myxoma or from arteriosclerotic plaques.

Endocrinopathic hypertrichosis, 220

Eosinophilic granuloma, 213

Ephelides, 254

Epidermis, 3

Epidermodysplasia verruciformis. A rare, apparently hereditary disease manifested by papulosquamous and warty lesions present at birth with no site of predilection. The prognosis for life is poor because of the eventual development of prickle cell epitheliomas from the lesions. *See* a defect in RNA replication.

Epidermolysis bullosa, 254, 292

Epidermophytid. A dermatophytid due to *Epidermophyton* infection.

Epidermophytosis. A fungus infection due to *Epidermophyton.*

Epiloia, 254, 283. A triad of mental deficiency, epilepsy and adenoma sebaceum.

Epithelioma, basal cell, 267
  calcifying, 284
  squamous cell, 269
Epulis. This term refers to any growth involving the gums.
Epulis, giant-cell. This is a solitary neoplasm or granuloma from the periosteum of the jaw bone in the gingival area.
Equipment, 335
Erosio interdigitale blastomycetica. A complex term signifying a monilial infection of the webs of the fingers.
Erysipelas, 121
Erysipeloid. A chancre-type infection on the hand occurring at the site of accidental inoculation with the organism, *Erysipelothrix rhusiopathiae*, seen in butchers, veterinarians and fishermen. A localized form runs its course in 2 to 4 weeks. A generalized form develops a diffuse eruption with occasional constitutional symptoms such as arthritis. A very rare systemic form exhibits an eruption, joint pains, and endocarditis.
Erythema ab igne (I-4). A marmoraceous-appearing redness which follows the local application to the skin of radiant heat such as from a heating pad.
Erythema elevatum diutinum. A persistent nodular, symmetrical eruption usually seen in middle-aged males with a rather characteristic histologic picture. This may be a deeper form of *granuloma annulare*.
Erythema induratum, 82
  infectiosum, 158
  multiforme, 80
    bullosum, 193
    in Arizona, 315
  nodosum, 81
Erythema of the ninth day. A morbilliform erythema of sudden onset appearing around the 9th day after the initiation of organic arsenic therapy for the treatment of syphilis. It may be accompanied by generalized lymphadenopathy and fever.
Erythema, palmar. Redness of the palms of the hands, which may be due to heredity, pulmonary disease, liver disease, rheumatoid arthritis, or pregnancy.
Erythema perstans, 80. Over a dozen entities have been described which fit into this persistent group of diseases that resemble erythema multiforme. The following entities are included in this group:
  Erythema annulare centrifugum (Darier); erythema chronicum migrans (Lipschutz), may be due to a tick bite for which Penicillin is effective therapy; *erythema gyratum perstans (Fox); erythema figuratum perstans (Wende); and erythema gyratum repens (Gammel).*
Erythrasma, 125, 168
Erythredema. *See* Acrodynia
Erythrodermas, 195, 294
Erythrodermia desquamativa. Another term for Leiner's disease.
Erythromelalgia. A rare disorder of hands and feet, most common in middle age; characterized by burning pain which is activated by exertion or heat and is refractory to treatment.
Erythroplasia of Queyrat, 282
Erythrose pigmentaire peribuccale. A rare condition of middle-aged women, characterized by diffuse brownish-red pigmentation about the

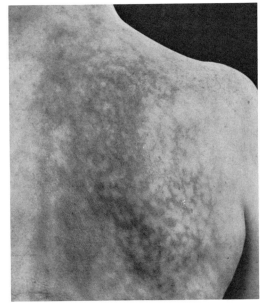

Fig. I-4. Erythema ab igne from a hot water bottle. (*K.U.M.C.*)

Erythrose pigmentaire peribuccale (*continued*) mouth, the chin and the neck with or without a slight burning sensation.
Espundia, 330
Exanthem subitum. Another term for roseola infantum or sixth disease.
Exclamation point hairs, 224
Exfoliative dermatitis, 195, 294

Factitial dermatitis, 217
Fall dermatoses, 25
Fat necroses of newborn, 295
Fat necrosis, subcutaneous, with pancreatic disease, 82. Histologic picture is quite characteristic.
Fatal granulomatous disease of childhood. A very rare, X-linked disease of males mainly characterized by eczematous lesions in infancy with progressive chronic granulomatous bacterial infections.
Female-pattern hair loss, 223
Fever blisters, 145
Fibroma, pedunculated, 260
Fibrosarcoma, 272, 284
Fifth disease, 158
Filariasis, 332
Fixed drug eruption, 68
Fluorouracil method, 265
Fogo selvagem, 334
Folliculitis, 116
  beard, 119
  decalvans, 119, 226
Folliculitis, perforating, of the nose (Fig. I-5). A folliculitis of the stiff hairs of the nasal mucocutaneous junction that penetrates deeply through to the external nasal skin. Unless the basic pathology is understood and corrected by plucking the involved stiff hair, the condition

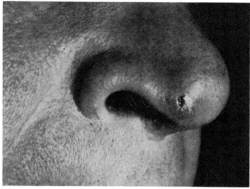

Fig. I-5. Folliculitis, perforating, of the nose. (*Dr. Chester Lessenden*)

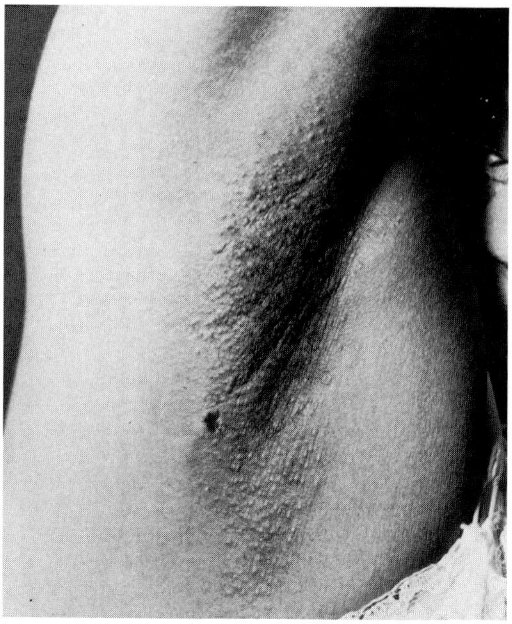

Folliculitis (*continued*)
   cannot be cured. The external papule can simulate a skin cancer.
Food testing, 10
Fordyce condition, 237, 283
Formulary, 33
Foshay test. A 48-hour intradermal test which, if positive, indicates that the person has or has had *tularemia.*
Fourth disease. Another term for Duke's disease.
Fox-Fordyce disease (Fig. I-6). A rare intensely pruritic, chronic papular dermatosis of the axillae and the pubic area in women. The intense itching is due to the closure of the apocrine gland pore with rupture of the duct and escape of the apocrine sweat into the surrounding epidermis.
Frambesia. *See* Yaws
Freckles, 254, 279, 286
Fröhlich's syndrome, 212
Frostbite. Exposure to cold can cause pathologic changes in the skin which are related to the severity of the exposure but vary with the susceptibility of the individual. Other terms in use that refer to cold injuries under varying conditions include *trench foot, immersion foot, pernio* and *chilblain. See* Chilblain.
Fungus diseases, 159. *See* Tinea
   elements, 159
   examination, culture, 11
      scraping, 11
   infections, Latin America, 328
Furuncle, 120
Fusospirochetal balanitis. *See* Balanitis, fusospirochetal

Galveston, Texas, 316
Gangosa. A severe ulcerative and mutilating form of yaws affecting the palate, the pharynx and nasal tissues.
Gardner's syndrome. An autosomal dominant trait with multiple osteomas, fibrous and fatty tumors, and epidermoid inclusion cysts of skin and multiple polyposes.
Gaucher's disease, 214
General paresis. A psychosis due to syphilitic meningo-encephalitis.
Genetic counseling, 250

Fig. I-6. Fox-Fordyce disease of axilla.

Genodermatoses, 249
   classification, 253
Gentian violet. A pararosaniline dye which destroys gram-positive bacteria and some fungi.
Geographic skin diseases, Central and South America, 321
   North America, 314
Geriatric state, 212, 303
Glands, sebaceous, 6
   infection, 121
   sweat, 6
Glandular appendages, 6
Glomus body, 5
   tumor, 5, 285
Glossitis, 237
Glossitis rhombica mediana, 238
Gonorrhea, 132, 143
Gonorrheal dermatosis. *See* Keratosis blenorrhagica and, 143
Gout, 256
Grain itch. Due to a mite, *Pediculoides ventricosus,* which lives on insects that attack wheat and corn. This mite can attack humans working with the infested grain and cause a markedly pruritic papular and papulovesicular eruption.
Granuloma. A tissue reaction due to several causes characterized by the presence of various combinations of the following cellular reactions: epithelioid cells, giant cells and necrosis, 1.
Granuloma annulare, 296 and Fig. I-7.
Granuloma, chronic cutaneous, 316
Granuloma faciale. Typically occurs as brownish papules or plaques, multiple or single, usually on the face, in middle age or older persons (usually males).
Granuloma, foreign body. A granulomatous reaction seen in the dermis due to the introduction, usually by trauma, of certain agents such as

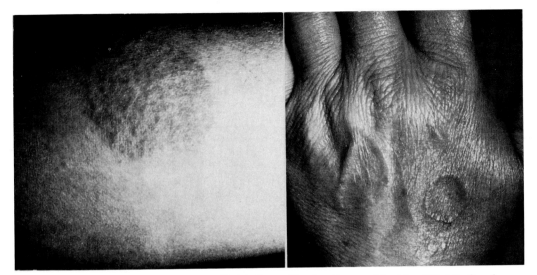

Fig. I-7. Granuloma annulare. (*Left*) On calf of a 7-year-old girl. (*Right*) On dorsum of hand. (*Dr. Chester Lessenden*)

Optic atrophy. Atrophy of the optic nerve due to syphilic involvement of the central nervous system of the tabetic type. Blindness is the end result.

Oral lesions, rare, 237

Orf. A viral infection characterized by a vesicular and pustular eruption of the mouth and the lips of lambs. Sheepherders and veterinarians become inoculated on the hand and develop a primary-type chancre lesion.

Oriental sore, 330

Oroya fever, 334

Osseous tumors, 285

Otitis, external, 74

Paget's disease, 283

Panniculitis, migratory, 82. In middle-aged women, lesions on legs enlarge rapidly.

Panniculitis, nodular, 82

Papilloma. An upward proliferation of the papillae which is seen histologically in nevus verrucosus, senile keratosis, seborrheic keratosis, verruca vulgaris and acanthosis nigricans.

Papillomatoses. Three forms of papillomatoses have been described and all are very rare.

Papular mucinosis. A rare disease characterized by deposition in the skin of mucinous material that forms papules and plaques. The skin lesions are probably part of a systemic dysproteinemia.

Papulosis, malignant atrophying (Degos' disease). A predominantly fatal disease with spotty vascular lesions and subsequent atrophy of the overlying tissues, affecting the skin, intestines and other organs including the brain, kidney and heart. It is differentiated from thromboangiitis obliterans and periarteritis nodosa.

Papulosquamous dermatoses, 97

Paracoccidioidal granuloma, 330

Paraffinoma. A foreign body granuloma due to the injection of paraffin into the subcutaneous tissue for cosmetic purposes.

Parakeratosis. An example of imperfect keratinization of the epidermis resulting in the retention of nuclei in the horny layer. In areas of parakeratosis the granular layer is absent.

Parapsoriasis. A term for a group of persistent macular and maculopapular scaly erythrodermas. An acute form with the synonym *pityriasis lichenoides et variolaformis acuta* (*Mucha-Habermann*) is now thought to be a distinct entity. (*See* Dictionary-Index.) One chronic form of parapsoriasis, *parapsoriasis guttata*, can resemble guttate psoriasis, pityriasis rosea or seborrheic dermatitis. This condition does not itch and persists for years. A variant of this type of parapsoriasis is *pityriasis lichenoides chronica* (Juliusberg) which is a form of guttate psoriasis with slightly larger scaly areas. Another chronic form of parapsoriasis, *parapsoriasis en plaque*, is characterized by nonpruritic or slightly pruritic scaly brownish patches and plaques. A high percentage of patients that are given this diagnosis terminate with mycosis fungoides.

Parasitology, 182

Parasitophobia, 183

Paronychia, bacterial, 178
    monilial, 178

Pediatric skin diseases, 287

Pediculosis, 183

Pellagra, 214, 247

Pemphigoid, 187

Pemphigus, benign mucosal pemphigoid, 187
    erythematosus, 188
    familial benign chronic, 186, 254
    foliaceus, 188, 334
    neonatorum, 115, 186
    vegetans, 188
    vulgaris, 187

Periadenitis mucosa necrotica recurrens, 237

Periarteritis nodosa, 73, 82, 173, 179, 212

Perlèche, 178

Pernio. *See* Chilblain *and* Frostbite

Petechiae, 84

Peutz-Jehgers syndrome, 201

Phobias, 217

Photosensitivity dermatoses, 244
    endogenous, 245
    exogenous, 244
    onycholysis, 234
    reaction, 68, 239

Phrynoderma, 214

Phthiriasis. Infestation with the crab louse.

Physical agents, dermatoses of, 239

Piebaldism, 254, 292

Pigmentary dermatoses, 198
    classification, 201

Pigmented purpuric eruption, 85

Pimples, 89

Pink disease. *See* Acrodynia

Pinta, 333

Pityriasis lichenoides et variolaformis acuta (Mucha-Habermann). This is an acute disease that appears as a reddish macular generalized eruption with mild constitutional signs including fever and malaise. Vesicles may develop and also papuloneucrotic lesion. This disease gradually disappears in several months. Histologically this is characterized by a vasculitis which differentiates it from the parapsoriasis group of diseases.

Pityriasis lichenoides chronica (Juliusberg). A form of guttate parapsoriasis.

Pityriasis rosea, 105

Pityriasis rubra pilaris, 254

Pityriasis simplex faciei, 296. A common disorder of children seen predominantly in the winter as a rather well-localized scaly oval patch on the cheeks. The end result is depigmentation of the area, but the normal pigment returns when the eruption clears up (usually in the summer). I believe this condition to be a mild form of atopic eczema.

Plasma cells, 3

Plummer-Vinson syndrome. A syndrome characterized by dysphagia, glossitis, hypochromic anemia and spoon nails in middle-aged women. The associated dryness and atrophy of the mucous membranes of the throat may lead to leukoplakia and squamous cell epithelioma.

Poikiloderma atrophicans vasculare. (Jacobi). *See* Atrophies of skin

Poikiloderma of Civatte, 201, 247, 307

Poikiloderma congenitale, 247. A rare syndrome characterized by telangiectasis, pigmentation, defective teeth and bone cysts. This may be similar to dyskeratosis congenita.

Poison ivy dermatitis, 52, 186

Polymorphic light eruption, 247

Pompholyx. *See* Dyshidrosis and 165

Porokeratosis. A rare disorder that begins as a small, slightly elevated, wartlike papule that

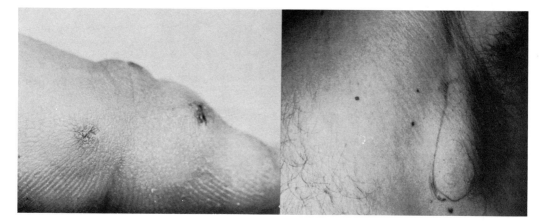

Fig. I-8. Primary chancre-type disease. (*Left*) Tularemic chancre on finger. (*Right*) Axillary adenopathy in same patient. (*Dr. Lawrence Calkins*)

Porokeratosis (*continued*)
slowly enlarges, leaving an atrophic center with a keratotic ridgelike border. The small individual lesions may coalesce. A disseminated form develops in middle-aged individuals on sun-exposed limbs.
Porphyria, 186, 245, 256
familial variegate, 245
Porphyria cutanea tarda, 245
Potassium hydroxide preparation, 10
Potassium permanganate. An oxidizing antiseptic usually used as a wet dressing in the concentration of 1:10,000.
Potassium permanganate bath, 191
Powder bed, 192
Prausnitz-Küstner reaction. A demonstration of passive sensitization of the skin of a nonsensitive individual. This is accomplished by the intradermal injection of serum from a sensitive patient into the skin of a nonsensitive individual. After 24 to 48 hours the atopen to be tested is injected intracutaneously into the previously injected site on the nonsensitive individual's skin. Passive transfer of the sensitivity is manifested by the formation of a wheal.
Precancerous tumors, 264
Pregnancy state, 210
Prickly heat, 7, 294, 320
Primary chancre-type diseases.
Anthrax
Blastomycosis, primary cutaneous type
Chancroid
Coccidioidomycosis, primary cutaneous type
Cowpox
Cutaneous diphtheria
Erysipeloid
Furuncle
Milker's nodules
Orf
Sporotrichosis
Syphilis (genital but also extragenital)
Tuberculosis, primary inoculation type
Tularemia (Fig. I-8)
Vaccinia
Protoporphyria, erythropoietic, 245, 256
Protozoal dermatoses, 182, 330
Proud flesh, 284

Prurigo nodularis. A rare chronic dermatosis, usually of women, consisting of discrete nodular pruritic excoriated papules and tumors scattered over the arms and the legs.
Pruritus ani, 75
essential, 72
generalized, 71
genital, 77
hiemalis, 71
senile, 72
Pseudoacanthosis nigricans, 255
Pseudochancre redux. A late, gummatous, syphilitic inflammation, occurring at the site of the original chancre.
Pseudoepitheliomatous hyperplasia, 270
Pseudopelade. *See* Alopecia cicatrisata
Pseudoxanthoma elasticum, 218, 254
Psoriasis, 97, *196*, 255
and arthritis, 218
nails, 232
Psychoses, 216
Puberty state, 210
Purpura, 84, 216
Purpura, senile, 85
stasis, 85
Purpura, thrombocytopenic, 85. May be idiopathic or secondary to various chronic diseases or a drug sensitivity. The platelet count is below normal, the bleeding time is prolonged, and the clotting time is normal, but the clot does not retract normally.
Purpuric eruption, pigmented, 85
Pyoderma gangrenosum, 212
Pyodermas, 114

Radiation, ultraviolet, 47
x-ray, 47
Radiodermatitis, 242
Radium therapy, 47
Rat-bite fevers. The bite of a rat can cause *sodoku* and *Haverhill fever*. Sodoku, caused by *Spirillum minus*, is manifested by a primary-type chancre and later by an erythematous rash. Haverhill fever, caused by *Streptobacillus moniliformis*, is characterized by joint pains and an erythematous rash.

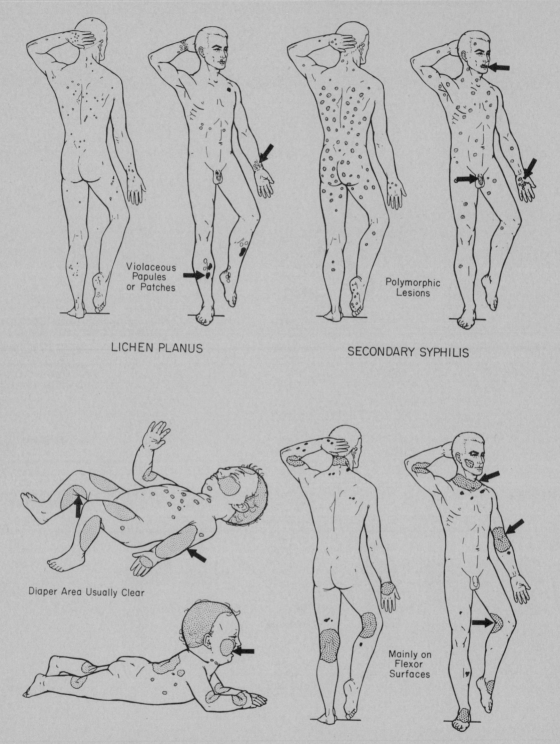

LICHEN PLANUS

Violaceous Papules or Patches

SECONDARY SYPHILIS

Polymorphic Lesions

Diaper Area Usually Clear

INFANTILE FORM of ATOPIC ECZEMA

Mainly on Flexor Surfaces

ADULT FORM of ATOPIC ECZEMA